Myth and (mis)information

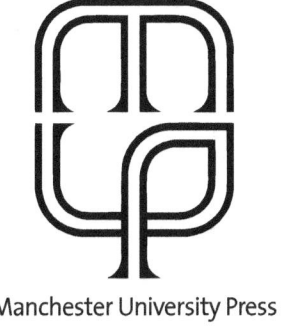

Manchester University Press

Myth and (mis)information

Constructing the medical professions in eighteenth- and nineteenth-century English literature and culture

Edited by

Allan Ingram, Clark Lawlor, Helen Williams

MANCHESTER UNIVERSITY PRESS

Copyright © Manchester University Press 2024

While copyright in the volume as a whole is vested in Manchester University Press, copyright in individual chapters belongs to their respective authors, and no chapter may be reproduced wholly or in part without the express permission in writing of both author and publisher.

Published by Manchester University Press
Oxford Road, Manchester, M13 9PL

www.manchesteruniversitypress.co.uk

British Library Cataloguing-in-Publication Data
A catalogue record for this book is available from the British Library

ISBN 978 1 5261 6682 1 hardback
ISBN 978 1 5261 9542 5 paperback

First published 2024
Paperback published 2026

The publisher has no responsibility for the persistence or accuracy of URLs for any external or third-party internet websites referred to in this book, and does not guarantee that any content on such websites is, or will remain, accurate or appropriate.

EU authorised representative for GPSR:
Easy Access System Europe – Mustamäe tee 50,
10621 Tallinn, Estonia
gpsr.requests@easproject.com

Typeset by
Cheshire Typesetting Ltd, Cuddington, Cheshire

Contents

Figures	vii
Contributors	ix
Introduction – Clark Lawlor and Helen Williams	1
1 'To level those monstrous Blotches or Pustules': skincare in Daniel Turner's *De Morbis Cutaneis* (1714) – Katherine Aske	23
2 Dr John Arbuthnot's literary treatment for false learning, pedantry and excess: from physic to metaphysics – John Baker	41
3 'The very women read it': medical self-fashioning, mythologies and (mis)information in George Cheyne MD's medical writings – Clark Lawlor	60
4 Studying in solitude: demythologising the masculine medical monopoly with Jane Barker's Galesia and Tobias Smollett's Sagely – Laurence Sullivan	77
5 'Take physic, Pomp': imagining dog doctors in eighteenth-century Britain – Stephanie Howard-Smith	96
6 'A man of common understanding': venereal disease, myth and reading as a protective practice in eighteenth-century Britain – Declan Kavanagh	117
7 Sir Anthony Carlisle's gothic (medical) intervention: carving the criminal body in *The Horrors of Oakendale Abbey* – Bethany Brigham	135
8 Mislabelling and the medical printer-publisher: demystifying the ephemera of Elizabeth Rane Cox (1765–1841) – Helen Williams	153
9 The uneasy relationship between traditional and orthodox medicine in the works of Elizabeth Gaskell – Barbara Witucki	174

10	Medical men recommend them: branded medicines and the myth of the medical moral economy *c.*1876–80 – Laura Robson-Mainwaring	193
11	Dissecting Venus: popular consumption of flap anatomies, 1890–1910 – Jessica M. Dandona	218
12	'You taught us that which you knew *not* to be the truth': the anti-vaccination medical doctor in Henry Rider Haggard's *Doctor Therne* (1898) – Carlotta Fiammenghi	240

Afterword – Allan Ingram   256

Bibliography   261
Index   285

Figures

1.1 Daniel Turner. Line engraving by George Vertue after Jonathan Richardson (1732). Wellcome Collection. Ref: 9296i. Public Domain. 27

5.1 Trade card of John Norborn (*c.*1790), British Museum (D,2.379). © The Trustees of the British Museum. All rights reserved. 99

5.2 After Henry William Bunbury, *The Dog Barber* (1771), etching, 22.4 × 13.8 cm, Metropolitan Museum of Art, New York, The Elisha Whittelsey Collection, The Elisha Whittelsey Fund, 2011. 109

5.3 James Bretherton after Henry William Bunbury, *The Dog Barber. La Francia* (1772), coloured etching, 24 × 15.8 cm, Wellcome Collection. Public Domain. 110

5.4 Thomas Rowlandson, *Tommy Stichwell, Cobbler and Dog-Doctor* (late 18th – early 19th century), pen, ink and watercolour over pencil, 24 × 30.25 cm, Lot 85, Old Masters, British & European Paintings, Wednesday 6 March 2019, Woolley & Wallis, p. 32. © Woolley & Wallis Salisbury Salesrooms. 111

8.1 Cox's Medical Labels, from the 1828 catalogue. Wellcome Library. Public Domain. 160

8.2 A medicine cabinet (h 22 cm × w 18 cm × d 16 cm), *c.*1850, sold by Graham Smith Antiques, complete with the booklet, 'Cox's Medical Cabinet', and the accompanying labels cut and stuck to the bottles. 165

10.1 A selection of trademarks registered in class three in the first issue of the *Trade Marks Journal* (3 March 1876). The National Archives, STAT 12/1/19. 200

10.2 Graph showing proportion of trademarks registered by professional medical practitioners. 201

10.3 Representation of the trademark 'Dr. Herbert Tibbits' Medical Battery', The National Archives, BT 82/54, no. 13383. 202
10.4 Advertisement for Dr Hank's Neuralgia & Nerve Mixture, *Chemist & Druggist*, 15 February 1881. Wellcome Library. 206
10.5 Representation of 'Spirolene' trademark, The National Archives, BT 82/54 no. 79,648. 208
10.6 Advertisement for Peptoleine, *Chemist and Druggist*, 15 December 1886, p. 128. 209
10.7 Representation of 'Zoolac' trademark, The National Archives, BT 82/46 no. 11,361. 210
11.1 William S. Furneaux (ed.) and Ethel Mayer (rev.), *Dr. Minder's Anatomical Manikin of the Female Human Body: An Illustrated Representation with Full and Descriptive Text* (New York: American Thermo-Ware Co., c.1905). Drexel University Legacy Center. 219
11.2 *Anathomia oder abconterfettung eines Weibs leib, wie er inwendig gestaltet ist* (Strasbourg: Jacob Frölich, [1544]). Wellcome Collection. 221
11.3 Furneaux (ed.), *Dr. Minder's Anatomical Manikin of the Female Human Body*. Drexel University Legacy Center. 227
11.4 Dr. Galtier-Boissière, *La femme: conformation, fonctions, maladies & hygiènes spéciales* (Paris: Schleicher Frères & Cie., Editeurs, [1905]). UCLA. 228
11.5 Adriani Spigelii, Tabula II, *Opera quae extant omnia. Ex recensione Joh, Antonidae vander Linden* (Amsterdami: Johannem Blaeu, 1645). Wellcome Collection. 229
11.6 Furneaux (ed.), *Dr. Minder's Anatomical Manikin of the Female Human Body*. Drexel University Legacy Center. 232
11.7 Furneaux (ed.), *Dr. Minder's Anatomical Manikin of the Female Human Body*. Drexel University Legacy Center. 233
11.8 Furneaux (ed.), *Dr. Minder's Anatomical Manikin of the Female Human Body*. Drexel University Legacy Center. 234

Contributors

Katherine Aske is a literature scholar working within the medical humanities, examining proto-dermatology in the long eighteenth century. Her doctoral thesis focused on physiognomy and the understanding of female beauty within eighteenth-century literature. She has published several chapters on these subjects, including an article in the *Journal for Eighteenth-Century Studies* examining cosmetics in Jonathan Swift's poetry. Aske completed a Postdoctoral Research Fellowship at Université de Bretagne Occidentale in 2016, working on the 'DIGITENS: Digital Encyclopaedia of European Sociability' project. She previously worked as a Senior Research Assistant for Northumbria University on the Sterne Digital Library, funded by the Arts and Humanities Research Council. She is now Lecturer in English at Edinburgh Napier University.

John Baker is a Senior Lecturer in English at the Panthéon-Sorbonne University in Paris. He contributed to the co-authored volume *Melancholy Experience in the Literature of the Long Eighteenth Century* (Palgrave/Macmillan, 2011) and is co-editor of *Writing and Constructing the Self in Great Britain in the Long Eighteenth Century* (Manchester University Press, 2019).

Bethany Brigham recently completed her PhD at Northumbria University, which was funded by the Arts and Humanities Research Council. Her doctoral thesis examined the presence of gothic trope, narrative and convention within medical writing surrounding anatomy in order to redefine the medico-gothic as a discourse mediated by a body of medical and gothic writers through the popular literary formats of the period 1790–1850. Her research sought to established a reformed understanding of the way in which the medico-gothic addressed ethical and social issues surrounding anatomy in order to reshape popular perceptions of medical practice and to reassess the distinction between medical 'fact' and gothic fiction. Her research seeks to reassess the cultural significance of ephemeral, obscure, anonymously or female-authored gothic texts and to recover marginalised narratives and experiences of medical practice and reform, particularly those of women and the working class. She acted as an associate of the British Association for Romantic Studies 'Gothic Women' project.

Jessica M. Dandona earned her PhD from the University of California at Berkeley in Art History and is Professor of Art History at the Minneapolis College of Art and Design. Her current book project is entitled *The Transparent Woman: Medical Visualities in Fin-de-Siècle Europe and the United States, 1880–1900*.

Carlotta Fiammenghi completed her PhD in Linguistic, Literary and Cultural Studies at the University of Milan, with a dissertation in English language and linguistics focusing on the media coverage of the debate surrounding the measles, mumps and rubella vaccine in the UK. She is currently a research fellow at the University of Brescia, where she is working on a project exploring public communication of governmental health institutions in Italy.

Stephanie Howard-Smith completed her PhD on the cultural history of eighteenth-century lapdogs at Queen Mary University of London in 2018. She is currently a Research Associate at the University of York. Her publications include an article on a 1760 London dog cull and a chapter on the circulation of porcelain pugs. Her current research focuses on canine health in Georgian Britain.

Allan Ingram is Emeritus Professor of English at the University of Northumbria. He has published books on Boswell, on Swift and Pope, and on eighteenth-century insanity and its representation, as well as edited collections of primary material on the relations between insanity and medicine. He has also published books on Joseph Conrad and on D. H. Lawrence. He edited *Gulliver's Travels* for Broadview Press (2012). He was Director of the Leverhulme Trust research project, 'Before Depression, 1660–1800', co-general editor of a Pickering & Chatto four-volume collection, *Depression and Melancholy, 1660–1800* (2012) and co-author of *Melancholy Experience in the Long Eighteenth Century* (Palgrave Macmillan, 2011). He was Co-director of the Leverhulme project, 'Fashionable Diseases: Medicine, Literature and Culture, 1660–1830' and co-edited a volume of essays, *Disease and Death in Eighteenth-Century Literature and Culture: Fashioning the Unfashionable* (Palgrave Macmillan, 2016); and he has been Co-director of the 'Writing Doctors' project. His latest book, which is part of the project, is *Swift, Pope and the Doctors: Medicine and Writing in the*

Early Eighteenth Century (Brill-Fink, 2022). He also co-edited the March 2023 issue of the *Journal of Eighteenth-Century Studies* to which he contributed the essay 'Medicating Georgia: Writing Doctors in the Old South'. He has served as co-editor for the journal *English*.

Declan Kavanagh is Senior Lecturer in Eighteenth-Century Studies (English) at the University of Kent. His study of masculinity and queerness in the period, *Effeminate Years: Literature, Politics, and Aesthetics in Mid-Eighteenth-Century Britain*, was published by Bucknell University Press in 2017, and he co-edited a special number of the *Journal for Eighteenth-Century Studies* on *Queer Swift: A Special Supplement* in 2020. He is currently working on libertinism and disability in the long eighteenth century.

Clark Lawlor is Professor of Eighteenth-Century and Romantic Literature at Northumbria University. He has published widely in the field of literature, science and medicine, and medical/health humanities, including *Consumption and Literature: The Making of the Romantic Disease* (Palgrave, 2006) and *From Melancholia to Prozac: A History of Depression* (Oxford University Press, 2012), as well as editing the volume *Literature and Medicine: The Eighteenth Century* (Cambridge University Press, 2021). He was Co-director of the Leverhulme Trust project 'Before Depression, ca. 1660–1800: The Representation and Culture of the English Malady' (2006–09) and Principal Investigator of the Leverhulme Trust major projects 'Fashionable Diseases: Medicine, Literature and Culture, ca. 1660–1832' and 'Writing Doctors: Representation and Medical Personality ca. 1660–1832' (2018–22).

Laura Robson-Mainwaring is the Health Records Specialist in the Collections Expertise and Engagement Department at The National Archives. She is a historian of the pharmaceutical industry, with a particular focus on the intersection between commercial and state bodies. In 2018 she published an article on the text found on pharmaceutical packaging as part of Palgrave's Literature and Medicine series. Her thesis, undertaken at the University of Leicester and funded by the Arts and Humanities Research Council and the Society of the Apothecaries, was on advertising, trademarks and packaging in the medical marketplace *c.*1870–1920.

Laurence Sullivan is a research partner at Northumbria University, having recently completed his PhD as part of the major Leverhulme-Trust funded project: 'Writing Doctors: Representation and Medical Personality ca.

1660–1832.' His research focuses on literary representations of women who practised domestic medicine during the eighteenth century, exploring the role medical self-help played in society, and how women could be empowered by being given the means to take ownership of their own health and that of those around them. He has forthcoming book chapters appearing in *Tobias Smollett After 300 Years: Life, Writing, Reputation* (Clemson University Press) and *The Oxford Handbook of Henry Fielding* (Oxford University Press), co-authored with Clark Lawlor.

Helen Williams is Associate Professor of English Literature at Northumbria University and a British Academy Innovation Fellow. She has published on eighteenth-century literature, the history of the book trades, and morbid and medical sociability. She is the author of *Laurence Sterne and the Eighteenth-Century Book* (Cambridge University Press, 2021), co-editor of John Cleland's *Memoirs of a Woman of Pleasure* (Broadview, 2018) and co-editor of Cleland's correspondence (Cambridge University Press, 2024). She is a Co-investigator of the Leverhulme Trust major project, 'Writing Doctors: Representation and Medical Personality ca. 1660–1832', and co-editor of the special issue of the *Journal for Eighteenth-Century Studies, Writing Doctors and Writing Health in the Long Eighteenth Century* (2023).

Barbara Witucki is Professor Emerita of English at Utica University, New York. She works in classical reception theory particularly as it manifests itself in the eighteenth- and nineteenth-century British and French novel. She has received fellowships from the National Endowment for the Humanities and the Center for Hellenic Studies, Washington, DC. Recent publications include: 'Goldsmith's *The Vicar of Wakefield* and Beccaria's *On Crimes and Punishments*', *Diciottesimo Secolo*, 4 (2019), 143–150, and 'The Tyranny of Tyrannies: Italian Culture in Burney's *The Wanderer; Or Female Difficulties*', in *Entangled Histories. Politics and Culture in 18th-Century Anglo–Italian Encounters* (Cambridge Scholars, 2019).

Introduction

Clark Lawlor and Helen Williams

In response to the coronavirus pandemic, the Centre for Countering Digital Hate (CCDH) published the report *Failure to Act* (2020), responding to widespread concern regarding the rise in false information about vaccination published across global media since 2019.[1] The World Health Organisation had already declared an 'infodemic'.[2] The blurring of fact and fiction had become a major concern. This was not, of course, the first 'infodemic' of medical (mis)information. Nor will it be the last. Infodemics, of macro as well as micro proportions, have always been around. When Oliver Goldsmith (1728–74) died after taking Dr James's Fever Powder, an array of products from the printing press both supporting and decrying Dr Robert James (1703–76) and his medicine proliferated in the marketplace. Printed advertisements authenticating eighteenth- and nineteenth-century medicines appeared alongside printed warnings against them, and booksellers participating in a growing medical marketplace made careers from selling and packaging the same medicines that the pamphlets they published criticised.[3] Very quickly, a media event – as we well know now – could spark debate at all levels of society about the use and (mis)use of (il)legitimate medical products.

The eighteenth and nineteenth centuries are particularly rich for a study of medical myth and (mis)information, considering the wealth of medical publications that emerged in that period. Towards the end of the seventeenth century, Britain had witnessed a turn from Latin to English vernacular as the standard language of medical expression.[4] No longer did a medical author need to have received an education for which the hallmark was a solid command of the Latin tongue, a fact which enabled women to participate in public discourse in growing numbers, as sales rather than sex began to determine a work's success.

The lapse of the Licensing Act in 1695 accelerated literacy rates over the next two hundred years and the rapid expansion of print culture ensured the relatively quick and widespread transmission of medical and quasi-medical information, not all of which could be verified. Through promotion and self-fashioning, medical practitioners were able to exploit the capacity of print to establish themselves as household figures, building up their practices and reputations.[5] Booksellers seized upon increased public literacy and greater purchasing power as opportunities for expanding their productions, thereby stimulating an appetite for science of all kinds and for works of medical utility. Readers were able to take increasing responsibility for their own and their families' health, bringing medicine into the home in an unprecedented way.[6] The public perception of medicine was shaped, among other factors, by poetry, the stage, fiction and the rise of the periodical press, where issues of personality, celebrity and the creative expression of the self were foregrounded. Celebrity doctors and new and emerging medical practices – among them vaccination – were by turns praised and lampooned, even condemned as sacrilegious, and the social, political and religious implications of the democratisation of medical knowledge were explored through literary forms such as poetic satire and science fiction and through innovations in the development of the book.[7]

The transmission and representation of medical (mis)information in the eighteenth and nineteenth centuries has much to contribute to any study of the cultural representation of disease and medicine. Too often there is an assumption that lay readers of the eighteenth and nineteenth centuries were simply a passive public being misled by an excess of unsubstantiated information. But as Wayne Wild has demonstrated, many readers were generally sceptical of medical authority and often non-compliant as patients. Our volume follows recent forays into lay audiences for medical publications, such as Wild's work, *Medicine-By-Post* (2006). Wild has traced the rhetoric of physicians in the eighteenth century as evidenced in their consultation correspondence. Rhetoric, as Wild defines it, signifies the language skills that 'produce belief', which is a key concern in medical matters, requiring the social and moral requisites of trust within the roots an early system of medical ethics.[8] Consultation letters were one of many means by which medical rhetoric was popularised, and then spilled over into the novel and other literary genres, mythologising illness and trauma for eighteenth- and nineteenth-century readers.[9] These reader-patients could be more or less receptive to the moment's medical rhetoric. In the eighteenth and nineteenth centuries, as today, patients challenged their physicians and, as Wild describes, 'they probed the knowledge and competence of their doctors by engaging in current medical jargon'. As Wild argues, 'Any study of rhetoric in doctor–patient letters must be sensitive to the tensions and the vying for authority that describe this complex relationship'.[10]

This was perhaps inevitable in a period which experienced a series of epidemics, including the influenza pandemic of 1782, the North American smallpox epidemic 1775–82, 1831–32 cholera, in 1836 and

1842 influenza, typhus, smallpox, measles, whooping cough and scarlet fever, and between 1846 and 1849 further epidemics of typhus, typhoid and cholera. Meanwhile, tuberculosis and venereal disease continued to cause deaths on a mass scale.[11] There was the debate about the workings of contagion between germ theorists and infectionists or 'miasmists', which, as Allan Conrad Christensen notes, 'was not conducted, however, on serenely rational, or scientific grounds'.[12] For Christensen, it marks the 'vulnerability of science, in its study of literal contagion, to a metaphorical contagion emanating from other discourses'.[13] It is precisely this metaphorical contagion or vulnerability that this volume proposes to address.[14]

English vernacular medical texts of the eighteenth and nineteenth centuries invite cross-comparisons with literary representations of health and medical practitioners in the period, to enrich the picture of medicine in the popular imagination and to provide important perspectives on those questions surrounding authenticity, agency, representation and accessibility that we might similarly ask about literature. The cross-fertilisation, or feedback looping, between these different forms of writing was significant in the construction of health and disease experience in these periods.[15] The popular imagination brings its own assumptions about illness that might contradict, confirm, or even help construct, professional ones. Literature's particular contribution to what we might call the construction and perception of the illness (or health) experience is in its ability to construct a narrative through time that provides a template for the reader: generic expectations of how to behave and what to expect. Literature, in the wider eighteenth-century sense, can act as a filter, or even crucible, for philosophies, theories and ideologies of medicine and related discourses that combine to produce the patient experience. However, scholarship on the construction of medicine and its practitioners in this period does not typically address questions of lies and falsehood, seeking rather to access a 'true' version of the past or to identify what the individuals of the past held to be true.[16]

There is a considerable body of scholarship on the issue of fakery and authenticity in fashionable disease and its representation, but this is generally focused on the way fashionable diseases were constructed via literature and art and the manner in which they might be appropriated by those who were not actually afflicted with them but exploited them for their cultural capital.[17] Our remit here is the transmission of medical information from a perspective broader than disease entities, although this research has aided our understanding of how apparent paradoxes can be produced and maintained through narrative and other cultural media. Quite often, as we shall see, our subjects embrace partial truths, outright untruths, and, as today, the media did not necessarily disseminate 'knowledge'. A fuller understanding of medical writing by and about different types of health practitioners can lay the foundations for better appreciating the literary and cultural effects of medical writing and creativity and their constructions of myth and (mis)information. This volume aims to fill some of these gaps in literary, cultural and medical scholarship and to show new ways in which the fields, and the interchanges between them, can progress and achieve a greater insight into a crucial aspect of eighteenth- and nineteenth-century life in the West. In particular, it is interested in the ways in which popular understanding of medical work and medical figures was not only informed but also misinformed, whether by dishonesty, false marketing, preconceived prejudice or through being made subordinate to non-medical literary ends such as comic or satiric productions or political or religious priorities.

From the very beginning of the period that this volume covers, fake news pervaded public cultures: Sir Richard Blackmore (1654–1729), noted medic, poet and essayist on matters medical and moral, provides a route into understanding the importance of the role of literature, and writing more generally, in the transmission of medical mythology and misinformation. Blackmore was a Modern in matters medical: he argued that knowledge needed to be based on the evidence of experiment, not on the received wisdom of the Ancients. A Whig in politics, devout Anglican in religion, and from a mercantile background, he rose to fame and was knighted as physician to royalty as well as – from the perspective of his detractors, who included Alexander Pope (1688–1744) – a bombastic epic poet who toadied to the monarchs of the day in both literature and medicine. Prolific in many genres, Blackmore published collections of essays ranging across a wide range of topics, including specific medical conditions such as consumption and gout, and literary ones, such as 'An Essay on the Nature and Constitution of Epick Poetry' (1717). His essays were aimed at the literati and were read by the notable writers and critics of the day, including Joseph Addison (1672–1719). Blackmore was keen to write in the vernacular to engage a wide audience and to transmit medical knowledge beyond a Latin- and Greek-based medical elite. In this he was in the vanguard of a movement that was gaining traction in the early eighteenth century, and supplies a context for our volume, both in the eighteenth century, but also leaning forward into the nineteenth, where the issues of truth and lies, information and misinformation, remain at least as crucial.

Most pertinently for our theme, Blackmore analysed the problematic relationship between writing, the author, and truth in the 'Of Controversial Writings' section of his 'Essay upon Writing' (1717).[18] Part of the difficulty with transmitting reliable information, for Blackmore, was the capacity of the writer to distinguish truth from falsehood, or the possession of

'Judgement', a quality that implied an innate intellectual prowess, hard study, and moral discrimination gained over time:

> IT is evident that Nature has bestow'd, on very few that Acuteness, Penetration and discursive Faculty, which are requir'd to qualify Men for Polemical Discourses; and those Persons whom Nature has furnish'd with Judgment and Capacity, must be accustom'd to read the most eminent Authors on Subjects of Controversy, and be well exercis'd and train'd to solid Reasoning, close Debates and Disputations, before their Pens will be accomplish'd for this difficult and important Province. (249)

By 'Polemical Discourses' Blackmore means writing that engages with (as the essay suggests) controversial topics, 'important' points of medicine, religion or politics (or even literary works that engage these topics) and that therefore require the highest powers of discrimination. Writing is key: 'Pens' must 'be accomplish'd for this difficult and important Province'.

Another part of Blackmore's problem is the difficulty of recognising Truth when lies look so convincing – and even beautiful:

> As Truth often lies entangled with such specious Mixtures of Falshood, that a sharp and distinguishing Taste is demanded to abstract and free it from opposite and repugnant Complications, and shew it in its pure and genuine Splendor; so Error has frequently such a plausible and shining Appearance, in which we meet with so many Lines and features, which imitate and resemble Truth, that it easily imposes on vulgar and credulous Understandings, tho it cannot escape the Observation and Discovery of Men of Sagacity and clear Judgment, long vers'd in detecting such Counterfeits and unmasking the Imposture; such able Writers with wonderful Readiness and Perspicuity, unravel difficult and knotty Subjects, and grapple with the Adversary with superior Strength, triumph in every Page, bear down all before them, and Spread the Field of Disputation with the Spoils of defeated Opponents. (249–250)

Blackmore was in the process of defending himself against Joseph Addison's accusation that he had written on for too long in his career and was, to use the modern term, past his sell-by date.[19] Part of Blackmore's agenda is to figure himself as just such an experienced author with 'sharp and distinguishing Taste' who is capable of differentiating between 'plausible and shining' Error and the Truth that it counterfeits. Blackmore fashions himself as one of the 'able Writers with wonderful Readiness and Perspicuity, [who] unravel difficult and knotty Subjects', and follows the logic of his heroic defence of Truth by taking on the masculine metaphor of the knight and warrior. Of course, he was a knight for reasons of medical prowess. It is he who can 'grapple with the Adversary with superior Strength, triumph in every Page, bear down all before them, and Spread the Field of Disputation with the Spoils of defeated Opponents'. This fantasy of himself as the noble defender of Truth is of a piece with Blackmore's devout Anglican faith, and conviction in the rightness of his own views. That it is a gendered fantasy is unsurprising, given his concept of writing in general, which requires a certain kind of education and confidence in one's place in the public sphere not often available to women, and certainly not in the same way as a man of the period.

In case we were in any doubt about the elite status of the true author, Blackmore continues the eulogy on such individuals (as himself), although he varies the metaphor:

> There are but few Disputants of this superior Rank in any Science; and happy are the Students in Theology and Philosophy, who have Wisdom enough to chuse and stick to these admirable Authors, or into whose Hands they fall by good Fortune or the prudent Advice of others. For these accomplished Masters, that by the resistless Light of their Reason, with great facility: penetrate and dispel the Mists and Error that hang upon and eclipse the Face of Truth, will in the Compass of a few Pages, convince and instruct them infinitely more than the shallow Productions of a light and volatile Genius, or the heavy and prolix Volumes of muddy Heads, who bewilder'd in their own undigested Notions darken the Disputation, confound the Reader by their insignificant Labour, and explain their Subject till it becomes unintelligible. (250–251)

This is an Enlightenment discourse, and here 'Science' means knowledge generally: 'the resistless Light of their [these admirable Authors'] Reason' dispels the 'Mists and Error that hang upon and eclipse the Face of Truth'.[20] Blackmore was a Modern, and championed experiment over received wisdom of the Ancients in medicine, and was identified as such in Jonathan Swift's *Battle of the Books* (1704) ('Bl – ckm – re, a famous Modern').[21] For Blackmore, the mission of the author, medical or otherwise, is to bring the light of reason where formerly there was scholastic darkness. To illustrate his point further, Blackmore switches to a medical logic: indigestion, the bane of physical health because it causes blockages in the circulation of the body's various systems (blood, spirits, formerly humours), afflicts those 'muddy Heads' who 'darken the Disputation' because they are unable to process the necessary ideas to enlighten the reader, and instead render 'their Subject ... unintelligible'.[22] At the opposite end of the bad author spectrum are 'the shallow Productions of a light and volatile Genius', not so much indigested as inadequately fed with any substantial ideas at all. Either way readers suffer from just such an overproduction of incomprehensible argument, unlike those of the 'accomplished Masters', who 'in the Compass of a few Pages, convince and instruct them'.

Truth, then, is a matter of literary style as well as content. The author who writes on 'Controversial Points' must 'to the strength, closeness and perspicuity of their Reasoning, add fine Temper and genteel Humanity. These Qualities gain immediately upon the Reader, and leave him prejudic'd in favour of the Disputant' (251). 'Deep and lasting Impressions' come from the good author's 'unobstructed good Sense' finding 'easy Admission to the Mind'. Again, the metaphor is military and manly:

> The Energy and convincing Force of a Polemical Writer, does not consist in the immoderate Heat and Fierceness of his Passion, but in the Strength and resistless Violence of his Arguments; not in big Words, arrogant Assurance and Airs of Authority, but in the commanding Force of his Demonstration. (251)

Controlled, 'resistless Violence' of logic and the 'commanding Force of his Demonstration' is Blackmore's preferred mode of argument, and one that assumes truth as the core than enables it to be 'resistless' (one of Blackmore's repeated and favourite terms here). Later in this volume we engage with alternative forms of medical and literary authority that work from a wider, feminine model of creativity, but here Blackmore is very much speaking from a traditional, patriarchal standpoint. Calm authority must be reinforced by a polite (in the powerful period sense of the term) and gentlemanly style:

> And as this gentle and well-manner'd Conduct is delightful and beneficial to the indifferent Reader, so it is most likely to gain upon the Opponent, who by such Candour, good Usage and respectful Expression, is more dispos'd to entertain and weigh the Evidence, and yield up the Cause to superior Reason. (251)

It is all very well to be in possession of the truth, but a masculine, militaristic command of rhetoric and register ('yield up the Cause'!) is needed to deliver that truth in a combative, 'controversial' mode.

Blackmore's conviction of a mainstream, Anglican and Whiggish medical truth based on empirical findings, as opposed to the wisdom of the ages, carries us forward into the Age of Enlightenment and the following centuries into scientific modernity. Writing, and writing in the vernacular, was key to going beyond the medical elite and into the hinterland of medical actors – midwives, apothecaries, cunning women, 'Lady Bountifuls', those in the country with the ability to learn medical techniques without botching them, those who could not afford elite medical care, and so on. To be sure, Blackmore held to a certain (masculine) model of truth and falsity, but he demonstrates the centrality of writing, creative and otherwise, to the construction of that knowledge. He sets in motion themes around the contestation of knowledge via the power of competing narratives that will remain crucial to the ensuing centuries, including our own, and foregrounds the need to analyse the process of writing as we seek for truth, however defined.

This collection, a product of the Leverhulme Trust-funded major research project 'Writing Doctors: Medical Representation and Personality, ca. 1660–1832' at Northumbria University, combines a diverse spectrum of scholarly approaches, from medical history to book history, exploring literary and scientific texts, such as recipes, satiric poetry, essays, anatomies, advertisements, and the novel, to shed light on the mythologisation and transmission of medical (mis)information through literature and popular culture throughout the eighteenth and nineteenth centuries. At the intersection of medical history and culture, the various chapters analyse the persuasive, promotional, and sometimes deceptive means by which myths about the medical professions proliferated in English literary culture of this period, from early eighteenth-century household remedies to the late nineteenth-century concerns with vaccination which continue to feel strikingly relevant since the outbreak of the coronavirus pandemic, and which make strong connections between our current climate of misinformation and that which flourished during the heyday of medical print culture in the eighteenth and nineteenth centuries.

This volume seeks to make direct links between social change and the mass availability and circulation of medical information beginning in the eighteenth century and expanding exponentially during the nineteenth, while positioning literary and print cultural forms as playing a pivotal role in how this information was received, interpreted and (often) distorted for an engaged public. At the same time, we situate emergent medical professions in relation to the contemporary marketplace and print culture.[23] While the volume addresses well-known figures like John Arbuthnot (1667–1735) and George Cheyne (1671–1743), it also includes lesser-known individuals, as in the medical publisher Elizabeth Cox (1765–1841). This approach enables us to deal with the mainstream, and the popular medical culture of the period, while also illuminating overlooked texts and writers, or, as in the case of Henry Rider Haggard (1856–1925), overlooked texts by figures who remain well known in the literary world but perhaps infrequently so closely considered, particularly in relation to medicine. Individual chapters also place prominent figures like Tobias Smollett (1721–71) and Elizabeth Gaskell (1810–65) in direct conversation with more obscure practitioners of domestic medicine, such as the women healers of the period.

Katherine Aske's chapter on early eighteenth-century skincare makes the important point that the relationship between elite professional medical advice and popular and domestic medical cures for minor skin ailments could be a blurry one and, for Daniel Turner (1667–1740), required a delicate balancing act in his attempt to negotiate the two. The professional medic needed to communicate the 'true' professional cure clearly and in the vernacular to a popular audience, who did not necessarily know Latin, while acknowledging/highlighting ineffective cures without losing the veneer of respectability. Turner's *De Morbis Cutaneis: A Treatise of Diseases Incident to the Skin* (1714) is the first treatise on this subject in English, which Aske uses to demonstrate the techniques by which Turner sought to dispel popular mythologies, or sometimes professional misdiagnoses and treatment, around skin health. Aske's chapter, like others in this volume, shows that medical truth is a contested entity in this period, as in our own, and that narrative and rhetorical ability was required to guide the intended audiences, popular or professional, towards the desired destination of the particular author. Skin is a crucial area of the body that invited a commerce between 'deeper' and more serious disease to be treated by professional medics and 'surface' blemishes and spots that beckoned quackery and popular mythological cures.

Turner, it transpires, was not above lifting and manipulating the work of others, sometimes popularising authors whom he had elsewhere criticised, unacknowledged: in this case William Salmon, who had translated George Bate's *Pharmacopoeia Bateana* (1688). In order to reinforce correct information (as provided by himself), Turner had to demonstrate, perhaps paradoxically, 'the interconnectedness of medical knowledge, and the necessity to engage with domestic and popular works in order to form a professional approach'. Elite medicine, if it wanted to speak to a wider audience than fellow medics, needed to reach out, and in so doing threatened its own validity. Patently this remains a problem in our own time, as we have seen with the coronavirus pandemic and the debates about following a supposedly unified scientific view, albeit Latin has been replaced by the specialised language of biomedicine.

John Baker discusses a world 'shot through with its spin, fake news, 'alternative facts', storytelling, scams, disinformation, conspiracy theories, propaganda, political lies' – as it happens, he is describing our own time, but points out that the early eighteenth century was very similar, and needed the treatment of a 'writing doctor' to cure, or attempt to cure, its ills. His chapter, 'Dr John Arbuthnot's literary treatment for false learning, pedantry and excess: from physic to metaphysics', takes the volume themes in their broadest sense, and includes the diseases of the nation as well as the individual, maladies that encompass medical myths and misinformation on a grand scale. Arbuthnot was both physician to the Queen and a member of the Scriblerus Club, a literary-satirical powerhouse of the Augustan age that included Alexander Pope and Jonathan Swift (1667–1745) as its primary members. Medicine and literature combined in the works of Arbuthnot, satirical or otherwise, to debunk quackery and charlatanism wherever he and his Scriblerian fellows found them.

Baker demonstrates that Arbuthnot interrogated the notion of lying via a pseudological mode, *The Art of Political Lying* (1712), parodying the logical method that the scientific part of his writings enacted so well. This chapter argues that Arbuthnot ranged through three 'domains and discourses, fact, fiction, and belief', which correspond to scientific, literary and religious writings, in order to expose truth and condemn falsehood across these areas. *The Art of Political Lying* and the *Memoirs of the Extraordinary Life, Works, and Discoveries of Martinus Scriblerus* (written around 1713–14) fall under the fictional and satirical category, whereas the later works, such as the poem *Gnothi Seauton, Know your self* (1734) were more concerned with philosophical reflections that led to a Christian explanation of matters of body, soul and wider society.

From one writing male doctor to another, Clark Lawlor's chapter '"The very women read it": medical self-fashioning, mythologies and (mis)information in George Cheyne MD's medical writing' discusses the ways in which the famous, and sometimes due to his colourful personal journey, infamous, Bath and London society physician Cheyne wrote popular medical essays (such as *An Essay of Health and Long Life* (1725)) and treatises that 'sold' the author himself as much as his methods. Cheyne did not have the generic range of Arbuthnot, but what Cheyne did, he did very well. Lawlor argues that Cheyne's mastery of writing in English, rather than Latin, allowed him to reach a much wider audience than fellow medics, although there were other factors in his successful self-fashioning. Improvements in print technology and distribution meant cheaper and easier production of his self-help works, as well as an expanding medical market. His ability to label his writing in an effective way in terms of genre, the simplicity of his treatments (regimens) and the way they fed into a religious aesthetic of slimness were crucial factors.

Cheyne uniquely debunked alternative, quack mythologies of health by promoting his own case and its cure, by himself. This bodily self-fashioning was described in his famous *English Malady* (1733), in which 'the Author's Case' eloquently detailed Cheyne's dissolute lifestyle, massive weight gain and what we might now approximately call depression, and then his dietary and general regimen treatment that normalised his lifestyle, weight and mental health. This sensational tale of physical and mental self-mythology played nicely into the new discourse of sensibility, which marked the suffering of the sensitive, possibly creative, individual as the price to pay for a superior intellect and morality underpinned by finer nerves. Lawlor also points out that self-fashioning is never as monologic as it sounds: often that fashioning is created as much by the 'other' (be it a publisher, audience, fellow medic or patient) as by the individual supposedly doing the intentional fashioning: a dialogical mythology of the self.

Laurence Sullivan's chapter 'Studying in solitude: demythologising the masculine medical monopoly with Jane Barker's Galesia and Tobias Smollett's Sagely' broadens the scope of who could participate in healthcare and its representation by examining the role of women in fiction. Sullivan argues that women could not only contribute to healthcare, but also do it better than male practitioners in some instances. Women may not have been permitted to enjoy a professional standing equal to that of Blackmore, but Jane Barker (1652–1732), whose brother was a licensed medic, had acquired knowledge via her relative's studies, but also through her own determination (and of course a good education that was not accessible to all women or men, depending on rank and individual family circumstances). Barker's novel, *A Patch-Work Screen for the Ladies* (1723), is unusual in that it features a semi-autobiographical character, Galesia, who treats the local community for diseases such as gout (Barker herself had devised a gout remedy that was actually marketed) and is respected for her expertise. Also unusual is Barker's interpolation of poetry into the novel, poetry that deals with the female perspective on healthcare as a giver rather than as a sufferer (the more common representation).

If Barker demythologises the masculine healthcare monopoly in her novel and practice as a female author and character, so does Tobias Smollett as a male physician and novelist. In his case, it is by means of his character Betty Sagely in *The Adventures of Roderick Random* (1748). Sagely, as the name suggests, is a wise woman who is isolated from her community by the apparently inevitable association of unmarried women practising healthcare with witchcraft. Smollett demonstrates, through Sagely's healing of the eponymous Roderick Random, that female healers are valuable contributors to the ecology of healthcare in the eighteenth century, despite the opprobrium heaped upon them by the male professional establishment. Both fictional and actual women (i.e. Barker herself) remain unmarried, an aspect of their identities that allows them to practise medicine to a specialised degree, as domestic duties might otherwise engage all their time and energy. Being a spinster is a mixed blessing, however: freedom from male control to some extent meant suspicion and social ostracism. Barker has to contend, as does Galesia, with mythologies of female incompetence created by the male profession, and Sagely too is shunned by her society even as she provides treatment for people's ills.

When we think of medical misinformation, we tend to think of medicine applying to humans, but Stephanie Howard-Smith's essay, '"Take physic, Pomp": imagining dog doctors in eighteenth-century Britain', demonstrates the importance of veterinary information and (often sexist) mythology about the owners as well as the medics. 'Dog doctors' was an insult, a term that arose through a cultural anxiety about the rise of dog and pet ownership as a leisure industry during the eighteenth century, and with it a veterinary market. As so often, women bore the brunt of this fear of a burgeoning consumerism representationally, specifically and inextricably in creative literature, although also to an extent in the visual arts in Britain and Europe. The lapdog was a symbol of useless canine luxury, an ornament to the equally useless elite woman, or worse, an instrument of sexual pleasure ('lap' dog!) gleefully depicted across literary genres and artfully hinted at in visual works. This exclusion of men from female pleasure no doubt exacerbated the worry that consumerism and its primary symbol, the consuming woman, were running amok and not susceptible to moral and male control. Dog doctors themselves were labelled as effeminate creatures, as effete as the dogs and their owners.

Creative literature is crucial here, for the powerful image created in novels, poems and plays (such as Francis Coventry's influential *History of Pompey the Little* (1751)) of women tending to their favoured pets rather than their children or husbands and paying extortionate amounts of money to quack dog doctors was difficult to shift for the profession. The absence of archival evidence only increases the importance of literary and visual materials for our understanding of the role of the dog doctors. Howard-Smith debunks the older myth that only elite women owned pet dogs, and positions dogs as a vital source of labour in the city and country, with important sporting functions as well. The rise of the culture of the sentimental also meant dogs were a form of companion beyond the economic, not unlike companionate marriage, although one might facetiously speculate that the dogs were more popular than the husbands. This image persisted throughout the nineteenth century, only to be replaced by 'a fresh myth – dogs received no specialist healthcare until the Victorian, Edwardian or even post-War periods', a myth that this chapter firmly contradicts.

Adopting a queer and disabilities studies perspective, Declan Kavanagh puts the emphasis very much on masculinity in his chapter dealing with the ways in which venereal infection challenged heteronormative and ableist mythologies, experiences and expressions in literary form. '"A man of common understanding": venereal disease, myth and reading as a protective practice in eighteenth-century Britain' takes three main instances of venereal infection from three different literary modes: William Buchan's (1729–1805) popular medical self-help advice in his *Observations Concerning the Prevention and Cure of the Venereal Disease* (1796), Tobias Smollett's eponymous character in *The Adventures of Roderick Random* (1748) and James Boswell's (1740–95) account of his own pox in his *London Journal* (1762–63). Buchan's philosophy of allowing men to take matters into their own hands (the implied sexual reference is deliberate in the case of Kavanagh and his subjects) and overcoming misinformation to cure themselves via knowledge gained by reading donated a form of male agency where none was forthcoming from rapacious quacks and charlatans, and where one's reputation might be damaged by wider exposure of a potentially embarrassing and often debilitating condition.

When it comes to novelistic representation, Smollett's Roderick Random, himself poxed, has the threat to his masculine identity, informed by both his autonomy in reputation and ability in agency, displaced by his sentimental care for Miss Williams, a woman who has also contracted venereal disease. Because Random has experience as an employee with the professional treatment of venereal disease and exposure to the dark arts of his former quack employer, he is able to treat Miss Williams and retain, in the process, his 'straight' masculine qualities of gallantry, self-possession and apparent physical integrity – we never see his 'leaky' vessel of a body for what it really is as all the representational mythology and information is directed at Miss Williams. The final instance, James Boswell's autopathography, if one can label it as such, in his *London Journal*, details Boswell's reclamation of his masculine physical, mental and reputational integrity by his demeaning rejection of the woman from whom he had allegedly received his infection – the opposite of the fictional Roderick Random's strategy of care. Boswell's anxiety about queering himself at all-too-intimate hands (when being treated) by his medical friend is mitigated by his splitting of the identity of Douglas into the professional doctor who might want to overcharge for treatment and the trusty friend minus such a medical identity. Venereal disease is a threat to the mythologies of compulsory able-bodiedness and heteronormativity, one that must be neutralised by various narrative strategies across these different genres.

Further pursuing eighteenth-century narrative strategies, Bethany Brigham, in her essay on the little-known but fascinating Minerva Press novel *The Horrors of Oakendale Abbey* (1797) by 'Mrs Carver', describes its engagement with the anatomy debates. Exploring its potential authorship by the surgeon and anatomist Sir Anthony Carlisle (1764–1840), Brigham demonstrates how the narrative is 'veined through with detailed medical knowledge' and plays into the debates of its moment, particularly by dealing with the politics of body snatching. While opening with gothic images of the walking dead, the novel soon assumes the style of the Radcliffean supernatural explained, when the protagonist learns that the abbey of the title has been repurposed as a vault for stolen corpses awaiting dissection. Brigham demonstrates how Carver/Carlisle manipulates the seeming excesses of the gothic genre to reflect the medical realities of late eighteenth-century England.

The Horrors of Oakendale Abbey captures a moment of uncertainty, when the growth in medical education throughout the eighteenth century also meant an increased demand for corpses for dissection. The Murder Act of 1752 permitted corpses of executed murderers to be donated to the London Company of Surgeons, combining criminality, ethics and anatomy in a bid to put a stop to a disturbing rise in body snatching as a lucrative underground business. However, body snatching continued to be a major source of anatomical subjects until the passing of the Anatomy Act by the UK Parliament in 1832. In the meantime, the anatomy debates continued, proposing imaginative alternatives to body snatching, and debating the propriety of both the theft and dissection itself. As a surgeon, Carlisle was unusual in promoting legislation to improve the supply of anatomical subjects. Until that point, the ethics of body snatching, dissecting criminals and of sourcing sufficient anatomical subjects in a largely Christian society continued to be debated at all levels of society. Brigham demonstrates how *The Horrors of Oakendale Abbey* unveils popular belief systems around death and dissection as a form of myth and misinformation that only further perpetuated body snatching and prevented legal reform. In Brigham's reading, the Minerva Press novel emerges as a gothic intervention uniquely placed to present the criminal body's centrality to the advancement of medical knowledge and as a viable solution to the 1790s anatomy debates.

From masculine mythology and self-empowerment we shift back to the provision of medical knowledge by women, as well as the subsequent erasure of, and misinformation about, that contribution. Part of the work of the 'Writing Doctors' project has been to recover and analyse female agency and writing in the creation of medical cultures: 'writing' can cover a multitude of modes of expression, however, and here we find that the world of printing is under-researched in this regard. The remainder of the volume also has a distinct focus on the ethics of medical practice. Helen Williams's chapter, 'Mislabelling and the medical printer-publisher: demystifying the ephemera of Elizabeth Rane Cox (1765–1841)', introduces us to Elizabeth Cox (née Rane) who, unusually, identified herself as a 'Medical Bookseller Labeller &c' in her will and made a major contribution to both medical knowledge and treatment in the nineteenth century. Cox owned a bookshop that also sold and loaned out medical books and branded medicines, and grew the business into a major player regarding the supply of printed medical information and carefully labelled medicines: Cox's institution had large influence on nineteenth-century medicine, but one that has been neglected until now. We have mostly lost her name and achievements because, Williams argues, she was misgendered as 'Messrs. Cox and Son', and given as 'Edward Fox' after her death, despite the fact that the real Edward Fox could not possibly have been old enough to be the actual author and owner of her works and business. In her own time,

Cox's name had become a brand, largely due to the efforts of Elizabeth rather than the husband from whom she inherited the business, Williams demonstrates: she was clearly a person of substance who commanded the respect of her market and was able to fashion an image that transcended her gender (although her son's alleged crime in forging 'a fraudulent plate for "Harvey's Fish Sauce" in 1811 or 1812' did temporarily dent her reputation).

Cox was printer-publisher of *Cox's Companion to the Medicine Chest* (c.1829), 'the most successful booklet of the nineteenth century', and vital to the spread of medical knowledge because, along with the coloured printed labels that Cox also provided in an innovatively detailed way, it allowed people to know exactly what was in the medicine chest, what it should be used to treat and in what quantity for each specific kind of patient. If Cox and others were not to provide preprinted and bespoke medical labels in both Latin and English, the results could be disastrous. Without such accurate information aimed at both the lay person and the practitioner (Cox knew her various markets) accidental poisoning could be a real possibility, and Williams outlines various cases in which the worst did happen. The apparently innocuous world of medicinal labelling was in practice one with very high stakes, and legal consequences.

The ethics of medical practice remain a key concern in Barbara Witucki's consideration of Elizabeth Gaskell's work, in which the novel emerges as an educational and politicised genre for writing about health. Witucki convinces us of the significance of Gaskell's novels as sources for the student of medical history, against a compelling backdrop of Gaskell's own familial medical networks. Perhaps surprisingly, given the extent to which Gaskell was embedded within medical sociability through a surgeon uncle, her literary representation of medicine tends toward a critique of its promised efficacy. Witucki notices how doctors and medical practice are obscured from the sight of the reader in many of Gaskell's works, particularly in *Mary Barton* (1848), where herbal remedies and women's healing become the focus of the narrative through the figure of Alice Wilson, domestic herbalist. Wilson's labour in the context of the harsh realities of daily life for the working poor in nineteenth-century Manchester sets up what becomes a common theme in Gaskell's fiction: a nostalgia for a traditional past free of the politics and bureaucracy of contemporary medical practice.

Perhaps most significantly, Witucki demonstrates how Gaskell's fiction works to query the profession's dependence on the formal qualifications of apprenticeship and to thereby question its accessibility and efficacy. Gaskell's novels of Victorian working life establish a distance between the people and the professional middle classes which works at the level of form as well as content, through which she gestures towards the myth of professional practice and reputation which can be democratising – in the case of illegitimate birth, for instance – but which continued to exclude women and the mill-working class.

Also considering the intersection of professional practice and reputation is Laura Robson-Mainwaring's chapter on medicines and trademark legislation. Robson-Mainwaring systematically demonstrates how this perceived distance between medical practitioners and their products has resulted in what has become a standard myth even extending to scholarship: that the medical profession did not engage in commercial trade in this period. Many nineteenth-century medicines, in fact, were registered by professionals keen to maintain reputations for objective transparency. The late nineteenth century saw the reappraisal of trademarks, which began to be considered an economic asset in commodity branding, providing consumers with a sense of the brand's credibility through provenance and mitigating against misinformation and mis-selling.[24]

The new culture of branding was perhaps appealing to medical practitioners, who were a far from homogeneous group, and some of whom may have wished to demonstrate ownership of a product without having to put their name to it. Robson-Mainwaring also topples the myth of patent medicines being associated with quackery. Her chapter sheds light on the competitive nineteenth-century medical marketplace, and in revealing that even the wealthiest professionals dabbled in commercial enterprise, dismantles the myth that the profession's core values delimited promoting commercial interests and obtaining intellectual property, and reveals a range of interpretations of the ethics of medical practice.

Jessica Dandona's chapter, like that of Robson-Mainwaring, provides an insight into the popular and material culture of nineteenth-century medicine, while also exploring its increasing popularisation for wider – and younger – audiences. Dandona recounts the history of nineteenth-century flap book anatomies, identifying colour lithography and halftone printing as technologies quickly transforming medicine into a visual enterprise which sought to both reveal and obscure reproductive histories. Produced in bright colours using dozens of superimposed images, flap anatomies were used by physicians, medical students and middle-class families in Britain and the United States. Works such as *Dr. Minder's Anatomical Manikin of the Female Human Body* (*c.*1905) opened medical discourse to lay communities, but in the process perpetuated an impossible ideal of health, youthfulness and fertility against which the bodies of living patients would be measured. Most dangerous of all was the way in which they were appropriated by the Physical Culture Movement, reproducing associations between classical aesthetics and notions of health, whiteness and reproductive fitness to support the 'science' of eugenics.

Flap anatomies perpetuated a myth of the 'anatomical body', articulated according to binary notions of normal and pathological anatomy, and transformed curiosity into knowledge, into power, through subjecting paper to intimate touch and a clinical gaze. Widely referencing classical art in order to avoid accusations of impropriety, but also to sanitise anatomisation and the process of decay, flap anatomies denied the unruly reality of the living, moving, dynamic flesh, and circumvented controversy by the careful construction of a sense of scientific objectivity which contributed to the growing discursive power of medicine.

We close with Carlotta Fiammenghi's reading of the little-known, and unique among Henry Rider Haggard's corpus of adventure stories, *Doctor Therne* (1898), a text he described as his 'only novel with a purpose'.[25] The story follows a medical doctor who publicly pretends to disbelieve the efficacy and safety of vaccines in order to run for Parliament as a Radical candidate. While the political impetus of *Doctor Therne* has led scholars such as Morton Norton Cohen to disregard it as propagandist,[26] Fiammenghi argues instead that its engagement with social and political reality invites reconsideration. Reading *Doctor Therne* against Haggard's *A Farmer's Year* (1899) for its approach to what Haggard identified as 'the Anti-Vaccination craze', Fiammenghi demonstrates that Haggard exploited the form of the novel to demonstrate the impact of the media and politics on medical matters, family life and – ultimately – social cohesion.

Fiammenghi identifies in Haggard's fiction echoes of anti-vaccination tracts and pamphlets popular at that time in Victorian England, such as John Gibbs's *Compulsory Vaccination Briefly Considered in its Scientific, Religious, and Political Aspects* (1856), providing a colourful snapshot of a media moment not unlike our own. Here, *Doctor Therne* provides a stark commentary on media influence while simultaneously reflecting on the power of literature – itself a form of media – to examine, interrogate and re-enact the complexities of medico-scientific and sociopolitical issues. Like the period's ephemera, Haggard makes a claim – or at least a hope – for the novel's influence on contemporary vaccination debates.

The concerns of Haggard's work resonate, as Fiammenghi demonstrates, with concerns perceptible in this, our coronavirus moment, as Allan Ingram further explores in his Afterword. Closing with this summation of the case studies we present, Ingram takes us on a tour of eighteenth- and nineteenth-century print media and culture, its myths and (mis)information, guiding us back to the present to see both the similarities and the disjuncts, and indicating how literary and cultural studies can shed light on medical matters including public health messaging, which in turn determines ideas about our bodies and communities. Throughout this volume, we explore some of the medical debates – on commercialisation and medical labelling – as well as public controversies, including the anatomy debates and rising anti-vaccination sentiment, that sparked a range of contributions across manuscript and diverse print sources. The cultures of misinformation that manifested around these topics feel particularly pertinent given the moment in which we present a volume that includes discussion of canonical and noncanonical creative as well as medical practitioners, and forms – from apothecary labels and flap books to Victorian novels – particularly well suited to demonstrate the diverse cultural media that conglomerate around, engage with, undermine and shape medical discourse in any given period.

In covering two centuries we are able to make connections between periods that are often addressed separately. But we must also acknowledge the limitations and gaps in existing scholarship, most obviously relating to race and colonialism, notwithstanding recent important interventions by Emily Senior and Suman Seth, among others.[27]

Nevertheless, we have expanded already growing fields, including queering and dis-abling eighteenth-century medical and literary discourses, emphasising the role of non-elite medical workers such as women involved in domestic medicine, non-human medicine, and the importance of the history of the book and material cultures, and forms of publication or manuscript not limited to the usually studied printed treatises or literary forms. As such, this volume includes much of interest for readers exploring the social history of medicine, as well as scholars of the literature and culture of the eighteenth and nineteenth centuries, contributing to our understanding of the phenomenon of writing about health and its wider social effects, whether it be representations of medical practitioners in literature and art, or creative works written by medical people.

Notes

1 Center for Countering Digital Hate, *Failure to Act: How Tech Giants Continue to Defy Calls to Rein in Vaccine Misinformation* (1 December 2020), available at https://counterhate.com/research/failure-to-act/, last accessed 5 April 2020.
2 World Health Organization, *Managing the COVID-19 Infodemic: Promoting Healthy Behaviours and Mitigating the Harm from Misinformation and Disinformation*, Joint statement by WHO, UN, UNICEF, UNDP, UNESCO, UNAIDS, ITU, UN Global Pulse, and IFRC (23 September 2020), available at https://www.who.int/news/item/23-09-2020-managing-the-covid-19-infodemic-promoting-healthy-behaviours-and-mitigating-the-harm-from-misinformation-and-disinformation, last accessed 5 April 2023.

3 Dorothy Porter and Roy Porter, *Patient's Progress: Doctors and Doctoring in Eighteenth-Century England* (Palo Alto, CA: Stanford University Press, 1989), p. 110. See also Helen Williams, *Laurence Sterne and the Eighteenth-Century Book* (Cambridge: Cambridge University Press, 2021), pp. 132–135.
4 See, for example, Eric Colman, 'The First English Medical Journal: *Medicina Curiosa*', *Lancet* 354:9175 (1999): 324–326; Audrey Eccles, 'The Reading Public, the Medical Profession, and the Use of English for Medical Books in the 16th and 17th Centuries', *Neuphilologische Mitteilungen* 75:1 (1974): 143–156; and Allen G. Debus, *The English Paracelsians* (New York: Watts, 1966).
5 On self-fashioning, see for example Giulia Rovelli, 'John Pechey (1654–1718) and the Popularization of Learned Medicine', *Writing Doctors and Writing Health in the Long Eighteenth Century*, Special Issue of *Journal for Eighteenth-Century Studies* 46:1 (2023): 59–73.
6 Elizabeth Lane Furdell, *Publishing and Medicine in Early Modern England* (Rochester, NY: University of Rochester Press, 2002); Ashleigh Blackwood and Helen Williams, Introduction, *Writing Doctors*, pp. 3–20.
7 On the figure of the celebrity doctor, particularly George Cheyne, see Michelle Faubert, *Rhyming Reason: The Poetry of Romantic-Era Psychologists* (London: Routledge, 2009); Katherine Richards, 'Medical Celebrity in Eighteenth-Century Britain', PhD thesis, West Virginia University (2018); and Wayne Wild, *Medicine-By-Post: The Changing Voice of Illness in Eighteenth-Century British Consultation Letters and Literature* (Amsterdam: Rodopi, 2006). On vaccination, see Stanley Williamson, *The Vaccination Controversy: The Rise, Reign and Fall of Compulsory Vaccination for Smallpox* (Liverpool: Liverpool University Press, 2007); Nadja Durcbach, *Bodily Matters: The Anti-Vaccination Movement in England, 1853–1907* (Durham, NC: Duke University Press, 2005); and Deborah Brunton, *The Politics of Vaccination: Practice and Policy in England, Wales, Ireland, and Scotland 1800–1874* (Rochester, NY: University of Rochester Press, 2008). On the democratisation of medical knowledge, see Roy Porter (ed.), *The Popularization of Medicine 1650–1850* (London: Routledge, 1992); Roy Porter, *Flesh in the Age of Reason: The Modern Foundations of Body and Soul* (New York: Norton, 2004); and Zachary Dorner, *Merchants of Medicines: The Commerce and Coercion of Health in Britain's Long Eighteenth Century* (Chicago, IL: University of Chicago Press, 2020). On literature and satire in this period, see Marie Mulvey Roberts and Roy Porter (eds), *Literature and Medicine During the Eighteenth Century* (London: Routledge, 1993); Allan Ingram and Leigh Wetherall Dickson (eds), *Disease and Death in Eighteenth-Century Literature and Culture: Fashioning the Unfashionable* (London: Palgrave, 2016); Clark Lawlor and Andrew Mangham (eds), *Literature and Medicine: The Eighteenth Century* (Cambridge: Cambridge University Press, 2021); and Clark Lawlor and Andrew Mangham (eds), *Literature and Medicine: The Nineteenth Century* (Cambridge: Cambridge University Press, 2021). On material cultural or book historical approaches to medical knowledge, see Anna Gasperini, *Nineteenth-Century Popular Fiction, Medicine and Anatomy* (London: Palgrave, 2019); Samuel J. M. Alberti, *Morbid Curiosities: Medical*

Museums in Nineteenth-Century Britain (Oxford: Oxford University Press, 2011); Catharine Coleborne, 'Exhibiting "Madness": Material Culture and the Asylum', *Health and History* 3:2 (2001): 104–117; Paula Bertucci, 'Shocking Subjects: Human Experiments and the Material Culture of Medical Electricity in Eighteenth-Century England', in Erika Dyck and Larry Stewart (eds), *The Uses of Humans in Experiment: Perspectives from the Seventeenth to the Twentieth Century* (Leiden: Brill, 2016), pp. 111–138; Helen Williams, 'Family Planning and the Long Eighteenth-Century Pocketbook', *Writing Doctors* 46:1 (2023): 113–133.

8   Wild, *Medicine-By-Post*, p. 10.
9   See, for instance, the Cullen Project, *The Consultation Letters of Dr William Cullen (1710–1790) at the Royal College of Physicians*, available at https://www.cullenproject.ac.uk/, last accessed 5 April 2023; Micheline Louis-Courvoisier, 'The Soul in the Entrails: The Experience of the Sick in the Eighteenth Century', in Rebecca Anne Barr, Sylvie Kleiman-Lafon and Sophie Vasset (eds), *Bellies, Bowels and Entrails in the Eighteenth Century* (Manchester: Manchester University Press, 2018), pp. 80–98; and Monika Class, 'Introduction: Medical Case Histories as Genre: New Approaches', *Literature and Medicine* 32.1 (2014): ii–xvi.
10 Wild, *Medicine-By-Post*, p. 9.
11 Allan Conrad Christensen, *Nineteenth-Century Narratives of Contagion: 'Our Feverish Contact'* (London: Routledge, 2005), p. 4.
12 Ibid.
13 Ibid.
14 See also Athena Vretos, *Somatic Fictions: Imagining Illness in Victorian Culture* (Stanford, CA: Stanford University Press, 1995).
15 See Clark Lawlor, *Consumption and Literature: The Making of the Romantic Disease* (Basingstoke: Palgrave, 2006), pp. 16, 84, and David Shuttleton's elaboration of the concept in 'The Fashioning of Fashionable Diseases in the Eighteenth Century', *Literature and Medicine* 35:2 (2017): 270–291 (at 279). Studying constructions of the medical profession in the period's English literature and culture fits into a broader scholarly interest in the role of the doctor in the medical and literary marketplace, as demonstrated by Anne Digby's *Making a Medical Living: Doctors and Patients in the English Market for Medicine, 1720–1911* (Cambridge: Cambridge University Press, 1994) and Tabitha Sparks's *The Doctor in the Victorian Novel: Family Practices* (Aldershot: Ashgate, 2009), to name just two period-specific studies.
16 Roberta Barker, 'Imaginary Invalids: The Symptom and the Stage from the Restoration to the Romantics' in Clark Lawlor and Andrew Mangham (eds), *Literature and Medicine: The Eighteenth Century*, pp. 70–88; David Shuttleton, *Smallpox and the Literary Imagination 1660–1820* (Cambridge: Cambridge University Press, 2007); Sari Altschuler, *The Medical Imagination: Literature and Health in the Early United States* (Philadelphia, PA: University of Pennsylvania Press, 2018); Noelle Gallagher, *Itch, Clap, Pox: Venereal Disease in the Eighteenth-Century Imagination* (New Haven, CT: Yale University Press, 2019);

Emily Senior, *The Caribbean and the Medical Imagination, 1764–1834: Slavery, Disease and Colonial Modernity* (Cambridge: Cambridge University Press, 2018); Tita Chico, *The Experimental Imagination: Literary Knowledge and Science in the British Enlightenment* (Stanford, CA: Stanford University Press, 2018); Sophie Vasset, *Murky Waters: British Spas in Eighteenth-Century Medicine and Literature* (Manchester: Manchester University Press, 2022).

17 See the many publications from the Fashionable Diseases Leverhulme Trust project, listed at http://www.fashionablediseases.info/, particularly Jessica Monaghan, 'Authenticity and Fashionable Disease in Eighteenth-Century Britain', *Literature and Medicine* 35:2 (2017): 387–408.

18 Richard Blackmore, 'Essay upon Writing', in *Essays upon several subjects. By Sir Richard Blackmore, Kt. M.D. and Fellow of the College of Physicians in London*, vol. II (London: Wilkins, 1717), pp. 241–287.

19 See Harry Solomon, *Sir Richard Blackmore* (Boston, MA: Twayne, G. K. Hall, 1980), pp. 157–159.

20 Blackmore also aspired to the Christian epic, hence his use of the word 'resistless', which echoes Milton's *Paradise Lost* Book 4, and is especially relevant to persuasion (rhetoric) via language, written or oral:

> 'Thence to the famous Orators repair,
> Those antient, whose resistless eloquence
> Wielded at will that fierce Democratie,
> Shook the Arsenal and ulmin's over *Greece*,
> To *Macedon*, and *Artaxerxes* Throne;' (ll. 267)

21 Jonathan Swift, 'The Battle of the Books', in Marcus Walsh (ed.), *A Tale of A Tub and Other Works*, The Cambridge Edition of the Works of Jonathan Swift (Cambridge: Cambridge University Press, 2010), pp. 137–164 (at p. 158). For the context, see Roger French, *Ancients and Moderns in the Medical Sciences: From Hippocrates to Harvey* (Aldershot: Ashgate, 2000).

22 See Rebecca Anne Barr, Sylvie Kleiman-Lafon and Sophie Vasset (eds), *Bellies, Bowels and Entrails in the Eighteenth Century* (Manchester: Manchester University Press, 2018); Hisao Ishizuka, 'From Hypo to Bile: The Rise and Progress of Biliousness in the Long Eighteenth Century', in Clark Lawlor and Andrew Mangham (eds), *Literature and Medicine: The Eighteenth Century*, vol. 1 (Cambridge: Cambridge University Press, 2021), pp. 113–143; Fredrik Albritton Jonsson, 'The Physiology of Hypochondria in Eighteenth-Century Britain', in Christopher E. Forth and Ana Carden-Coyne (eds), *Cultures of the Abdomen: Diet, Digestion, and Fat in the Modern World* (Basingstoke: Palgrave Macmillan, 2005), pp. 15–30; Jonathan Andrews and James Kennaway, 'Experiencing, Exploiting, and Evacuating Bile: Framing Fashionable Biliousness from the Sufferer's Perspective', *Literature and Medicine* 35:2 (207): 292–333; William F. Bynum, *Gastroenterology in Britain: Historical Essays* (London: Wellcome Institute, 1997); Ian Miller, *A Modern History of the Stomach* (London: Pickering & Chatto, 2011).

23 Digby, *Making a Medical Living*; David Gentilcore, *Medical Charlatanism in Early Modern Italy* (Oxford: Oxford University Press, 2006); Mark Jenner and

Patrick Wallis (eds), *Medicine and the Market in England and its Colonies, c.1450–1850* (Basingstoke: Palgrave Macmillan, 2007); Roy Porter, *Quacks: Fakers and Charlatans in English Medicine* (Stroud: Tempus, 2000); Kevin P. Siena, 'The "Foul Disease" and Privacy: The Effects of Venereal Disease and Patient Demand on the Medical Marketplace in Early Modern London', *Bulletin of the History of Medicine* 75:2 (2001): 199–224.

24 Alan Mackintosh, *The Patent Medicines Industry in Georgian England: Constructing the Market by the Potency of Print* (Basingstoke: Palgrave, 2017).

25 Henry Rider Haggard, *The Days of My Life* (London: Longman, 1911), pp. 346–347.

26 Morton Norton Cohen, *Rider Haggard: His Life and Works* (New York: Walker and Company, 1968), p. 219.

27 Senior, *The Caribbean and the Medical Imagination*; Suman Seth, *Difference and Disease: Medicine, Race, and the Eighteenth-Century British Empire* (Cambridge: Cambridge University Press, 2018); Rana A. Hogarth, *Medicalizing Blackness: Making Racial Difference in the Atlantic World, 1780–1840* (Chapel Hill, NC: University of North Carolina Press, 2017); Deirdre Cooper Owens, *Medical Bondage: Race, Gender, and the Origins of American Gynecology* (Athens, GA: University of Georgia Press, 2017); Alan Bewell, *Romanticism and Colonial Disease* (Baltimore, MD: Johns Hopkins University Press, 1999); Mark Harrison, *Medicine in an Age of Commerce and Empire: Britain and its Tropical Colonies 1660–1830* (Cambridge: Cambridge University Press, 2010); Christobal Silva, *Miraculous Plagues: An Epidemiology of Early American Narrative* (New York: Oxford University Press, 2011); Richard Wrigley and George Revill (eds), *Pathologies of Travel* (Amsterdam: Rodopi, 2000); Ole Peter Grell, Andrew Cunningham and Jon Arrizabalaga (eds), *Centres of Medical Excellence: Medical Travel and Education in Europe, 1500–1789* (Farnham: Ashgate, 2009); Pratik Chakrabarti, *Materials and Medicine: Trade, Conquest and Therapeutics in the Eighteenth Century* (Manchester: Manchester University Press, 2010); Pratik Chakrabarti, *Medicine and Empire, 1600–1960* (Basingstoke: Palgrave Macmillan, 2011).

1

'To level those monstrous Blotches or Pustules': skincare in Daniel Turner's *De Morbis Cutaneis* (1714)

Katherine Aske

The skin represents a boundary between our invisible insides and our visible body. Throughout history, this boundary, how it appeared, and what it could reveal about the body, has been a crucial source of medical knowledge, in domestic and professional healthcare alike. As Kevin Siena and Jonathan Reinarz have argued, medical interpretations of the skin have never been 'disinvested of enormous and complex meaning'.[1] With such an observable subject matter, advice and treatments for the skin circulating within domestic manuals, pharmacopeia and medical treatises throughout the seventeenth and eighteenth centuries created sites of exchange and interaction between domestic, popular and professional sources of knowledge. Patients, even with little medical knowledge, could identify whether their skin needed treatment, perhaps from a quick check in their remedy book, a chat with their local apothecary or nearest wise woman, or possibly a visit to a medical professional – although an accurate diagnosis may have been harder to come by. Within these spheres of medical practice, the skin provided a common ground, a macrocosm, as well as a microcosm of information about the human body and the individual. Whether a simple pimple or a dangerous rash, the signs on the skin and, most importantly, how they were interpreted, remain to this day an important indicator of the body's health and state. For the early eighteenth century, with medical knowledge continuing to advance through print, the skin was the site where professional and domestic treatment collided, and yet research into the origins of dermatological treatment in this period remains underdeveloped.[2] This chapter explores the professionalisation of medical skincare in print and considers its interaction with common practices, accusations of mistreatment, and the representation (and misrepresentation) of professional medical opinion.

Treating the skin, as early eighteenth-century licentiate Daniel Turner argued, was not as simple as it appeared, and should therefore not be undertaken by 'any of his Readers, unless Professors of the same Art'.[3] In *De Morbis Cutaneis: A Treatise of Diseases Incident to the Skin* (1714), the first English medical treatise dedicated to the study of the skin, Turner took it upon himself to save his readers from 'forged Tales or bawdry Stories', the 'Shams' designed to sell 'Quack-Medicines' by those 'publishing almost as many Lyes as Lines', and to correct the myths and misinformation circulating in the 'delusive Arts of Quackery'.[4] Here I consider Turner's approach to the professional medical remedies for the skin included in several of his case studies. The presentation of medical knowledge in *De Morbis Cutaneis* reveals the value Turner placed on professional experience, and his active distrust of alternative or inexperienced medical knowledge, particularly from women. This distrust had been voiced in an earlier publication, *Apologia Chyrurgica, A Vindication of the Noble Art of Chyrurgery* (1695), where Turner, then a practising surgeon, called out the 'gross Abuses offer'd thereunto by *Mountebanks, Quacks, Barbers, Pretending Bone-setters*' and female physicians he calls 'Petticoat Pretenders'.[5] With his *Apologia*, Turner addressed a growing need to correct the 'Causes of Contempt of Chyrurgeons', and expressed his desire to separate the work of professionals from the 'Fraudulent Practices' of 'Pretenders'.[6] Although less direct in its accusations, the same concerns – including protecting the public from being 'spoyl'd by the workmanship of a Woman' – can also be found in *De Morbis Cutaneis*.[7]

Turner's treatise on the skin was published at a time when tensions between the trifactor of medical practitioners in London were particularly high; that is, the apothecaries or chemists, who prepared, and from 1704, could legally prescribe medicines;[8] the surgeons, who treated the external body; and the physicians, some of whom were university educated, while self-proclaimed doctors were commonly referred to as empirics. The relationship between members of the Royal College of Physicians and apothecaries had been troubled for much of the seventeenth century, and the news in 1687 that the college was intending to provide a public dispensary and free treatment to the poor caused further pressure, as apothecaries feared for their livelihoods.[9] This tension finally came to a head in 1704, with the landmark case between apothecary William Rose and the college, who accused Rose of prescribing medicine without a physician. The House of Lords decided in favour of Rose, and the precedent awarded apothecaries the right to diagnose patients and prescribe medicines. However, unlike members of the college, they could not charge for their consultation services.[10] The ever-present conflicts between medical practitioners, alongside the increasing availability of medical advice in print and over-the-counter remedies, meant that negotiating medical diagnosis and treatment with the public was increasingly complicated and, above all, inconsistent. Much like their patients, practitioners held widely varying knowledge and experience. This was further exacerbated by domestic knowledge of treatments – what Turner vulgarly refers to as 'some old Wives Salve[s]' – found in home remedy books or handed down in handwritten family collections. These widely varying sources of medical information and knowledge were continually at odds with that of the university-educated physicians, who were keen to keep themselves and their reputations, distinct.[11] Turner sat somewhat awkwardly in this group. He was an accomplished surgeon, but he aimed for elite status through the acquisition of a physician's medical degree. In 1711, Turner removed himself from the Barber-Surgeons Company and was admitted to licentiate by the Royal College of Physicians. A licentiate was an alternative medical qualification, given to 'such other Persons Skilled in Physick, who by reason of their being Foreigners, or their not being admitted Doctors in one of Our Universities, ... yet, may, notwithstanding, be serviceable to the Publick'.[12] Although not the coveted title of MD, the licentiate was a clear recognition of Turner's extensive medical knowledge and skill without a university degree. Yet, according to Philip Wilson, Turner wrote to Yale University in 1722 and requested that they grant him a medical degree in exchange for twenty-five of his publications. Yale gave him an honorary degree in absentia (despite not actually having a medical school at that time) and Turner went down in history, being awarded the first ever medical doctorate by Yale.[13] While the College of Physicians failed to recognise Turner's MD, that did not prevent him from using the title, and signing his name 'Daniel Turner, M.D., of the Royal College of Physicians', from 1724.[14]

De Morbis Cutaneis was Turner's first publication as a licentiate. With the treatise, Turner demonstrated his knowledge and reputation by compiling works of historic and modern doctors to treat various ailments of the skin. As Turner was already battling with his reputation as an established surgeon and his recent move into the physicians' creed, *De Morbis Cutaneis* attempted to bridge the gap, demonstrating his skills in both internal and external medicine. According to Emily Cock, the skin, for Turner, marked the 'theoretical boundary' between the jurisdictions of surgeons and physicians.[15] In this sense, Turner was out to prove himself as qualified as any physician, and in the 1724 preface to the second edition of his treatise *Syphilis* – the first time he uses 'Turner, M.D.' on the title page – he claimed that through '*twelve Months in an* Hospital *of Sick People, you will, with the Knowledge of a few* simple Medicines, *become a much better* Curer of Diseases, *or a more knowing* Physician *therein, than if you were to spend seven times seven Years in the* Schools *or* Colleges *of a* University'.[16] While Turner was always quick to point out the 'gross abuses' of pretenders, he was also, somewhat incongruously, adamant that medical experience was what really counted, and he continued to prove his own extensive practical knowledge through publications.

Professional medical treatises, especially those published (mostly) in English, straddled a complex ground. To participate in the popular medical market, infiltrated with cheap, fast medicines and false promises, qualified doctors would have to demonstrate their knowledge while making their publications accessible enough to convince their readers – many of whom would not have read Latin – to avoid potentially dangerous pretenders and to consult an experienced doctor. Negotiating this relationship in print was a mammoth task, risking both professional judgement and lumping oneself with the quacks and the vernacular medical writers Turner so vehemently discredited. But it would also mean poor sales if the wrong balance were struck. Fortunately for Turner, he was a prolific writer. At almost four hundred pages, *De Morbis Cutaneis* was predominantly aimed at fellow professionals, but its accessible English case studies and medical information by no means limited its readership.[17] *De Morbis Cutaneis* went through five editions between 1714 and 1736, and the text covered numerous diseases of the skin, including examples of patient treatments, the maternal imagination[18] and venereal disease, with detailed descriptions as well as remedies. The accessibility of Turner's publication is particularly evident in three of his case studies, concerning smallpox, shingles and freckles, where his treatment of these more commonly known and therefore more widely (mis)treated skin issues, demonstrates his negotiation of professional and popular readerships.

Poxes and petticoats

In his chapter on '*the* Small-Pox, *and other* cutaneous *Eruptions from malignant Fevers*', Turner includes an example 'recorded by *Borellus*', the French chemist and physician Pierre Borel, of a 'Beautiful Noble Woman' with smallpox, who 'was desirous to have a Remedy that might either prevent or get out the Marks'.[19] He explains that, in pandering to her request, 'an imprudent Physitian' ordered a 'cold Cataplasm, by which the Remains of the Disease being driven in upon the Brain, she soon receiv'd her Death instead of her expected Beauty'.[20] Attributing this example to the potential dangers of inexperienced physicians, and in turn, the countless cosmetic treatments claiming to treat or cover the ravages of smallpox, Turner suggests that any treatment or 'secret Powder' that 'could hinder the coming out of the *Small-Pox* … without any prejudice to Health' is an 'absolute Impossibility'. Instead, he suggests that 'the best Way is to do nothing at all to the Face to keep it from pitting: Because Oyls, Liniments, &c. only make the white Scurff longer in coming off'.[21] However, to appeal to those readers who might face the same apprehensions as the ill-fated

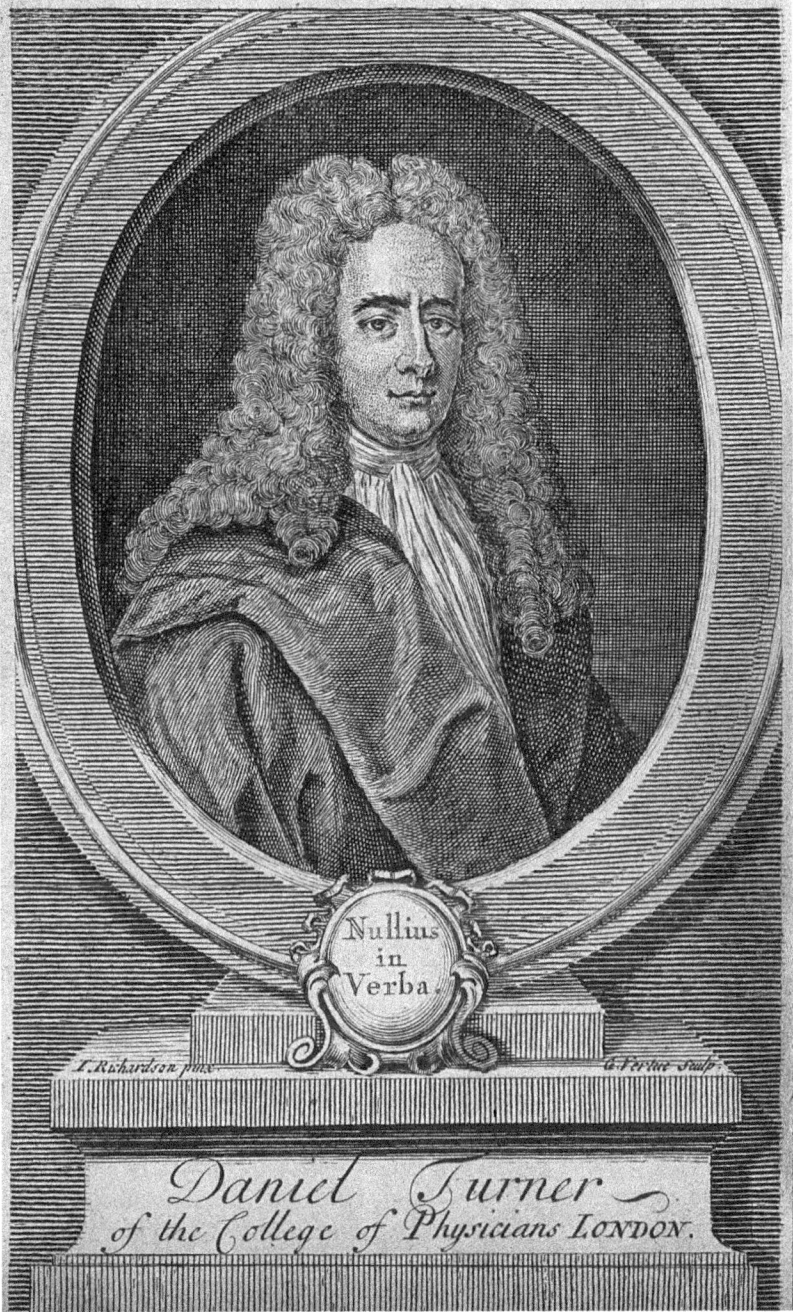

Figure 1.1 Daniel Turner. Line engraving by George Vertue after Jonathan Richardson 1732. Wellcome Collection. Ref: 9296i. Public Domain.

noblewoman, Turner recommends, 'when the Scabs are all off, to smooth the Skin and recover the Complexion' with a range of cosmetic remedies. While he delineates the remedies in Latin, a common practice that would help to avoid any uneducated attempts at recreation, he does include English directions, adding another layer of inconsistency to Turner's views on the unqualified application of medical treatments.

While Turner clearly engages with popular medical knowledge, not only to correct but also to educate and to demonstrate his own prowess, his case studies often involve examples of misdiagnosis or mistreatment that he subsequently corrects. His description of the beautiful noblewoman suggests she might have lived had she sought proper medical advice (and perhaps not let her vanity cloud her judgement). However, in his chapter 'Of the Herpes', Turner includes an example of how a professional medical opinion could be sought, but also abused. Turner writes of a woman with spots on her thigh. Unlike a previous example of a 'Merchant's Man' with a similar issue, he describes this 'Servant-Maid' with details of her physical appearance: she is 'of a fine Skin, and clear Complexion (being red-hair'd)'. Concerned about the 'burning Heat and tingling in her Thigh', and 'apprehensive' that the spots might be smallpox, Turner claims:

> I was called in, and admitted to view the Thigh, which I found overspread with miliary Eruptions, discharging great Plenty of purulent Matter: When I told her Mistress it was the Shingles, she said she was willing to satisfie me for my Visit, and accordingly did so, saying, now she knew the Distemper, she had a Remedy which she doubted not would cure her. I bid her be advis'd in what she did, since by improper Application the young Woman might be indanger'd.[22]

Having diagnosed the disorder, Turner expresses his apprehension in the mistress's cure, and its 'improper Application'. Nevertheless, he leaves the young woman in the hands of her mistress, only to be called back to the house sometime later.

Turner purposefully includes the 'Experiment' to which the patient had been exposed, 'made with the Blood of a black Cat (for it must be of no other Colour) which was smeared on the Parts'. To further incite the reader's disgust, he claims that the blood 'was taken from the Cat's Tail, being cut off for this Purpose', and suggests that the remedy 'was try'd only once' because 'the Anguish was so increased that the poor Wench would not suffer them to go to Work again'. Turner reports that with the

> Limb looking also black, and smelling strong, they were frightened, as believing the same mortifyed; and by a Friend they made Interest to me, that I would not resent their Usage of me, but come to them again, which I did; and perceiving what had been done, with some warm Milk I gently bath'd the

Parts, and got off the Blood, incompassing the whole Limb with my Cerate, letting her Blood and ordering a Bolus of *Lenitive Elect*. With *Pulv.Rhab*. and *Crem Tart*. to be taken the next Morning.²³

Keen to undermine women's domestic medical knowledge, Turner presents his treatment of the leg as careful and educated, gently removing the blood, applying and prescribing prepared purging medicines.

The shingles remedy from which Turner claimed to save this young woman had been included in Hannah Woolley's seventeenth-century popular domestic medicine book, *A Supplement to The Queen-like Closet* (1674). The *Supplement* was one of her final publications, and Woolley was a well-established household name by the 1670s. Claiming 'I have been *Physician* and *Chirurgion* in my own House to many', and vowing to share only those receipts 'wherein People cannot easily Erre', her popularity and educated advice allowed Woolley to make a living from being an author.²⁴ Her works went through numerous editions, covering all things domestic, from cooking and medicine to education and conduct, and her recipes and remedies would have been frequently copied into domestic manuscripts and family cookbooks.²⁵ *A Supplement* was an extended edition of *The Queen-like Closet* (1670), the most famous of her books, and even translated into German.²⁶ Although the original was more focused on culinary recipes, the *Supplement*, a text directed to 'all Ingenious Ladies', offered much more guidance on medical treatments, and listed the following advice for the shingles:

Take a Cat, and cut off her Ears, or her Tail, and mix the Blood thereof with a little new-Milk, and anoint the grieved place with it Morning and Evening for three days; and every night when the Party goes to Bed give her or him two spoonfuls of Treacle-water, to drive out the venom.²⁷

Earlier versions of the gruesome cure are listed in remedy books for both shingles and measles, but only use the cat's ears.²⁸ While neither Woolley's, nor other versions of the cure, mention the colour of the cat, Turner has likely embellished his description here with the specification of a 'black Cat' to invoke an element of superstition or witchcraft. Black cats had long been associated with evil, and the sacrificial and brutal nature of this animal blood-cure can be seen as an additional way to distance the remedy from Turner's professional and careful approach of bloodletting and prescription medicine, despite the similarity of his application of 'milk' to the area and the follow-up treatment of a laxative medicine. In the presentation of this case study, with the mistress's misinformed remedy and his own correction of the error, Turner indicates, while also undermining, the widespread medical knowledge of women in the domestic sphere. No doubt considered by Turner as a 'Petticoat Pretender', Woolley had a significant impact on domestic medical knowledge for women. As Keir Waddington has suggested, with women's importance in the home, 'they were expected to practise some form of medicine as a domestic art and had an active role in looking after the sick'.[29] Treatises like Woolley's, purposefully advertised to women as guides in sundry domestic duties, presented medicine as accessible. Anne Stobart claims that such recipes were copied down, shared, tried and tested even as printed material became more available, and that 'these two formats were not necessarily different in content'.[30] However, as Turner here implies, experience is key. The mistress knew a supposed cure for shingles but was unable to diagnose the disorder – and even once she knew, administered an ineffective, outdated and potentially dangerous treatment. In fact, many printed remedy books listed a simple recipe and directions for application but relied on the reader's knowledge to diagnose a pimple from a shingle, or a rash from a case of scabies. Turner, however, in his carefully organised treatise, insured that his remedies were preceded by descriptions and explanations of each skin issue, making the text more accessible than many circulating medical books at the time. But in his framing of this 'Experiment', Turner, while engaging with and fully acknowledging domestic medical knowledge, does so to present professional medicine – guarded by Latin and supported by fellow doctors – as the safest means of diagnosis and treatment.

However, Turner, perhaps unknowingly, endorses an extremely morbid cure himself. In the cosmetic remedies Turner recommends for the case of the beautiful noblewoman's smallpox, he describes one that early modern French physician, Lazare Rivière, 'praiseth'. It includes oil of egg yolks, and gives the option of adding either water made from milleflorum (a type of lily), or cow dung collected in the month of May, 'with which the Face is to be washed, and after anointed with *Axungia humana*'.[31] The final ingredient, *Axungia humana*, is human fat.[32] Although by no means a common ingredient, and often listed in its Latin phrasing, human fat was used as a medical ingredient well into the eighteenth century. Pierre Pomet's *A Complete History of Druggs* (1712), a title from the same publishers as *De Morbis Cuteanis*, suggests that 'Human Fat or Grease' could be readily bought in Paris from 'the publick Executioner'.[33] The inclusion of this ingredient casts Turner's presentation of the cat's blood cure in a somewhat hypocritical light. It suggests that there is a blurred line between the dismissal of 'old Wives'' remedies and an active advocation of the similarly outdated or barbaric, verging on cannibalistic, treatments of well-known, if not antiquated, physicians.

Bate and blotches

In addition to the professional treatment of shingles and smallpox, Turner also addresses some minor ailments of the skin's surface in his chapter on 'Diseases incident to the Skin of the Face, such as Redness, pustulary Eruptions or Pimples, Freckles, &c.'. While such issues may seem beneath the call of a physician, and treatments for pimples and freckles could be found readily available from apothecaries or listed in most healthcare books, Turner defended their professional treatment. He writes, 'I cannot think the Task below the Dignity of a Physician' to 'level those monstrous Blotches or Pustules, with other Breakings out, that so much disfigure'.[34] Where beauty and medicine have enjoyed a long and complex relationship, one responsible for many of the quick cures Turner warns against, his inclusion of treatments for these 'Blemishes' entwines the realms of public and professional dermatological knowledge. Attempting to bring the treatment of pimples and freckles under the jurisdiction of a physician, Turner draws on the remedies of established physicians, using medical language and Latin references to further stress that topical treatments should be treated as seriously and as professionally as internal medicines.

Turner's chapter on facial skincare is extensive, but here I will focus on a specific case study concerning freckles. Claiming the incident was from his own experience, Turner details a female patient with facial burns, and suggests that after his treatment and upon removing her bandages, he noticed 'several yellow Specks' on the fabric, which he 'easily conjectur'd' were freckles. He examines them under his 'Glass', finding each 'rugged and unequal in its Superficies, of Colour tawny, or a muddy Yellow'. But after his examination, he explains:

> I had the Curiosity, picking several of them off the Skin with the Point of a Needle, to lay them lightly on my Tongue, where I perceiv'd (at least fancy'd so) a perfect bitter or cholerick Taste, confirming me in the Opinion that they are very probably certain Particles of Bile effused from the capillary Vessels of the Skin, and not finding Passage through the Cuticle, are there dry'd by Heat into those *Guttlae* or little Drops and Specks, shining through the same of a golden or yellow Colour. Be this as it will, it is certainly a common, and I think true, Remark, that yellow and red-hair'd Persons are most troubled with them: tho' few or none we may suppose will make this Gentlewoman's Experiment (how infallible soever) to get rid of them.[35]

In the detailed description of what freckles were believed to be, and his experience of viewing them under a microscope, Turner demonstrates what his professional knowledge could bring to this commonly regarded skin 'issue'. He then lists some 'less painful or hazardous' methods to remove these unwanted marks.[36]

Within a list of cures for freckles, written in Latin, Turner includes several remedies from the work of seventeenth-century English medical physician, George Bate. Bate was trained at Oxford University, became an

MD in 1637 and was a Fellow of the Royal College of Physicians from 1640 until his death in 1669. With several direct and indirect references to Bate's posthumous *Pharmacopoeia Bateana*, published in Latin by his apothecary James Shipton in 1688 and 1691, Turner positions Bate as a renowned and reliable source of medical knowledge.[37] Advising 'An excellent Medicine' for removing freckles, Turner includes 'the *Savanetta Cosmetica* of *Bate* prepared thus':

> *Rx Sapon. Ven ℨij. Solve in Suc. Limon ℨj. Addendo Ol. Amygd. amar. Tart. p. Deliq. d ℨss. Misce & insoletur dum Unguenti spissitudinem acquirit, quotidie agitando: demum adde Ol. Rhod. gut. vj. & reservetur Usui.*
>
> With this the Parts are to be anointed over Night, and washed next Morning with the Water of Bran or Lupines.[38]

Turner added these English directions to the original *Savanetta Cosmetica* from Bate's 1688 publication, which, like most pharmacopeia, simply lists the remedy and offers no further direction for its application.[39] In the second edition of Bate's text from 1691, Shipton only makes some slight adjustments to the quantities for this recipe, and still does not include any directions.[40] While most of Turner's recipes appear in abbreviated Latin, a common practice for professional medical publications, he does often balance their potential inaccessibility with English descriptions. That said, Turner's Latin is not an exact copy of Bate's. His reference to Venetian soap (made from olive oil) is '*Sapon. Ven*' rather than '*Smegm. Venet*', and he has halved the quantity of lemon juice, but otherwise the ingredients are the same, including the cheaply available tartar (a biproduct of wine making) and almond oil, as well the much more expensive oil of rhodium, an essential oil made from rosewood, which has antiseptic properties.[41] While it is surprising that Turner would not have copied the recipe exactly, considering he does attribute this treatment to Bate, it is possible that he has made educated adjustments to update the Latin, lessen the astringency of ointment and reduce the quantity produced.[42]

However, in 1694 *Pharmacopoeia Bateana* had been translated by the notorious medical empiric and author William Salmon, revealing the mysteries of its Latin recipes. Salmon's translation extended the second edition of Bate's *Pharmacopoeia* considerably, adding detailed uses and applications.[43] Salmon claimed that Bate's popular book, selling over 'Six thousand' copies in only a few years, deserved to be translated into English.[44] Even more of a household name than Woolley, Salmon was a very popular medical writer. Often signing himself 'M.D.', and being one of the 'Pretenders' Turner was so wary of, Salmon practised medicine in his own surgeries, provided care for those turned away from hospitals and spoke out about the Royal College's monopolisation of the medical profession.[45]

For his presentation of the recipe for '*Savanetta Cosmetica*, A beautifying Soap or Ointment', Salmon, like Turner, added what it was used for, and what it did to your skin:

> Bate.] *Rx Venice Soap ʒij. dissolve it in Juice of Limons ʒij. add Oil of bitter Almonds, Oil of Tartar per deliquium, A. ʒj. mix, and insolate so long, till it comes to the thickness of an Ointment, stirring it well every day. Lastly, add Oil of Rhodium, gut. vj. vel q.s. and make an Ointment.*
> Salmon.] § 1. It clears the Skin and makes it white, soft and smooth, freeing it from Pimples, Breakings out, Scurf, Morphew, Sun burning, and other Defedations.
> § 2. It is reported, that if it be spread thick upon a Cloth, and laid upon the Face, or other parts of the Skin troubled with Lentils, Freckles, and the like, it will take them away; but it ought to lie on two days, and to be renewed two or three times, or till the scurf Skin seems to come off, which it will do in a little time with the discolouring or spots upon it, which I have sometimes seen.[46]

What is most striking in the comparison of these versions of the *Savanetta Cosmetica* is Salmon's very similar experience to Turner's with the gentlewoman's freckles, where he suggests that after using this soap on a 'Cloth', the top layer of skin will come off 'with the discolouring or spots upon it'. This is Salmon's addition, with the claim that 'it is reported', and it appears nowhere in Bate's original or Shipton's second edition. Whether Turner may have inadvertently repeated a similar example for the removal of freckles, if he had read Salmon's translation, or if this was simply a commonly believed myth about the nature of freckles, it remains uncertain, but the similarities in their descriptions are noteworthy.[47] While the potential borrowing of materials from a renowned quack by a respectable licentiate would be too embarrassing to admit, there is another more convincing example in Turner's chapter.

Under the same topic of freckles, Turner cites another of Bate's recipes, which includes the same oils of tartar, almond and rhodium which 'have generally answer'd my Patients Expectation':

> In the Use of this, the Oil of Tart. is to be increased or diminish'd according to the Fineness or Coarsness of the cuticular Fabrick, or as the Patient can bear it: It sufficeth if it raise the outward *Lamina*, which you will perceive to peel off in a thin Scale or Scurf; after which some common Pomatum may be used: in the Author's Words, it will excite a little Smart and Twinging for the present, but goes off again without other Detriment or Inconvenience.[48]

Although Turner often omits the titles of Bate's formulae, this is his *Oleum Cosmeticum*. Again, the Latin recipe from 1688 simply lists the ingredients without any further instructions.[49] In Shipton's second edition, he slightly alters the quantities, and simply adds '*Ad cutem detergendam & erugendam*', which, with the possible misspelling of *erigendam*, translates as 'to clean and raise the skin'; but neither of Bate's Latin editions mention any discomfort.[50] Salmon presents the recipe thus:

> IV. *Oleum Cosmeticum,* A beautifying Oil.
> Bate] Rx *Oil of Bitter Almonds ℥iv. Oil of Tartar* per deliquium *℥ij. Oil of Rhodium, gut. iv. mix them. S. A.*[51] It cleanses the Skin and smooths it.
> Salmon.] § I. It brings off the Skin, but by degrees; it makes not the Face raw, but makes it fall off in a manner of a Scurf. ... § 3. It ought to be used three or four times a day, or oftener, and to be continued for five or six Weeks more or less, as you see occasion. It will smart a little, but without any other detriment, and at length leave the Skin very smooth, clear, and white.[52]

Where Turner writes 'in the Author's Words, it will excite a little Smart', 'but goes off again without other Detriment', the wording is so similar, that it is not only likely that Turner has read Salmon's translation, but also that he has used this edition as a source for Bate's treatments. With an English copy already available of Bate's text, in its fourth edition by the time *De Morbis Cutaneis* was published, Turner likely drew from this work, but included the ingredients in Latin, making them inaccessible to most of his readers. In doing so, Turner elevates his work above the common man's dispensatory, while claiming to save his readers from the same translations he himself has presented as the work of a renowned physician.

Turner makes no allusions to Salmon in *De Morbis*, who died a year before the treatise was published. However, in the aptly named *The Modern Quack* (1718), written anonymously by 'a London physician', but later attributed to Turner, he directly criticised Salmon's medical skills and publications:

> he was a good *Chymist*, but like them, *Empirical, Immethodical,* and entirely unacquainted with Rules of Art; he was neither *Surgeon* nor *Apothecary*, nor would either of those Corporations ever admit him a Member of their Societies, much less the *Royal College of Physicians*, altho' he pretended to be a great Proficient in all three; he was, indeed, a great friend to the *Paper Manufacture*, large quantities of which he wasted in his Collections and Transcripts from other Writers; nor can it be said truly, that he was ever the real Author of one good Book, tho' he spoiled a great Number by his foolish *Translations, Alterations, Additions, Comments, Explanations,* or *Annotations.*[53]

Despite such accusations, Salmon's works were so popular that his name continued to be used on medical publications even after his death. Turner's claim that experience is more significant than education does not seem to apply to those outside of the respectable medical 'Societies', and he continually reinforced the hierarchy he fought so hard to climb. Turner's work, perhaps inadvertently, demonstrates the interconnectedness of medical knowledge, and the necessity to engage with domestic and popular works to establish a professional approach to medicine. On the other hand, *De Morbis* also shows the extent of Turner's hypocrisy and his own self-interestedness, challenging and subsequently upholding the value of a university medical degree. Equally, the misrepresentation of Turner's recipes as his own (or as Bate's), puts in a different light his questioning of whether Salmon 'was ever the real Author of one good Book'. Such misinformation highlights the complexities of reputation for medical practitioners in the eighteenth-century marketplace, and the degree to which individuals, their credentials and their works could be mythologised and misrepresented by either themselves or their readers.

Conclusion

Turner's ground-breaking text exemplifies the precarious and yet concomitant relationship between professional, popular and domestic medical treatment of the skin. His treatise illustrates a calculated presentation of medical information in Latin, not only to establish authority by including references to renowned doctors like Bate, *Borellus* and Rivière, but also to distinguish a hierarchy of knowledge. While the reproduction of medical remedies is nothing new, there is an elitism guiding Turner's presentation of medical information, reframing and advocating expert treatments over their 'foolish *Translations*'. In this way, Turner continually underlines the potential dangers of patients treating symptoms without expert medical advice. He ardently believed that topical treatments could enter the body through the pores, becoming internal medicines, which only a trained physician should administer. The fine balance between accessibility and inaccessibility in Turner's case studies allows the reader, and the potential patient, to participate in a medical dialogue without providing a means for self-medication – reinforcing the necessity of consulting a doctor or trained professional for diagnosis and cure.

Alongside Turner's direct engagement with domestic remedies there is an overarching issue that the presentation of medical knowledge and its attribution to a perceived reliable source was of far greater significance than the actual treatments – whether or not they involved cat's blood or human fat. Although many of the domestic remedies for skincare in this period often included the same essential oils and ingredients that Turner recommends, he continues to discredit their unqualified administration and instead works to underpin his treatments for these common skin issues with professional backing and examples of his experience. Ultimately, Turner's treatise not only promoted the work of educated practitioners, but also demonstrated a necessity to acknowledge the significance of popular medical culture in professional practice. Although research into the medical history of the skin currently remains underdeveloped, further examination of the ways skincare remedies were shared and presented within medical resources, whether in manuscripts, domestic publications or commercial advertisements, could help to unpick this blurred hierarchy of knowledge, and reveal how treatments for common skin issues developed into the origins of dermatology.

Notes

1 Jonathan Reinarz and Kevin Siena, 'Scratching the Surface: An Introduction', in Jonathan Reinarz and Kevin Siena (eds), *A Medical History of Skin: Scratching the Surface*, Studies for the Society for the Social History of Medicine, 10 (London: Routledge, 2016), pp. 1–15.
2 Although the subject of skin in the eighteenth century has been carefully explored by Barbara Duden, Philip Wilson and Jonathan Andrews and others, there has been little exploration of the ways proto-dermatological remedies reveal avenues of medical knowledge exchange. See Barbara Duden, *The Woman Beneath the Skin: A Doctor's Patients in Eighteenth-Century Germany*, trans. Thomas Dunlap (Cambridge, MA: Harvard University Press, 1998); Philip Wilson, *Surgery, Skin and Syphilis: Daniel Turner's London (1667–1741)* (Amsterdam and Atlanta, GA: Rodopi, 1999); and Jonathan Andrews, 'History of Medicine: Health, Medicine and Disease in the Eighteenth Century', *Journal for Eighteenth Century Studies*, 34:4 (2011): 503–515. See also Katherine Aske, 'Sharing Skincare Secrets in Eighteenth-Century Popular Culture', in Katherine Aske et al. (eds), *Participation, Collaboration, Association: Communities, Exchanges, Politics and Philosophies in the Eighteenth Century* (Paris: Honoré Champion, 2023), pp. 179–192.
3 Daniel Turner, 'To the Reader', *De Morbis Cutaneis* (London: R. Bonwicke et al., 1714), unpaginated.
4 Turner, 'To the Reader', unpaginated.
5 Daniel Turner, *Apologia Chyrurgica, A Vindication of the Noble Art of Surgery* (London: J. Whitlock, 1695), title page, pp. 106–107.
6 Turner, *Apologia*, p. 117. See also Roy Porter, *Quacks: Fakers & Charlatans in English Medicine* (Gloucestershire: Tempus, 2003).
7 Turner, *Apologia*, p. 108.
8 A 1704 ruling from the House of Lords. See Janet Foster and Julia Sheppard (eds), 'Society of Apothecaries Archives', *British Archives*, 4th edn (Basingstoke: Palgrave, 2002), pp. 462–463. See also Penelope Hunting, *A History of the Society of Apothecaries* (London: Worshipful Society of Apothecaries of London, 1998), p. 153.

9 See Sarah Gillam, 'Sir Samuel Garth's poem, "The Dispensary"', *Royal College of Physicians Blog*, 22 September 2017, available at https://history.rcplondon. ac.uk/blog/sir-samuel-garths-poem-dispensary, last accessed 3 November 2023.
10 See Stuart Anderson, *Pharmacy and Professionalization in the British Empire, 1780–1970* (Switzerland: Palgrave Macmillan, 2021), pp. 40–41.
11 See Roy Porter, *The Greatest Benefit to Mankind* (London: Harper Collins, 1997), pp. 288–289.
12 [Anon.], [Broadside], *The Catalogue of the Fellows and Other Members of the Royal College of Physicians* (London: The Statutes of the College of Physicians, 1696).
13 See Philip K. Wilson, 'Turner, Daniel (1667–1741)', *Oxford Dictionary of National Biography* (January 2008), available at https://doi.org/10.1093/ref:odnb/27844, last accessed 13 January 2023.
14 The titles from the Royal College, that is, Doctor, Fellow and Licentiate, went somewhat unmonitored, according to a 1747 address to the College of Physicians: 'I would advise every regular Physician, who is an Author, to style himself M.D. *Oxon*. [Dr. George Bate] or M.D. *Cantab* [Dr. Thomas Fuller]. And then we should not have the Publick impos'd on by every paltry hunger-bitten Scribbler with an M.D. tagg'd to the End of his Name. – If a Dissenter publishes, let him sign *Licentiate of the College of Physicians*, which would be a distinguish'd Mark of Credit to himself, and at the same time contribute to the main End of discountenancing your M.D. Tricksters, and rend those two Letters ineffectual to the carrying on any longer the low Cunning of such Impostors'. See A. Z., *An Address to the College of Physicians, and to the Universities of Oxford and Cambridge* (London: M. Cooper, 1747), p. 18.
15 Emily Cock, '"He would by no means risque his Reputation": Patient and Doctor Shame in Daniel Turner's *De Morbis Cutaneis* (1714) and *Syphilis* (1717)', *Medical Humanities*, 43:4 (2017): 231–237 (at 231).
16 Daniel Turner, *Syphillis: A Practical Dissertation on the Venereal Disease* (London: R. and J. Bonwicke et al. 1724), Preface.
17 The text was advertised under its English subtitle, 'A Treatise of Diseases incident to the Skin, in Two Parts', in the *Post Boy*, 10 November 1713, issue 2888.
18 Turner's thoughts on the maternal imagination caused somewhat of a dispute, and they were discredited (although not by name) by fellow member of the College of Physicians, Dr James Blondel in his publication *The Strength of Imagination in Pregnant Women Examin'd* (London: J. Peele, 1727). Turner responded with a separate publication, entitled *The Force of the Mother's Imagination upon her Foetus in Utero* (London: J. Walthoe et al., 1730), as a response to Blondel's dismissal.
19 Turner, *Morbis*, p. 68.
20 Ibid., p. 68.
21 Ibid., p. 68.
22 Ibid., pp. 53–54.

23 Ibid., pp. 53–54. A lenitive electuary is a premade laxative or purging medicine often including senna, and this example also includes powdered rhubarb [*pulv. Rhab.*] and cream of tartar [*Crem Tart.*].
24 Hannah Woolley, *A Supplement to The Queen-like Closet* (London: Richard Lownds, 1674), unpaginated.
25 See David B. Goldstein, 'A Guide to Ladies: Hannah Woolley's Missing Book emerges from the Archives', *Shakespeare and Beyond Blog*, 29 March 2019, available at https://shakespeareandbeyond.folger.edu/2019/03/29/a-guide-to-ladies-hannah-woolley-missing-book/, last accessed 17 October 2023.
26 See Teri Moores, 'Woolley, Hannah (*c*.1623–after 1677)', in Cathy Hartley (ed.), *Historical Dictionary of British Women* (London: Europa, 2003), p. 465.
27 Woolley, *A Supplement*, p. 47. Treacle-water was a common medicine, and often cited as an *alexipharmic*, or an ingredient that could create a purging or laxative effect in order to cleanse the body of 'venom' or infection.
28 See Ralph Williams, *Physical Rarities* (London: J. M. for George Calvert, 1651), p. 149; and Johann (John) Schröder, *Zoologia: or, The History of Animals as they are Useful* (London: E. Coats, 1659), p. 26. Williams is listed as a 'Practitioner in Physick and Chyrurgerie' and Schröder is titled 'Dr. of Physick'.
29 Keir Waddington, *An Introduction to the Social History of Medicine: Europe Since 1500* (Basingstoke: Palgrave Macmillan, 2011), p. 171.
30 Anne Stobart, *Household Medicine in Seventeenth-Century England* (London: Bloomsbury, 2016), p. 30.
31 'Ol. Ex Vitel. Ovorum; also the Aq. Milleflorum seu è Stercore Vaccino, Mense Maio destillata'. Turner, *Morbis*, p. 68. See also Lazari Rivirii, *Praxis medica cum theoria* (Leipzig: Matthiam Trinkberg, 1660), p. 365.
32 The same ingredient is listed as a cure for a fracture in the second edition of Turner's *The Art of Surgery* (London: C. Rivington, 1732), p. 179.
33 Pierre Pomet, *A Complete History of Druggs* (London: R. Bonwicke et al. 1712), p. 229. Pomet, a French pharmacist, is listed as 'chief Druggist to the present French King'.
34 Turner, *Morbis*, p. 163.
35 Ibid., p. 176.
36 Cures for freckles were widespread, but remedies suggesting they could be washed away began to face criticism as medical knowledge of the skin advanced. For example, Nicolas Andry de Bois-Regard claimed that 'Some pretend to have particular Secrets for curing Freckles; but these only consist in applying to the Face corrosive Waters, which make the Scarf-skin peel off, and afterwards leave the Face just as they found it: which is not surprising, because the Freckles have not their Seat in the Scarf-skin; it is in the Skin itself'. See Nicolas Andry de Bois-Regard, *Othopaedia: or, the Art of Correcting and Preventing Deformities in Children* (London: A. Millar, 1743), pp. 120–121.
37 Elizabeth Lane Furdell, 'Bate, George [pseud. Theodorus Veridicus] (1608–1668)', *Oxford Dictionary of National Biography* (January 2008), available at https://doi.org/10.1093/ref:odnb/1661, last accessed 13 January 2023.

38 Turner, *Morbis*, p. 177. 'Dissolve two ounces of Venetian Soap in one ounce of Lemon Juice, add Oil of Bitter Almonds, Oil of Tartar half an ounce, mix and place in the sun until a thick ointment, stir daily and finally add six drops of Oil of Rhodium, and reserve for use' (my translation).
39 George Bate, *Pharmacopoeia Bateana* (London: Sam Smith, 1688), p. 97. '*Savanetta Cosmetica. Rx. Smegm. Venet. ℥iii. Solve in succ. limon. ℥ii. adde ol. Amygd. amar. ol. [Tartarum] ri p. d. a ℥i. m. & tamdiu insolentur donee in Unguenti spissitudinem pervenerint, sing. diebus probe agitando. Tum adde ol. st. Rhodii gt.vi, vel q. s. f. ung.'
40 George Bate, *Pharmacopoeia Bateana* (London: Sam Smith, 1691), p. 143. '*Savanetta Cosmetica. Rx. Smegm. Venet. ℥ij. solve in succ. limon. ℥ij. adde ol. Amygd. amar. ol. [Tartarum] ri p. d. ā ℥i. m. & tamdiu insolentur donee in Unguenti spissitudinem pervenerint, sing. diebus probè agitando. Tum adde ol. st. Rhodii gt.vi, vel q. s. f. ung.'
41 Incidentally, Bate's *Pharmacopoeia* was reissued in Latin in 1719 by Thomas Fuller, and the main ingredient has been updated to 'Sapon. Venet.' See George Bate, *Pharmacopoeia Bateana*, with additions by Thomas Fuller (London: John Innys, [1719]), p. 178. Prices are listed in Robert Pitt, *The Craft and Frauds of Physick Expos'd* (London: Tim Childe, 1702). 'Spirit of Tartar ... Six Pence the Ounce' (p. 112); 'Oyl of Sweet and Bitter Almonds ... three pence the Ounce' (p. 109); oil of rhodium, 'One Shilling and Six Pence the Dram' (p. 111). Eight drams were the equivalent of one ounce. For more information on the use of these ingredients in skincare remedies, see Aske, 'Sharing Skincare Secrets'.
42 Turner notes the astringency of lemon juice in a subsequent cosmetic remedy, which can be made 'with or without the Juice of Lemon, if the Place will not suffer it by Reason of its Tenderness' (*Morbis*, p. 178).
43 See Philip K. Wilson, 'Salmon, William (1644–1713)', *Oxford Dictionary of National Biography* (November 2021), available at https://doi.org/10.1093/ref:odnb/24559, last accessed 13 January 2023. See also M. Geshwind, 'William Salmon, Quack-Doctor and Writer of Seventeenth-Century London', *Bulletin of the History of Dentistry* 43 (1995): 73–76.
44 'That if whilst it wandred thro' the World in an unknown Tongue (as to the Vulgar) and was a Stranger, it became so desirable and acceptable; how much more, if we indulg'd it, by making it a Free Denizon [citizen], or Native of our own'. See George Bate, *Pharmacopoeia Bateana: or, Bate's Dispensatory*, with additions by William Salmon (London: Sam Smith and Benj. Walford, 1694), Preface. Sam Smith was the publisher of both of Bate's Latin editions of *Pharmacopoeia*.
45 Wilson, 'Salmon, William'.
46 Bate, *Pharmacopoeia Bateana: or, Bate's Dispensatory* (1694), p. 876.
47 Additionally, Turner refers to 'that great Physician Dr. *Bate*', and the recipes 'found in his Dispensatory set forth by *Shipton*', *Morbis*, p. 137. While this could simply be an issue of terminology, Salmon titled Bate's *Pharmacopoeia* as *Bate's Dispensatory*, and the authorship was still listed under George Bate.
48 Turner, *Morbis*, p. 177.

49 '*Ol. Cosmeticum. Rx [Oil] Amygd. amar. ℥iiii. [Oil of Tartar] ri p. d. ℥ii. [Oil] Rhod. gt. 4. m. s. a.'. Bate, *Pharmacopoeia Bateana* (1688), pp. 71–72.
50 Bate, *Pharmacopoeia Bateana* (1691), p. 104. My translation.
51 S. A. is shorthand for *Secundum Artem*, meaning according to practice or art, and highlighting the additional direction from Shipton.
52 Bate, *Pharmacopoeia Bateana: or, Bate's Dispensatory* (1694), p. 876.
53 A London Physician [Daniel Turner], *The Modern Quack* (London: J. Roberts, 1718), pp. 124–125. Although its authorship remains uncertain, the tone of the publication is very similar to Turner's *Apologia*. Like his accusatory claim that men are 'spoyl'd by the workmanship of a Woman', *The Modern Quack*'s preface details a very similar derogatory phrase 'trying first of all some old Wife's Receipt, has cost many a poor Miser [what next to his Money is of the dearest value to him], I mean his Life' (unpaginated). The use of phrasing like 'frauds', 'abuses' and 'pretenders' is also similar to *Apologia*. Moreover, the text includes a supplementary 'List of all the several Members of the College of Physicians' and their residences in London. 'D. Turner in *Bishopsgate-Street*' is included in the long list of names specifically grouped as 'Dr.', which, according to the following note, has omitted 'the several Dignities and Divisions into Fellows, Honorary Fellows, &c.', and includes only those 'who have a Right to Practice' by their 'Examination at the Censors Board being found qualif'd' (p. 156). As Turner was never recognised as an MD by the Royal College, it is very likely that this publication was of his own creation to (anonymously) establish his position as a 'qualif'd' doctor.

2

Dr John Arbuthnot's literary treatment for false learning, pedantry and excess: from physic to metaphysics

John Baker

I caught Uncle Percy's eye. It had swivelled round at me with a dumb, pleading look in it, as if saying that suggestions would be welcomed.

'How would it be,' I said – well, one had to say something, 'if you told her the truth?'

'The truth?' he repeated dazedly, and you could see he thought the idea a novel one.

Joy in the Morning, P. G. Wodehouse

'an Air of Truth'

There exist at least three time-honoured paths credited with leading to knowledge and truth which can be termed fact, fiction and belief. They are not watertight classifications, and not only is there overlap between the categories themselves but one can surmise that everyone partakes to some degree of all three, although the balance within any individual can be radically different, itself fluctuating and uncertain over time. To gain access to knowledge and truth there is, then, the religious and faith-based path, the path of literature in the form of stories, allegories, poetry, drama, etc., which require what Coleridge called 'that willing suspension of disbelief for the moment, which constitutes poetic faith',[1] where 'truth' is revisited, refashioned and revealed by fiction, imagination and indirect expression, and thirdly, of course, there is 'natural philosophy', modern science itself based on empiricism, observation and verification. The Coleridge quote conflates the three in an oblique and economical fashion. The 'suspension' 'for the moment', shows that the action is both temporary and voluntary. It is thus the act of a free agent. The reference to 'disbelief' suggests that one can discriminate between fact and fiction, that one knows what is what, and is ready of one's own free will to embrace the movement and contours of the fiction proposed and thus, again temporarily, to agree to believe what one knows to be a fabrication.

How is this shifting balance, this *triangulation*, construed and disposed in the writings of Dr John Arbuthnot?

I must,[1] then, plead guilty at the outset to the exercising of a certain latitude in tweaking the notion and theme of medical representation and misrepresentation. In several respects Arbuthnot fits the bill. He is quintessentially a 'writing doctor', but his writings taken as a whole can leave the reader perplexed given the range of the subject matter he addresses – more often than not far from the medical beaten track – and the reader can be further disoriented by the contrast between the sober, rational and scientific focus and style of some works, and the playful, parodic and satirical character of others. I will suggest here that Arbuthnot offers a holistic appraisal and diagnosis of human ills, taking into account the moral, intellectual and spiritual, as well as the physical infirmities inherent to the human condition in general and, more specifically, to Augustan society.

This chapter will focus on a selection of works – informative, satirical and poetic – which illustrate Arbuthnot's thematic, stylistic and linguistic choices in seeking out remedies, and applying a literary treatment for what he, along with the Scriblerian fraternity, saw as a threatening and rampant intellectual affliction and distemper of the age. The age was threatened by the encroachment of 'the great empire of Dulness' which Alexander Pope's *Dunciad* was to explore and 'celebrate'.[2] The disorder is difficult to name in literary-medical terms, but its symptoms include pride, false learning, overreaching, pedantry and excess. Among those commonly affected were *virtuosi* and antiquarians, and Arbuthnot and his fellow Scriblerians propose through their written works a treatment at times as radical as the illness itself which takes the form of lampooning, parodying, allegorising and satirising. Like, in a sense, is treated with like, but with a vengeance. Jonathan Swift's peculiar medicine could be drastic, as could Pope's. As George Orwell, a great admirer of Swift, albeit a critical one, wrote in his imaginary interview with the latter, 'even I can't help feeling that you laid it on a bit too thick'.[3] Arbuthnot's powders and potions tended to be more measured. These treatments are applied, then, at times with care and a certain restraint, at others the medicine is more purgative, and is administered in large dollops, but in both cases they are dispensed with humour and delectation.

The Scriblerus Club was a close-knit association of writers and friends who met up regularly for a short period in the final years of Queen Anne's reign and, by all accounts, Arbuthnot was a leading light, acknowledged as such by the members themselves. There is much in the Scriblerian agenda to commend it to the modern reader, and in particular in today's world. The present period, a 'post-truth' age (for some), shot through with its spin, fake news, 'alternative facts', storytelling, scams, disinformation, conspiracy theories, propaganda, political lies, etc., seems a peculiarly apposite moment to revisit the club. Writing on John Arbuthnot presents several acknowledged problems. One concerns the still uncertain attribution of some works; a second, identifying the precise nature of his contributions to the collective *Memoirs of the Extraordinary Life, Works, and Discoveries of Martinus Scriblerus*, and indeed to other Scriblerian works. A third challenge arises from the breadth of Arbuthnot's own interests, and the very different domains of knowledge he explored. It is fair to assume, and critics generally do, that much of the inspiration and, in places, the detail of the collaborative *Memoirs*, given Arbuthnot's wide-ranging interests in particular in the medical and scientific fields, as well as the tone and humour of the work, can, necessarily tentatively, be attributed to Arbuthnot, even if Pope was responsible for the final polishing, ordering, evening out, and indeed publishing of the work in 1741. By the time the *Memoirs* were published, four of the six members of the Scriblerus Club had died: Thomas Parnell (1679–1718), Robert Harley (1661–1724), Lord Treasurer in the Tory government (1711–14), Earl of Oxford and Mortimer, John Gay (1685–1732) and Arbuthnot himself (1667–1735). Swift was in poor physical and mental health and died in 1745, Pope in 1744. The work was, then, a partially posthumous publication. But 'the Scriblerian spirit'[4] was to continue in its written expression well beyond the meetings of the Scriblerus Club proper, which often took place at Arbuthnot's lodgings at St James's Palace in 1713 and 1714. The masterpieces emanating from that group of friends and literary accomplices are Swift's *Gulliver's Travels* (1726) and Pope's mock-epic *The Dunciad* (1728–43) in its various elaborations and editions.

The Scriblerians explore both the resources and the misuses and abuses of language. Swift's *Gulliver's Travels* exploits throughout the destabilising reversibility of signs, how the words on the page can signify one thing but are to be understood as meaning the opposite. Richard Sympson, a cousin of Captain Lemuel Gulliver (himself previously a surgeon), who was, at Gulliver's behest, to publish *Travels into Several Remote Nations of the World*, in his note to the reader presenting the author, writes, 'There is an Air of Truth apparent through the whole; and indeed the Author was so distinguished for his Veracity, that it became a Sort of Proverb among his Neighbours at Redriff, when anyone affirmed a Thing, to say, it was as true as if Mr. *Gulliver* had spoke it'.[5] The message to the gentle reader is clear: 'Don't believe a word of what you are about to read'. Part 4 of *Gulliver's Travels*, 'A Voyage to the Country of the Houyhnhnms' is, among other things, a wonderfully skewed treatise on lying and falsehood. The nature of lying is ingenuously described by Gulliver himself:

And I remember in frequent Discourses with my Master concerning the Nature of Manhood, in other Parts of the World; having Occasion to talk of *Lying*, and *false Representation*, it was with much difficulty that he comprehended what I meant; although he had otherwise a most acute Judgment. For he argued thus; That the Use of Speech was to make us understand one another, and to receive Information of Facts; now if any one *said the Thing which was not*, these Ends were defeated; because I cannot properly be said to understand him; and I am so far from receiving Information, that he leaves me worse than in Ignorance; for I am led to believe a Thing *Black*, when it is *White*, and *Short*, when it is *Long*. And these were all the Notions he had concerning that Faculty of *Lying*, so perfectly well understood, and so universally practised, among human Creatures.[6]

What then is the nature of lying? Is it not an affront to truth? Is it a natural tendency, an aberration, or even a talent? Cannot someone be said to be a 'good' liar? To what extent can it be considered as a moral ill, and why? Whatever the answers may be, lying is a recurring theme in the early decades of the eighteenth century, and both Swift and Arbuthnot were to focus on the art, i.e. the techniques, of political lying. In a sense lying is the stuff of fiction itself as characters and events, however 'true to life' they may sound and appear, remain fictitious, and figments of the writer's and, by transferral, the reader's imagination, the reader being a willing accomplice in the make-believe.

The nature and essence of learning, knowledge and truth were a constant source of preoccupation, exchange, debate and antagonism in the Restoration period and the early decades of the eighteenth century, a period John Locke called, with more than a dash of irony, 'this our knowing Age'.[7] What did true knowledge consist of? What were its foundations and purpose? The key role language played in the transmission and representation of knowledge was similarly under close and critical scrutiny. For Locke, as for the Scriblerians after him, the limits of what we can aspire to know, and the nature of the language used to convey knowledge, are of vital importance.

John Arbuthnot, elected Fellow of the Royal Society in 1704, Fellow of the Royal College of Physicians in 1710, appointed Physician Extraordinary to Queen Anne in 1705 and Physician-in-Ordinary in 1709, was the author of medical treatises on aliments and diet (1731), and the effects on health of the air we breathe (1733), among his many other writings. Lester M. Beattie nonetheless chose to entitle his critical study, *John Arbuthnot, Mathematician and Satirist* (1935).[8] The perhaps surprising title is a justified one in that Arbuthnot presents himself first and foremost as a mathematician, despite spending almost all his professional life as a practising physician. In his 1701 letter to a young friend, *An Essay on the Usefulness of Mathematical Learning*, mathematics is presented as the cornerstone of all sciences, the foundation of all 'useful' and serious knowledge. In the course of the letter, Arbuthnot runs through the various fields of human enquiry arguing that in each case, to carry out any meaningful study, at least some grasp of mathematics is indispensable. As Beattie writes: 'The areas of verifiable knowledge to be annexed by a mathematically entrenched method seemed to him boundless'.[9] Among the spheres of knowledge passed rapidly in review he mentions astronomy, mechanics, chronology, geography, history, military affairs, navigation, politics and trade, and, of course, medicine, but also the arts such as painting, music and architecture: 'In all Ages and Countries, where Learning hath prevailed, the *Mathematical Sciences* have been looked upon as the most considerable branch of it'.[10] He goes on to set out the benefits of mathematical reasoning: 'The advantages, which accrue to the Mind by *Mathematical* studies, consist chiefly in these things: 1*st*. In accustoming it to *attention*. 2*dly*. In giving it a habit of *close* and *demonstrative reasoning*. 3*dly*. In freeing it from *prejudice, credulity,* and *superstition*'.[11] Here Arbuthnot sets out his epistemological stall and states that 'truth' is to be established by scientific method and enquiry. Lest the addressee and the reader at large be tempted to suppose that this in some way sidesteps or disqualifies religion, Arbuthnot hastens to add, while putting Roman Catholicism on a par with superstitious belief:

> How great an enemy *Mathematicks* are to superstition, appears from this, That in those Countries, where *Romish Priests* exercise their barbarous Tyranny over the minds of Men, Astronomers, who are fully perswaded of the motion of the Earth, dare not speak out: But tho the *Inquisition* may extort a Recantation, the Pope and a general Council too will not find themselves able to perswade to the contrary Opinion. Perhaps, this may have given occasion to a calumnious suggestion, as if *Mathematicks* were an enemy to Religion, which is a scandal thrown both on the one and the other; for truth can never be an enemy to true examined Religion, which appears always to the best advantage, when it is most examined ... On the contrary, the Mathematicks are friends to Religion; inasmuch as they charm the passions, restrain the impetuosity of imagination, and purge the Mind from error and prejudice. Vice is error, confusion and false Reasoning; and all truth is more or less opposite to it.[12]

These quotations and this essay serve to establish Arbuthnot's scientific credentials and standpoint, as well as his position that natural philosophy and religion are in no way antithetical.

Unpacking a pack of lies

The majority of Arbuthnot's published writings veer back and forth between two poles, two modes of discourse. The first consists of providing information and fact based on observation and the available data on subjects related to Arbuthnot's own diverse interests (mathematics, probability theory, numismatics, etc.) and his medical and scientific background, with the avowed intention of conveying 'useful', verifiable knowledge. The second is, in appearance, diametrically opposed in that it gleefully muddies the waters of clear perception in its roundabout and upside-down use of language and logic, and delights in going down the sinuous and disfiguring paths of satire, parody, the burlesque and allegory. The latter partakes of the *pseudological*, which the *Oxford English Dictionary* defines variously as the (systematic) making of false statements, the art of lying, and/or a pretended branch of knowledge. In both matters, the essential tools are epistemological and linguistic. They are employed either to expound on a given subject in a rational manner, or to confound, distort, debunk and amuse. There is convergence in that both, in accordance with their peculiar idiom, and in their own manner, can be said to target truth and knowledge.

Arbuthnot's *The Art of Political Lying* (1712),[13] published anonymously, had at least two precursors: Swift's own paper, the *Examiner*, on the same theme (Thursday, 9 November 1710) and, closer in time, the announcement of another sham work, first mentioned in the *Plain Dealer*, XIII (5 July 1712), and then fleshed out the following week with the title 'Proposals for printing by Subscription, A General History of the Lyes rais'd by the W—s since the Beginning of last Winter, in 6 Vols., in Folio' in the *Plain Dealer* XIV, 12 July 1712.[14] Arbuthnot's proposals in *The Art of Political Lying* concerning the time of publication and the call for subscriptions, are accompanied with detail: addresses of coffee houses where the subscriptions can be paid, prices, and the promise of a price reduction for multiple subscriptions – the equivalent of the modern 'buy two, get one free' – 'Two Volumes in 4to' etc., are all more than strikingly similar to those in the *Plain Dealer*. Arbuthnot contents himself with a mere two volumes, the first of which we are invited to believe has been 'carefully perus'd' by the author-cum-reviewer who generously gives the reader a fulsome abstract.

The Art of Political Lying clearly falls into the second of the literary categories mentioned above, and is a bottomless pit. The whole apparatus of the paratext – in fact the whole work is a paratext, a preparation for something which doesn't exist, and never will – is all a cheat. From top to bottom, inside and out, the proposal is a pack of lies. And yet the language is exact and the abstract itself clearly organised and conducted. The scalpel is handled with precision, care and a moderation all the more convincing in its eschewal of excess. Leslie Stephen referred to the work as 'one of the best specimens of the ironical wit of the time'.[15] Swift, curiously, in a letter to Esther Johnson, wrote of the pamphlet "tis very pretty, but not so obvious to be understood'.[16] It is indeed a work with many twists and turns.

Arbuthnot calmly and systematically anatomises the stratagems and techniques of political lying in eleven chapter abstracts, making the practice of lying that one might normally expect to be presented as morally wrong and dishonest, and to be condemned outright, into a banal manoeuvring of the representation of facts and events, a way of going about things like any other, perfectly normal and acceptable, but requiring the acquisition of certain skills, an apprenticeship, and the application of guidelines. Arbuthnot picks up on several points that Swift had developed in the *Examiner*, the reference to the genealogy of lying, and the metaphor of the mirror. Swift's politically motivated and, again, unsigned paper begins with a frontal attack on the Whig Junto, and a reference to Satan as the grand master of mendacity, a master who, we are led to believe, has been surpassed in particular by the doings of the Whig administration of the past two decades. He makes lying various in nature and in its genealogy. One form of lying is referred to as a monster, and then as a goddess: 'This Goddess flies with a huge *Looking-glass* in her Hands, to dazzle the Crowd, and make them see, according as she turns it, their Ruin in their Interest, and their Interest in their Ruin'.[17] Arbuthnot takes his cue from Swift but elaborates on it, referring to lies and truth as the two faces of a mirror (a '*Plano-Cylindrical Speculum*'), the plain side being the surface fashioned by God, and reflecting plain truth, and the Cylindrical Figure, the work of the Devil:

> The plain side represents Objects just as they are; and the Cylindrical side, by the Rules of Catoptricks, must needs represent true Objects false, and false Objects true; but the Cylindrical side being much the larger Surface, takes in a greater Compass of visual Rays. That upon the Cylindrical side of the Soul of Man depends the whole Art and Success of *Political Lying*.[18]

False representations are thus privileged and have the upper hand. The second chapter explains that political lying is not an aberration but is defined as '*The Art of convincing the People of* Salutary Falshoods, *for some good End*'.[19] Political lying is a perfectly natural predisposition that, being normal and ingrained, can be nurtured and refined. What Arbuthnot provides is a reader-friendly user's manual, a conduct book for budding or confirmed politicians, a practical handbook to excel in 'that Noble and Useful Art of *Political Lying*'.[20] This *vade mecum* for politicians at no point openly broaches the question of whether lying is good or bad, right or wrong, moral considerations being beside the point. The only real question is when and how to lie, how to take people in, and best get away with it.

The reviewer's tongue remains firmly lodged in his cheek throughout this 'mock proposal'.[21] If Arbuthnot carefully avoids the invective and propaganda present in the Tory propaganda newspapers the *Examiner* and the *Plain Dealer*, he nonetheless damns the Whigs with praise. They are guilty not of lying (which is no offence), but of overdoing it. All is sweetness and light where the mechanics and techniques of best-practice lying are exposed and all is for the best in the best possible world of mendacity. Not the least of the ironies of the pamphlet is its length. Beattie notes: 'Only the first of the two volumes is outlined; but that is done on a large scale, with particulars for all the eleven chapters, so that the abstract amounts to a full-length essay'[22] by the anonymous provider of the abstract '*who has with great Care perus'd the* Manuscript'.[23] But the lie of lies, of course, is the fact that the work so meticulously anatomised and detailed is itself a fiction. No such work exists. No first volume has ever been carefully perused. The summary is a *mise en abyme* of its very subject, a faithful reflection of an inexistent object. The whole enterprise is thus a mirror of the theme; it is just one great big lie.

The treatise advances in a deliberate mist, weaving a web of doublespeak. Not only are political lies 'not wrong' but they are also indeed an absolute right. It is the fundamental nature and purpose of politics to be deceitful. Thus, in the third chapter, the author examines 'the Lawfulness of *Political Lying*' and introduces various unlikely categories such as 'private Truth' and 'oeconomical Truth':

> He shews, that the People ['People' here, of course, means 'men', and men of certain means: the propertied classes] have a Right to private Truth from their Neighbours, and œconomical Truth from their own Family; that they should not be abused by their Wives, Children, and Servants; but, that they have no Right at all to *Political* Truth: That the People may as well all pretend to be Lords of Mannors and possess great Estates, as to have Truth told them in Matters of Government.

Here Arbuthnot ratchets up the argument; it is simply preposterous to think that there is a right to political truth – i.e. it is the fundamental nature and purpose of politics to be deceitful.

The maze and intricacy, the cumulative effect of the argument and examples Arbuthnot provides (and this is no doubt what Swift was referring to when he found it 'not so obvious to be understood'), are boosted by a final turn of the screw in chapter eleven devoted to 'one simple Question', a return to the image of the distorting mirror: '*Whether a Lye is best contradicted by Truth, or another Lye*. The Author says, that considering the large Extent of the Cylindrical Surface of the Soul, and the great Propensity to believe Lyes in the generality of Mankind of late Years, he thinks the properest Contradiction to a Lye, is another Lye'.[24] Here again Arbuthnot logically, absurdly and symmetrically is treating like with like.

'that inviolable *Regard to Truth*'[25]

From these enlightened proposals it is a short step to a work of erudite misrepresentation on a more panoramic scale. *Memoirs of the Extraordinary Life, Works, and Discoveries of Martinus Scriblerus* is the collective, extravagant masterwork left by the Scriblerus Club. In itself a digest of the excesses of false learning, it traces the life of Martinus, 'this Prodigy of our Age',[26] son of the antiquary Cornelius and Mrs Scriblerus, from his conception, through his education, to his maturity, travels and disappearance. Christopher Fox writes that 'the Scriblerians portray in Martinus's story a veritable pedant's progress'.[27] As with Lemuel Gulliver, the reader is assured from the outset of the veracity of the narrative by the anonymous narrator. Thus we learn that, even in the womb, Martinus-to-be was marked out for an illustrious destiny: 'on a particular day, he was observed to leap and kick exceedingly, which was on the first of April, the birth-day of the great *Basilius Valentinus*. The Truth of this, and every preceding Fact, may be depended upon, being taken literally from the Memoirs'.[28] In July 1714, Swift encouraged Arbuthnot in his contribution to the embryonic Scriblerus project of debunking false learning and denouncing both modern trends in scholarship and the overattachment to ancient knowledge:

> To talk of Martin in any hands but Yours, is a Folly. You every day give better hints than all of us together could do in a twelvemonth; And to say the Truth, Pope who first thought of the Hint has no Genius at all to it, in my Mind. Gay is too young; Parnel has some Ideas of it, but is idle; I could putt together, and lard, and strike out well enough, but all that relates to the Sciences must be from you.[29]

George Aitken notes, 'The *Memoirs* are excellent in their kind, and the mock gravity is admirably maintained. Arbuthnot was the most learned of the wits of the time, and the piece is full of out-of-the-way knowledge. Many parts, too, involved an intimate acquaintance with medicine which he alone, of the members of the club, possessed'.[30] The space the project opened up allowed Arbuthnot's imagination to have a field day and the *Memoirs* focus in several chapters on Martinus's medical training concerning diseases of both the body and of the mind. And yet if there is not more on supposed medical misrepresentations and abuses, Kerby-Miller suggests this may be due to Pope's 'drastic editing and revising';[31] or perhaps a more likely explanation could be that Arbuthnot was temperamentally loath to descend into the already crowded and animated arena of medical disputations and pamphlet wars with his medical colleagues.

One of the fleetingly evoked 'Discoveries and Experiments' concerning the 'History of the Progress of Martinus in the Studies of Physick' is intriguing and has contemporary relevance.

> One of the first was his Method of investigating latent Distempers, by the sagacious Quality of *Setting-Dogs* and *Pointers*. The success, and the Adventures that befel him, when he walk'd with these Animals, to smell them out in the Parks and public places about London, are what we would willingly relate; but that his own Account, together with a *List of those Gentlemen and Ladies* at whom they made a *Full Sett*, will be publish'd in time convenient.[32]

This promised publication was again, unsurprisingly, never to materialise. The image of dogs running around, setting and pointing, sniffing out illnesses among the fashionable ladies and gentlemen strolling in London's parks as if they were game does provide an entertaining image, but it is now known that dogs' olfactory capabilities are remarkably various, effective and highly developed. Not only are they used to smell out explosives, arms and drugs, but their olfactory prowess is also a subject of medical research as they can identify various diseases including some cancers and, more recently, Covid 19.[33] That setters and pointers among other breeds are used to hunt is common knowledge, but I have been unable to identify if the transferral here to using scent as a means of detecting illness was indeed a topical issue for physicians in the early eighteenth century. However this may be, this particular example of 'misrepresentation' can, with hindsight, be said to have backfired. The boundaries between fact and fiction can at times, and in the course of time, become blurred, and fiction (or satire) can morph into fact.

One real-life character who enjoys the dubious privilege of appearing in the *Memoirs* under his own name is Dr John Woodward (1665–1728), himself an eminent natural philosopher, physician, geologist and antiquarian, a polymath like Arbuthnot, who can be viewed as Arbuthnot's outlandish alter ego. Arbuthnot's discretion and self-effacement contrast markedly with Woodward's 'egomania'.[34] He figures in the *Memoirs* on three occasions, as antiquary, physician and geologist, in references to the 'Ancient Shield, so famous through the Universities of Europe',[35] rolled out for the imbroglio of Martinus's christening and then purchased in the narrative by Dr Woodward, to 'Dr. Woodward's *Universal Deluge-water*', and as an advocate of 'vomition' as a treatment for smallpox.[36] But he is recognisable also in the traits of character of both Cornelius Scriblerus and his son, Martinus. Roy Porter sums up his contemporaries' appreciation of his personality as follows: 'In character he was a conceited, vain, stubborn man; querulous, hot-tempered, contemptuous of his fellow-workers'.[37] Angus Ross points to Woodward's scientific shortcomings: 'Woodward was a serious thinker with a fatal penchant for rushing into rash conclusions'.[38]

It would be inexact to say Woodward and Arbuthnot crossed swords as Woodward never entered into open dispute with Arbuthnot and did not respond to Arbuthnot's ironic rebuttal of his 1695[39] work which fuelled the Deluge controversy. Arbuthnot published his critical account, *An Examination of Dr. Woodward's Account of the Deluge* in 1697. However, Woodward did literally cross swords with Dr Richard Mead in the courtyard of Gresham College in 1719 when the so-called smallpox wars were raging, where the possible cures for smallpox, purging and vomiting, and then inoculation, were hotly disputed.[40] There is an echo of Woodward's implacable obstinacy to be found in the description of Cornelius: 'he reckon'd it a point of honour never to be vanquish'd in a dispute; from which quality he acquir'd the title of the *Invincible Doctor*'.[41]

The 'mock gravity' of the *Memoirs* identified by Aitken ensures a steady, leisurely, agreeable tone while the burden remains delightfully unhinged. At the same time, correspondences are made that reflect the preoccupations of the age. Diet is a constant concern and source of study for physicians of the time, notably George Cheyne, and Arbuthnot followed the trend in publishing in 1731 *An Essay concerning the Nature of Aliments*. He published *An Essay concerning the Effects of Air*, a topic also explored by Cheyne, in 1733, and had intended to continue with other non-naturals which neither his health nor time allowed him to do.

With Cornelius, the take on diet, a vignette of a few lines, is clearly more whimsical than Arbuthnot's extensive, didactic and rational treatise. Cornelius, to the dismay of Martinus's nurse who 'has a longing desire to a piece of beef', explains the risks that she would be running for Martinus's health, and proceeds to give her a short lecture in which he associates various victuals with moral flaws he attributes to various European peoples. In Cornelius's eyes diet is linked to national character:

> Consider, Woman, the different Temperaments of different Nations: What makes the English Phlegmatick and melancholy but Beef? what renders the Welsh so hot and cholerick, but cheese and leeks? the French derive their levity from their Soups, Frogs, and mushrooms: I would not let my Son dine like an Italian, lest, like an Italian he should be jealous and revengeful: The warm and solid diet of Spain may be more beneficial, as it might endue him with a profound Gravity, but at the same time he might suck in with their food their intolerable Vice of Pride. Therefore Nurse, in short, I hold it requisite to deny you at present, not only Beef, but likewise whatsoever any of those Nations eat.[42]

The poor nurse ends up having to make do with 'Butter mix'd with Honey'. Later, Martinus applies his talents to the diseases of the mind, which provides the authors of the *Memoirs* with the opportunity for a passing swipe at Woodward:

> But being weary of all practice on *foetid Bodies*, from a certain niceness of Constitution, (especially when he attended Dr. Woodward thro' a Twelvemonth's course of Vomition) he determined to leave it off entirely, and to apply

himself only to diseases of the *Mind*. He attempted to find out Specifics for all the *Passions*; and as other Physicians throw their Patients into sweats, vomits, purgations, &c. he cast them into love, hatred, hope, fear, joy, grief, &c. And indeed the great Irregularity of the Passions in the English Nation, was the chief motive that induced him to apply his whole studies, while he continued among us, to the Diseases of the Mind.[43]

Martinus lists four observations which underpin his own holistic physic, treating the soul and the body as interdependent. The first two are as below:

Ist, He observ'd that the Soul and Body mutually operate upon each other, and therefore if you deprive the Mind of the outward Instruments whereby she usually expresseth that Passion, you will in time abate the Passion itself, in like manner as Castration abates Lust.

2dly, That the Soul in mankind expresseth every Passion by the Motion of some particular Muscles.[44]

There follows a litany of emotional ills and corresponding physical remedies. Two cases, however, prove to be beyond the reach of even Martinus's science. Both mobilise such a number of muscles that it proves impossible to find a remedy: affectation and laughter. Of the former we read: 'But there were two Cases which he reckon'd extremely difficult. First, *Affectation*, in which there were so many Muscles of the bum, thighs, belly, neck, back, and the whole body, all in a false tone, that it requir'd an impracticable multiplicity of applications'.[45]

The concluding chapter of the *Memoirs* yields a detailed prospect of Martinus's achievements and exploits *'made and to be made, written and to be written, known and unknown'*,[46] as the chapter heading has it, drawing up a composite picture of what the Scriblerians saw as false learning and quackery. A further eccentricity of Martinus's is related here concerning 'his extraordinary practice of *Physick*. From the Age, Complexion, or Weight of the person given, he contrived to prescribe at a distance, as well as at a Patient's bed-side. He taught the way to many modern Physicians to cure their Patients by *Intuition*, and to others to cure *without looking on them at all*'.[47] The reference again is brief and sketchy but ties in with the long-running professional war between apothecaries and physicians. Kerby-Miller quotes a passage from *Some Memoirs of Dr John Radcliffe*, which illustrates the background to what one could imagine to be pure fantasy on the part of the Scriblerians, but is grounded in fact:

The Apothecaries, and other Smatterers in the Art of Pharmacy, had in order to draw People to them, gave out, that they could as well cure People at a Distance, as by Personal Attendance, of all manner of Human Maladies, by a sight of their Water; which would be of great Use to Patients, who, by Reason of their Infirmities, could not apply for Relief to theirs [i.e. them]; or, of their Poverty, could not pay for Visits at their own Homes.⁴⁸

A woman brings a urinal to Radcliffe to learn what her husband's sickness is, and how to cure it. They live four miles away. The good doctor enquires as to her husband's profession. She replies that he is a shoemaker. The doctor then empties the urinal into a chamber pot, urinates in it, hands it back to the lady and tells her to return to her husband and inform him that if he is capable of making a pair of boots for the doctor by observing the doctor's water in the urinal, the doctor will in return prescribe a cure for his distemper. The example may appear, like the earlier 'Setting-Dogs and Pointers' vignette, to be simply far-fetched but the analysis of urine in laboratory tests is of course a staple of modern medical practice. Henry Connor, in his brief history of uroscopy in medieval times – the observation of urine collected in a *matula*, a bladder-shaped clear glass flask – cites a reference to footwear that predates the Radcliffe story: 'Thomas Linacre (?1460–1524), the founder and first president of the College of Physicians of London, was said to have ridiculed those who were "too ready to carry about the patient's urine, expecting they would be told all things from the mere speculation of it", sarcastically suggesting that they bring the patient's shoe instead and "he would prophesie full as well over that"'.⁴⁹ But as Andrew Wear notes, 'Taking the pulse and uroscopy were two specialised skills which enabled the practitioner (and occasionally a lay person) to assess the state of a patient and make a diagnosis'. He goes on to say that 'uroscopy, if used as the sole means of diagnosis and in the absence of the patient, was attacked by physicians as the fraudulent practice of empirics'.⁵⁰

'O Truth divine!'

In his last published work, *Gnothi Seauton, Know your self* (1734),⁵¹ a pocket-sized philosophical poem of 137 lines, Arbuthnot revisits the Delphic maxim Γνῶθι σεαυτόν. He delivers in verse – this being the only poem of substance he was to write – a poetic coda. After his medical and critical writings, and his satirical and parodic works, Arbuthnot chooses to make a closing statement, affirming and explicating his Christian belief.

The poem is a precious and unexpected document. It is precious because there exists an autograph MS,⁵² a version of the poem that has been revised and improved on before the publishing of its definitive printed version of 1734. There is no external proof, but there is internal evidence that the poem was at the very least influenced by Pope's *An Essay on*

Man (1733–34), not only because of the date, the poetic form, and the chosen theme, but also because of the clear echo of certain lines and ideas. It is precious also because of its at once personal, philosophical and religious nature. It is unexpected because Arbuthnot chose poetry to compose this testament, the tailpiece of his writings.

One finds in the poem the same qualities as in Pope, the Augustan balancing act, a similar concision and precision, the symmetry; the same pervasive presence of, and taste for, paradox and antithesis, the moral didacticism, the occasional wagging finger of warning and reprimand; the same common-sense advice, and insights into the human condition. In short, the same optimistic and buoyant pessimism. It is a further and final condemnation of vanity and overreaching, and an acknowledgement and acceptance of one's own limits, of the limits of human knowledge (Locke again), and the confines, as Pope and Arbuthnot see them, of the human situation. Through this quest, Arbuthnot seeks a solution to the riddle that is humankind, a remedy for, and an understanding of, our moral ills. He believes he has found it in the Christian God. It is a lucid, economical, accessible and accomplished exercise in containment.

The opening passage is busy with questions, five in the first couplet, and recalls questions of personal identity, central to the *Memoirs*, and which Christopher Fox has examined in detail in his study on Locke and the Scriblerians, but offers no answers:

> What am I? how produc'd? and for what End?
> Whence drew I Being? to what Period tend?
> Am I th' abandon'd Orphan of blind Chance;
> Dropt by wild Atoms in disorder'd Dance?
> Or from an endless Chain of Causes wrought?
> And of unthinking Substance, born with Thought?
> By Motion which began without a Cause,
> Supremely wise, without Design, or Laws.
> Am I but what I seem, mere Flesh and Blood;
> A branching Channel, with a mazy Flood?
> The purple Stream that through my Vessels glides,
> Dull and unconscious flows like common Tides:
> The Pipes thro' which the circling Juices stray,
> Are not that thinking I, no more than They:
> This Frame, compacted with transcendent Skill,
> Of moving Joints, obedient to my Will;
> Nurs'd from the fruitful Glebe, like yonder Tree,
> Waxes and wastes; I call it Mine, not Me:
> New Matter still the mould'ring Mass sustains,
> The Mansion changed, the Tenant still remains:
> And from the fleeting Stream repair'd by Food,

Distinct, as is the Swimmer from the Flood.
What am I then? (1–23)

Arbuthnot proceeds in an orderly, disorderly fashion. The questions crowd upon him. Some are rhetorical and contain the seeds of their own destruction. Despite the use of the first-person singular, Arbuthnot seems, at least at first, to be embarking on an objective rather than a subjective mission. In lines three to eight Arbuthnot aligns questions all of which are, the reader is to understand, self-evidently absurd. This is the poet's very summary rebuttal of Epicureanism. This somewhat hectic opening gambit is foregrounded by the use of terms in lines three and four of negative connotation: 'abandon'd orphan', 'blind', 'wild', 'disorder'd'. He asks in a tone that is bemused and scornful, dismissive, rather than perplexed, whether Man could be:

... from an endless Chain of Causes wrought?
And of unthinking Substance, born with Thought?
By Motion which began without a Cause,
Supremely wise, without Design, or Laws. (5–8)

Then, however, moving from the abstract and the metaphysical, the physician-poet Arbuthnot examines the body, and in particular the circulation of the blood, a fluid in a state of constant flux, in search of the origin and home of the 'I' that makes a being an individual with a specific, enduring identity. Everything here is elusive – gliding, straying, branching, 'a mazy Flood', 'common Tides', movement which, while active and unceasing, seems to lack direction. If the blood is found wanting, in that it fails to provide an answer, so does the body itself. Like other natural phenomena it lives and dies, waxes and wanes, a 'mould'ring Mass'; a transient ever-changing entity, 'I call it mine, not Me'. Both the body as substance, and the circulating blood, in their impermanence and mutability translate an essential ontological insecurity and anxiety.

All again is motion, but to what end? Arbuthnot here is the physician but also the philosopher, seeking something solid, dependable, unchangeable. Man remains separate from the body that houses him, 'distinct as is the swimmer from the flood' (22). After this animated and apparently unavailing beginning, Arbuthnot finds himself none the wiser and, having cleared the ground, back at square one: 'What am I then?' (23).

The philosophers offer Arbuthnot no consolation. Religion alone provides an answer of sorts. And the personal 'I', imploring and petitioning God to show the way forward, is the emotional apex of the poem, the turn. Arbuthnot brings the whole poem on the unsatisfactory, 'jarring', human condition, torn between conflicting desires and extremes, to a finally resigned, if perplexing and inconclusive, conclusion:

> In vain thou hop'st for Bliss on this poor Clod,
> Return, and seek thy Father, and thy God:
> Yet think not to regain thy native Sky,
> Born on the Wings of vain Philosophy;
> Mysterious Passage! hid from human Eyes;
> Soaring you'll sink, and sinking you will rise:
> Let humble Thoughts thy wary Footsteps guide,
> Regain by Meekness what you lost by Pride. (130–137)

In his last letter to Pope, written from Hampstead where he had moved to breathe a more healthy air to relieve his asthma, Arbuthnot wrote: 'And I make it my Last Request, that you continue that noble *Disdain* and *Abhorrence* of Vice, which you seem naturally endued with, but still with a due regard to your own Safety; and study more to reform than chastise, tho' the one often cannot be effected without the other'.[53] Where Arbuthnot puts the emphasis on reform, Pope in his reply explains his position of personalising satire if he feels it serves a purpose: 'it is as impossible to have a just abhorrence of Vice without hating the vicious, as to bear a true love for Virtue without loving the Good. To reform and not to chastise, I am afraid is impossible ...' .[54] Despite the difference of nuance, and it is a difference that is visible in the potency of the satires of Pope, Swift and Arbuthnot, the Scriblerians did share a common reforming and not only reactionary ethos. Arbuthnot displays in his serious works, on aliments, on air, on mathematics, and coins, however derivative they may be, a firm attachment to scientific methodology and empirical enquiry. In his satires, individual and collective, he holds up a distorting but always entertaining mirror to denounce and ridicule what he sees as the excesses of the time. In his final work it is his religious faith that he chooses to highlight, a more intimate apprehension of knowledge, in his quest for truth that he chooses to finalise and publicise in poetic form. In all three domains and discourses, fact, fiction and belief, Arbuthnot is unceasingly questioning, sifting, paring down, to see what, of truth, remains in the crucible. Through his holistic and plural approach, he remains to the end a physician of the body, of the mind, and of the soul, seeking out truth and knowledge, proposing remedies after a fashion, be they medical, satirical, didactic or poetical, and exploring the paths of fact, fiction and belief to do so.

Notes

1 Samuel Taylor Coleridge, *The Collected Works of Samuel Taylor Coleridge: Biographia Literaria or Biographical Sketches of My Literary Life and Opinions*

(1817), vol. II, ed. James Engells and W. Jackson Bate (Princeton, NJ: Princeton University Press, and London: Routledge & Kegan Paul, 1983), chapter 14.
2 Alexander Pope, *The Dunciad*, ed. James Sutherland (London: Methuen, 1963), p. 54.
3 George Orwell, *Essays*, ed. Peter Davison (London, New York, Toronto: Everyman's Library, 2002). 'Imaginary Interview: George Orwell and Jonathan Swift', *BBC African Service*, 6 November 1943, p. 452.
4 Charles Kerby-Miller (ed.), *Memoirs of the Extraordinary Life, Works, and Discoveries of Martinus Scriblerus*. Written in Collaboration by the Members of the Scriblerus Club: John Arbuthnot, Alexander Pope, Jonathan Swift, John Gay, Thomas Parnell and Robert Harley, Earl of Oxford (New Haven, CT: Yale University Press, 1950; Reissued New York: Russell & Russell, 1966), p. 41.
5 Jonathan Swift, *Gulliver's Travels* (1726), edited with an introduction by Paul Turner (Oxford and New York: Oxford University Press, 1986), p. xl.
6 Ibid., p. 242.
7 John Locke, 'The Epistle to the Reader', *An Essay concerning Human Understanding*, ed. Peter H. Nidditch (Oxford: Clarendon Press, 1975), pp. 6–14, at p. 9.
8 Lester M. Beattie, *John Arbuthnot, Mathematician and Satirist* (Cambridge, MA: Harvard University Press, 1935).
9 Ibid., p. 208.
10 John Arbuthnot, *An Essay on the Usefulness of Mathematical Learning: in a Letter from a Gentleman in the City to his Friend in Oxford* (Oxford: Peisley, 1701), p. 2.
11 Ibid., p. 3.
12 Ibid., pp. 8–9.
13 John Arbuthnot, *Proposals for Printing A very Curious Discourse, in Two Volumes in Quarto, Intitled, ΨΕΥΔΟΛΟΓΙΑ ΠΟΛΙΤΙΚΗ; or, A Treatise on the Art of Political Lying, with An Abstract of the First Volume of the said Treatise* (London: Printed for John Morphew, near Stationers-Hall, 1712).
14 Beattie tracks the evolution of, and interaction between, these publications. See Beattie, *John Arbuthnot*, pp. 288–298.
15 Leslie Stephen, 'Arbuthnot, John', in *Dictionary of National Biography*, vol. 2 (London: Smith, Elder, and Co., 1885–1900).
16 Jonathan Swift, *Journal to Stella*, ed. Harold Williams (Oxford: Blackwell, 1974), letter LVI, London, 12 December 1712.
17 *The Examiner*, No. 14, Thursday 9 November 1710, in *The Examiners for the Year 1711* (sic) (London: Printed for John Morphew, 1712), p. 81.
18 Arbuthnot, *Art of Political Lying*, p. 7.
19 Ibid., p. 8.
20 Ibid., p. 6.
21 Kerby-Miller, *Memoirs of Martinus Scriblerus*, p. 72.
22 Beattie, *John Arbuthnot*, p. 292.
23 Arbuthnot, *Art of Political Lying*, p. 6.
24 Ibid., p. 21.

25 Kerby-Miller, *Memoirs of Martinus Scriblerus*, p. 165.
26 Ibid., p. 166.
27 Christopher Fox, *Locke and the Scriblerians: Identity and Consciousness in Early Eighteenth-Century Britain* (Berkeley, Los Angeles, London: University of California Press, 1988), p. 82.
28 Kerby-Miller, *Memoirs of Martinus Scriblerus*, p. 97.
29 Angus Ross (ed.), *The Correspondence of Dr John Arbuthnot* (Munich: Fink, 2006), Letter of Jonathan Swift to Arbuthnot, 3 July 1714, p. 182.
30 George A. Aitken, *The Life and Works of John Arbuthnot M.D., Fellow of the Royal College of Physicians* (Oxford: Clarendon, 1892), p. 58.
31 Kerby-Miller, *Memoirs of Martinus Scriblerus*, p. 272.
32 Ibid., p. 130.
33 'Animal sniffing is an innate behaviour, and canine olfactory acuity is over 100 000 times stronger than human acuity. Animal sniffing (by dogs and rats) has been used for centuries for detecting people, and since the twentieth century animals have also detected weapons, bombs, narcotics and food, for example, at borders and airports. According to a recent literature review, animals have been used as diagnostic tools in various fields of medicine, such as recognizing diabetic ketoacidosis in emergency rooms and scent detection of various human tumours and metabolic diseases'. E. Cambau and M. Poljak, 'Sniffing Animals as a Diagnostic Tool in Infectious Diseases', *Clinical Microbiology and Infection* 26:4 (2020): 431–435, at 432.
34 Roy Porter, 'John Woodward: "A Droll Sort of Philosopher"', *Geological Magazine* 116:5 (1979): 335–417, at 339.
35 Kerby-Miller, *Memoirs of Martinus Scriblerus*, p. 103.
36 Ibid., pp. 102–104, 130, 168.
37 Porter, 'John Woodward', p. 339.
38 Ross, *The Correspondence of Dr John Arbuthnot*, p. 53, n. 49.
39 John Woodward, *An Essay toward a Natural History of the Earth and Terrestrial Bodies, especially Minerals: as also of the Sea, Rivers, and Springs: with an Account of the Universal Deluge: and of the Effects that it had upon the Earth* (London: Printed for Richard Wilkin, 1695).
40 See Sophie Vasset, 'Medical Laughter and Medical Polemics: The Woodward–Mead Quarrel and Medical Satire', *XVII–XVIII* (*Autour du rire / Laughing Matters*) 70 (2013): 109–133.
41 Kerby-Miller, *Memoirs of Martinus Scriblerus*, p. 125.
42 Ibid., p. 106.
43 Ibid., p. 130.
44 Ibid., p. 131.
45 Ibid., p. 132–133.
46 Ibid., p. 166.
47 Ibid., p. 168.
48 John Radcliffe, *Some Memoirs of the Life of John Radcliffe, M.D.* (London: Printed for E. Curll, 1715), p. 12. See Kerby-Miller, *Memoirs of Martinus Scriblerus*, p. 344.

49 Henry Connor, 'Medieval Uroscopy and its Representation on Misericords – Part 1: Uroscopy', *Clinical Medicine* 1:6 (2001): 508.
50 Andrew Wear, *Knowledge & Practice in English Medicine, 1550–1680* (Cambridge: Cambridge University Press, 2000), p. 120.
51 John Arbuthnot, *Gnothi Seauton. Know Your Self* (London: J. Tonson, 1734). The poem was originally published anonymously. It first appeared under Arbuthnot's name in the first volume of the three-volume *A Collection of Poems. By Several Hands*, printed by Robert Dodsley in 1748 (196–202). Following the airing of doubts and self-doubt about the nature of humankind and the human predicament in the opening section of the poem, Arbuthnot in an apostrophe to God finds succour and a tranquillity of sorts through his reading of the Bible – 'the sacred Text, / The Balm, the Light, the Guide of Souls perplext:' (85–86) – and affirms his religious faith:

> O Truth divine! enlightned by thy Ray,
> I grope and guess no more, but see my way;
> Thou cleardst the Secret of my high Descent,
> And told me what those mystick Tokens meant. (91–94)

52 John Arbuthnot, 'An *English* poem by Dr. Arbuthnott. *Autograph*', British Library London, Department of Manuscripts, Add.MS.22625, f.31. The poem was first printed under Arbuthnot's name in 1748.
53 Ross, *The Correspondence of Dr John Arbuthnot*, Letter 183, Arbuthnot to Alexander Pope, Hampstead, 17 July 1734, p. 385.
54 Ibid., Letter 184, Alexander Pope to Arbuthnot, 26 July 1734, p. 386.

3

'The very women read it': medical self-fashioning, mythologies and (mis)information in George Cheyne MD's medical writings

Clark Lawlor

I never wrote a Book in my Life but that I had a Fit of Illness after'
George Cheyne to Samuel Richardson, 7 July 1741[1]

Dr George Cheyne (1672–1743) was a master of self-mythologisation, or self-fashioning, to use a cognate term. He was perhaps the most successful self-publicising medic of his time – doctor to the literati like Samuel Richardson and Alexander Pope, and author of best-selling medical self-help manuals such as the *Essay of Health* and the *English Malady*, in which he made the generic innovation and ultimate act of self-fashioning by taking the role of both doctor and patient in his autobiographical, yet artfully constructed, 'Case of the Author'. In her 'Medical Celebrity in Eighteenth-Century Britain', Katherine Richards, extending celebrity theory into the eighteenth-century medical realm, argues that 'for medical practitioners to be celebrities – there must be a representation of a public and private self that captured people's interest'.[2] This is not the only element necessary for celebrity, but it is clear that Cheyne generated such an interest in his private life in one fell swoop, with the paradoxical effect of making him an everyman – and woman – as well.

The apparent paradox at the core of this essay is the fact that Cheyne had the aim of making useful and accurate medical information available to a wide audience via the medium of print and an accessible style in the vernacular, but at the same time fashioning an image of himself, partly by creating a mythology of his own case study – literally of his own body or 'crazy carcase'. I will explore the way in which Cheyne became a fashionable and effective writing doctor by rewriting medical information in a more engaging and comprehensible style, and by exploiting his own ailments in a new form of medical self-fashioning, but building on the achievements of previously innovative medics writing in the vernacular, such as Sir Richard Blackmore (1654–1729). Key to this fashioning and fashionability was Cheyne's choice of language and genre, and his shaping of that genre to his own innovative creative vision of medical writing. Although Cheyne was concerned to mythologise a certain aspect of his own character, he was also attempting to provide good medical information that would correct the misinformation being peddled, as he saw it, by other medics who denied the efficacy of his 'milk and seed' diet. Concentrating on Cheyne's career up to and including the publication of the *English Malady* (1733), we will focus particularly on those writings aimed at a more general audience, including *An Essay on the Gout* (1720) and *An Essay of Health and Long Life* (1724), as well as the *English Malady* itself. As we will see, Cheyne's medical theory stressed the superior nervous systems of certain types of people, usually the upper and middling sort, including the literati and himself, in a form of widely approved medical misinformation, despite the fact Cheyne also believed it, and considered himself to be supplying the most relevant and up-to-date form of medical knowledge in a literary form the people would understand.

Cheyne and writing in English

Cheyne benefitted from the efforts of those doctors, like Sir Richard Blackmore, who campaigned for the use of the vernacular rather than Latin to spread medical knowledge to a much wider constituency than the narrower professional circle).[3] Blackmore, who I discuss elsewhere, to take a notable example of a champion of writing medical works in English, saw such a shift as part of Enlightenment progress, a spreading of knowledge that would be of benefit both to nation and Church. Blackmore was also a successful poet, author of the best-selling *Creation: A Philosophical Poem* (1712), as well as many medical tracts in English on subjects such as the gout, consumption and the spleen. He had fought a battle on several fronts to ensure the legitimacy of publishing in English, and so successful was this Queen's physician that Cheyne rarely reflected on this shift into the vernacular by the time he came to popular authorship, and seems to have taken it for granted.

Latin had its place, but Cheyne did not take for granted the need to write in a style that engaged the new audience made possible by writing in English. Form and content needed to interact, however: Cheyne's major innovation was to self-fashion his public persona by crossing the boundary between the private sphere and the public. By showing his own vulnerability as a patient, his own 'Case' (which also meant body), he was able to extend his appeal to his target audience.

Who was Cheyne's audience? Initially he engaged in internecine medical disputes, defending his patron in the Scottish medical world, Archibald Pitcairne, against professional rivals. Fellow doctors, and perhaps their potential lucrative patients of the Scottish upper orders, were the primary recipients of arguments about the nature of fevers. These arguments dragged Cheyne into a form of medical satire that quickly descended into ad hominem insults and attacks on the reputations of Pitcairne's enemies, a move that Cheyne soon regretted and later recanted in print.

Cheyne's conception of his true audience became at once more capacious and yet more specific when he started to practise in England, encouraged by his patron Pitcairne, and by the examples of successful migrant Scottish medics like Dr John Arbuthnot (1667–1735), member of the Scriblerus Club (with Alexander Pope, Jonathan Swift and John Gay), literary satirist in his own right, and Physician-in-Ordinary to Queen Anne from 1709. Cheyne and Arbuthnot were contemporaries and friends as students at Marischal College, Aberdeen, and Arbuthnot later introduced Cheyne to many of the literati who would become his patients. Through a wider audience, and because of a wider audience, Cheyne would resist the mythologies that kept medical knowledge – and ultimately health – hidden from public view.

An Essay of Health and Long Life

By the early 1720s Cheyne had begun to build a practice, partly thanks to the sway of Arbuthnot and other influential patrons, treating those who could afford his services: members of the aristocracy, including the Court, and the increasingly wealthy middling sort who were making money from trade rather than the land. Cheyne moved more or less permanently to Bath from London in 1718, but kept in contact with his London circle and lucrative patients. This relocation to the increasingly fashionable location of Bath Spa, with its integrated leisure and health industries catering both to the fashionably ill and the fashionably well, prompted Cheyne's shift to writing popular medical works rather than technical pieces. The first work of note was *An Essay on the Gout* (1720), Cheyne's first attempt at a popular work that duly gained a wider readership and acclaim for its accessible style and content, including a message of temperance in diet and lifestyle that was also criticised. Dr Robert Hale, who – along with many others – had no intention of giving up red wine and meat, attacked the *Essay on the Gout* as a mercenary production more akin to a Grub Street money-making exercise than a worthy attempt to improve the health of the God-fearing Christian.[4]

The suspicions of his enemies were confirmed with the publication of *An Essay of Health and Long Life* (1724), Cheyne's most popular work, which doubled down on the broad prescriptions of the gout essay and encouraged a 'low' vegetarian diet with the emphasis on denial of those rich foods and strong drinks that the modern, civilized and sophisticated lifestyle forced on the unsuspecting fashionable person, and this time it was more than gout that could ensue if one did not fall into line with Cheyne's methods.[5] Exercise such as horse-riding was advised, as were various hygienic habits (but no knowledge of bacteria at this time was possible).[6] Again, the *Essay* began life as advice to an individual patient, in this case Sir Joseph Jekyll, and was intended to help him 'Conduct his Health for the future' and to enable him to continue 'the great Business he is engaged in' (*EH*, p. xi). Again Cheyne wrote up his private prescription into a public essay, and one in which Cheyne is clear about his audience: 'The Robust, the Luxurious, the Pot-Companions, the Loose, and the Abandoned, have no Business here; their Time is not yet come', but those 'very learned, ingenious, and even Religious Persons, who being weak and tender (as such generally are), have suffered to the last for want of a due Regimen of Diet, and other Directions of Health'. Cheyne was the man to supply the necessary self-help manual for the polite sort, who consist of the 'Sickly and the Aged, the Studious and the Sedentary, persons of weak Nerves and Gentlemen of the Learned Professions' (*EH*, p. xiv). The target audience was not suffering because of their lack of interest in being healthy, or their loose morals, but because they knew no better and needed the correct information to realise that they had to change the habits of a so-called civilized or 'sophisticated' lifestyle.

An Essay of Health and Long Life was massively popular, ran to ten editions by 1745, and was still being reprinted as late as 1813. As with *An Essay on the Gout*, it was fashionably controversial, and inspired many satires, critiques from medical professionals, and anecdotes at the time. Cheyne had now established himself, via his authorial medical self-fashioning, as one of the most important medics of his day. His advice for preventing disease and promoting health via personal regimen, personal self-management, was one of the main models for the also popular poem *The Art of Preserving Health* (1744) by Dr John Armstrong.[7]

Cheyne had a gift for literary writing, and his aphoristic, epigrammatic talents are evident from the beginning of his *Essay of Health*, which is worth quoting at length:

> It is a common saying, That every Man past Forty is either a Fool or a Physician: It might have been added, that he was a Divine too: for, as the World goes at present, there is not any Thing that the Generality of the better Sort of Mankind so lavishly and so unconcernedly throw away as Health, except eternal Felicity. Most Men know when they are ill but very few when they are well. And yet it is most certain that 'tis easier to preserve Health than to recover it, and to prevent Diseases than to cure them. Towards the first, the means are mostly in our Power: Little else is required then to bear and forbear. But towards the latter, the Means are perplexed and uncertain; and

for the Knowledge of them the far greatest Part of Mankind must apply to others, of whose Skill and Honesty they are in a great measure ignorant, and the Benefit of whose Art they can but conditionally and precautiously obtain. A crazy Constitution, original weak Nerves, dear-bought experience in Things helpful and hurtful, and long Observation on the Complaints of others who came here for relief to this universal Infirmary, BATH, have at last (in some measure), taught me some of the most effectual Means of preserving Health and prolonging Life in those who are tender and sickly and Labour under chronical Distempers. (*EH*, pp. 1–3)

Cheyne begins with an appeal to common-sense wisdom that amuses as it engages his readership, and then expands upon it to reinforce the message about the importance of health. He adds a beautifully balanced Augustan aphorism of his own, that would not be amiss in a line of Pope's poetry: 'Most Men know when they are ill but very few when they are well', and repeats that see-sawing symmetrical rhythm and content by adding 'it is most certain that 'tis easier to preserve Health than to recover it, and to prevent Diseases than to cure them'. The opposition of 'Ill' to 'well' is inverted to that of 'preserve', 'recover', and then again to 'prevent' versus 'cure'. This elegant Augustan prose continues to connect general, accepted truths to his audience's experience, but then takes the original turn of introducing his own 'crazy Constitution' into the equation, a prelude to the fuller examination of his 'crazy Carcase' in the 'Case of the Author' in the *English Malady* (*EH*, p. xvi). Cheyne was a master of the catchy phrase, combined with the ability to drive home his key point, as he does when he lands on 'chronical Distempers' at the end of this finely crafted paragraph. So memorable was Cheyne's writing that 'Ephraim Quibus M.D.' (John Martyn) mimicked him as 'Meteorus ... swollen with epithets' when satirizing in a letter 'the method of writing Cases in Physick and Surgery' in *The Grub St Journal* (no. 8, 26 February 1730).[8]

Part of the self-fashioning in *An Essay of Health* is the autobiographical Preface, which in some senses looks forward to the new genre he creates in the *English Malady*, wherein he becomes the case study himself and causes the readers to identify with him, to perceive the fashionable sufferer of nerves as 'a way to be', to use Ian Hacking's concept.[9] It was here that Cheyne shifted his style away from his role as witty and controversial defender of his patron, Pitcairne, by recanting his former indelicacies and instead became more of a man of feeling, a sentimental, sensible (in the widest sense of the term), sufferer of the nerves, one with whom his patients could identify or even wish to emulate.

Cheyne abandoned his former emphasis on obscure mathematics because they 'leave a Stiffness, Positiveness, and Sufficiency on weak Minds, much more pernicious to Society, and the Interests of the Great End of our Being', failing to inspire the true fellow feeling that the new medicine of sensibility was to encourage: to 'sweeten the Temper, or mend the Heart'. Politeness was now the driver, and Cheyne to become more and more an 'amiable humourist', as Stuart Tave has argued.[10] Now he was to 'heartily condemn and detest all personal Reflexions, all malicious and unmannerly Turns, and all false and unjust Representations, as unbecoming Gentlemen, Scholars, and Christians' (*EH*, p. vii). This new genre, at one with the requirements of the turn to the culture of sensibility, required a new style with 'as little Subtilty and Refinement ... as the Present state of Natural Philosophy could admit' – overcomplication would alienate the wider audience of fellow feelers that Cheyne was attempting to engage (*EH*, p. xv). Cheyne was 'often contented with plain and obvious Facts to account for Appearances, and the Cautions thence deduced; when according to the Humour of the present Age, I might have run into refined Speculations of Metaphysicks, or Mathematicks' (*EH*, p. xvi).

For Cheyne to self-fashion as an appealing medical writer, his style had to diverge from the common herd: other medical authors failed to provide 'the Perspicuity and natural Way of convincing the ingenious, sickly and tender Sufferers, so necessary to make them chearfully and so readily undergo such severe Restraints; which I take to be the most difficult Part of such a Work, and which I have Laboured with my utmost Power to supply' (*EH*, p. xvii). This new art of medical persuasion had practical consequences for treatment: patients might be fed proper medical information, but it had to arrive in a rhetorically effective manner otherwise it might as well be useless mythology and quackery.

Genre and, relatedly, marketing were crucial factors in Cheyne's move away from more academic, medical writings better suited to a career in academe (as could have been the case earlier in his medical progress), and a vital marker of genre and its practical business at the booksellers is the title of the work in question. Apparently, the *Essay of Health* was initially called 'A Treatise of Sanity and Longevity', but Nathaniel Hooke, Cheyne's friend, reports that 'the Sale of a book may be hurt a great deal by an ill-chosen title. Dr Cheyne's bookseller absolutely refused to print his book on health unless he would change the title'.[11] The bookseller was James Leake, a new force on the Bath scene who was keen to cash in on the medical market for accessible advice in the vernacular, and as such highly aware of the effects of labelling his wares. 'A Treatise' implies an academic, technical form of publication that is very much intended for a specialized, possibly Latin and Greek-speaking, audience (and many of these works were written in Latin and heavy in citation of original Greek). The change of title from 'Treatise' to 'Essay' allowed Cheyne access to a labelled genre familiar to a wide readership (and opened up a direct comparison with the *Spectator* tradition) and a genre that assumed the English language as its primary mode. Essays, as accessible forms of writing, appealed to both men and woman.

We must pause to refine the concept of self-fashioning here: Cheyne was persuaded – forced even – to change the title of his work by the bookseller, a coercive act that was entirely to the benefit of Cheyne's image as a popular medical author, a man of the people (albeit a certain type of person). Again, self-fashioning is not entirely dictated by self-willed interiority – that is an illusion. In dialogue with external literary and cultural forces, Cheyne's authorial status is improved. Self-fashioning is never just about personal vision, but about how the individual moves through their particular historical environment – in this case, the publishing and print culture of the early eighteenth century. What benefitted Cheyne made profit for the publisher too.

There was precedent for the popular medical essay as well: Sir William Temple wrote his 'Essay of Health' (1702) that Cheyne would certainly have read.[12] The more relaxed, gentleman-scholarly tone of Temple's work provided a starting point for Cheyne, and the very form of the essay itself allowed a more free-flowing, exploratory form and content. Gold dust for the researcher into the tangible effects of popular medical essay writing is Lord Balmerino's annotated copy of Cheyne's *Essay of Health*, which is full of useful comments (both to Balmerino and to us), many of which were made while Balmerino made his way round Europe on a combination of Grand Tour and health tour.[13] The study of travel for health and literature remains rather undercooked, but it was often the case that the two, health and culture, were combined, including closer to home at Bath. Clearly Balmerino viewed Cheyne's *Essay* as sufficiently portable and easy to understand, so much so that he was prepared to haul it around Europe, and to consult it regularly for practical advice.

Cheyne's move towards widening medical advice was of a piece with a more general call to the popularization of hitherto elite knowledge, a move made concrete in Addison's argument in the *Spectator* – itself a vehicle for the dissemination of information to a wider constituency – that 'Philosophy' should be brought 'out of Closets and Libraries, Schools and Colleges, to dwell in Clubs and Assemblies, at Tea-Tables, and in Coffee-Houses' (*Spectator* 10). It is here that Alexander Pope's satirical comment, 'The very women read it', about William Wollaston's *Religion of Nature Delineated* (1724), comes in. For Pope, popular works such as Wollaston's and Cheyne's trivialize and misrepresent important and masculine discourses that should be kept away from those who are unable to critique or handle such knowledge. Women read Wollaston and then 'pretend to be charm'd with the beauty which they generally think the least of. They make as much ado about truth, since this book appeared as they did about health when Dr Cheyne's [*An Essay of Health and Long*

Life (1724)] came out; and they will doubtless be consulted in the pursuit of one, as the other'.[14] If nothing else, Pope proves Cheyne's ability to achieve fashionability across the genders.

The role of women in Cheyne's readership has been discussed by George Rousseau and David Shuttleton, with Shuttleton following Ginnie Smith's argument that 'Though impossible to prove, it seems probable that Cheyne's works had a particular appeal to female readers allotted the traditional roles of domestic carers and nurses, at a time when many middle-class households did a certain amount of doctoring at home'.[15] No doubt more research remains to be done on this subject, but Pope's complaint – antifeminist though it is – could be masking the practical popularity of Cheyne's works aimed at an audience of both genders, not merely the aristocratic male like Balmerino. As George Rousseau has argued, the presence of works of natural philosophy in Cheyne's proposed 'Catalogue of Pamela's Library', which was a pet project that Cheyne had urged on his friend Samuel Richardson for the eponymous heroine of his novel, *Pamela*, proves that women were a legitimate part of the market for popular works of science.[16]

We should remember that Cheyne's literary works were reinforcing a rising cult of personality, or celebrity, inculcated by Cheyne's direct interactions with his patients. As his Bath practice burgeoned in the early 1720s, so did his quasi-religious message of abstinence and self-management. One unlikely convert was Lord Hervey (he of Pope's scurrilous attack in the *Epistle to Dr Arbuthnot*), who was Cheyne's patient from 1724. Hervey bantered with Cheyne as Cheyne did with his patients in his quest to keep them on the dietary straight and narrow:

> If you were as just to my practice as I am to your doctrine, it would be impossible for you, whilst I always acknowledge and rever you as the great Aesculapius of this age and country, to speak of me as an apostate, a heretic or even a schismatic to your medical religion. In order therfore to set you right, and to let you know who is one of your most pious votaries, I write this letter to let you know the method I am in.[17]

The metaphor of Cheyne's 'medical religion' is thoroughly exploited here by Hervey, who was responding with mock shock to Cheyne's accusations (themselves framed as bantering good humour) that Lord Bateman (dedicatee of *The English Malady*) was reverting to his former ways. Likewise, poet and politician Lord George Lyttelton found 'the Immortal Doctor Cheney' to be 'the greatest Singularity, and the most Delightful I ever met with. I am not his patient, but am to be his Disciple, and to see a Manuscript of his which comprehends all that is necessary, salutary or useful either of Body or Soul'.[18] Hervey and Lyttelton's words have a tinge of irony that prevents them from being totally subsumed by the cult of Cheyne, but their enthusiasm in the modern sense is clear enough. Polite badinage with their esteemed doctor was that of equals, not of income necessarily, nor even of social rank, but Cheyne's celebrity and the charisma that went with it, as well as a clear message delivered in an accessible and entertaining manner, enabled such elegant and subtle interactions.

The ladies were drawn into Cheyne's cult of personality as well. Hester Thrale provided a ringing endorsement of Cheyne's rhetorical powers when she, again with a certain amount of mocking self-awareness, announced that 'few books carry so irresistible a Power of Persuasion with them as Cheyne's do: when I read Cheyne I feel disposed to retire to Arruchar in the Highlands of Scotland – live on oat bread and Milk, and bathe in the Frithe of Clyde for seven years'.[19] This was in 1790, many years after Cheyne's death, but still carrying an idealist primitivism that chimed well with Rousseauvian and Romantic tenets of a retreat back to Nature from the physical as well as moral corruptions of civilization. Cheyne himself was not advocating winding back the clock to living as his ancestors had done, but more regarded nervous diseases as the price to pay for an advanced and fashionable lifestyle. The key point for us here, however, is the sheer force of Cheyne's writing to 'convert' his readers, however remote – as in the case of Thrale – to his theory and practice.

The English Malady

The publication of *The English Malady*, with its appended 'Case of the Author', in 1733 marked a step forward in Cheyne's self-fashioning in print.[20] It is the most studied of Cheyne's works, partly for the simple reason that Cheyne put himself on public display as both patient and medic, the disease and the cure as it were:

> perhaps it may not be quite useless to some low, desponding, valetudinary, over-grown Person, whose Case may have some Resemblance to mine: which every one's has in some degree, that has a mortal Tabernacle subject to, and afflicted with nervous Disorders, by a mistaken Regimen, or hereditary Misfortune; and I have, on that Account, written this in a plain narrative Stile, with the fewest Terms of Art possible, without supposing my Reader, or shewing myself, to have look'd ever into physical Book before, thinking this Manner and Stile might be most instructive and beneficial to common valetudinary Readers (*EM*, pp. 362–363).

This was self-fashioning in a new genre, one that we might call the popular medico-autobiographical self-help manual, although one that picked up on elements of puritan autobiography, but without the interest in affairs of the soul beyond the affirmation that a healthy physical regimen would certainly assist the mind and soul (these two terms were shifting gradually, with the soul being displaced by mind) in their own well-being.[21] Style, in this case 'a plain Narrative stile', was crucial; without the understanding of a wider audience, 'common valetudinary Readers', Cheyne's message would not result in action. Technical vocabulary should be eschewed as far as possible, with 'physical Book' in this instance meaning a book about medicine. Readers needed to understand that Cheyne was like them, and they could be cured, just as he had cured himself.[22]

The longer title is *The English Malady: or, a Treatise of Nervous diseases of all kinds: as spleen, vapours, lowness of spirits, hypochondriacal and hysterical distempers ... with the Author's Own Case at Large*. We note that the title relegated the more technical generic term 'Treatise' to a secondary status, perhaps to reinforce Cheyne's academic credentials as opposed to 'essay', and foregrounded the much catchier and inclusive name of the cluster of nervous diseases – the English Malady.

But what did this term, and the subtitle, mean? With the (uneven) displacement of humoral theory by hydraulic and mechanical conceptions of the body prompted by the discoveries of William Harvey and Isaac Newton, terms like the 'vapours' became more metaphorical than medically accurate, and were inserted into the constellation of 'nervous' disorders now thought of as relating to the functioning (or malfunctioning) of circulating fluids (like blood) or to ill-defined 'spirits' conveying messages to different parts of the body. Where bad diet and lifestyle in humoral theory resulted in vapours ascending to the brain because the spleen had failed to regulate the balance of the black bile, thus resulting in a clouded mind and mental diseases, mechanical-hydraulic explanations substituted blocked pipes and channels, the putrid products of which would equally result in mental illness as well as physical. Much depended on where the blockage was, and what kind of things were causing it. Cheyne's message, simply put, was to avoid blockages by living a healthy lifestyle, the cornerstone of which was a healthy 'milk and seed' diet.

Why the English Malady? This was part of the cleverness of Cheyne's manipulation of his own image and that of the genre aimed at patient self-help. This instruction manual was also an endorsement and flattery of the refined, polite and intelligent sufferer of these nervous diseases. The malady was English because the English were the most advanced of countries in matters of religion, politics and manners, but such a success brought with it problems, not least the responsibilities associated with a modern, enlightened Englishness:

> The moisture of the Air, the variableness of the Weather (from our Situation amidst the Ocean), the Rankness and Fertility of Our Soil, the Richness and

> Heaviness of our Food, the Wealth and Abundance of our Inhabitants, (from the Universal trade), the Inactivity and Sedentary Occupations of the better Sort (among whom this evil mostly rages) and the Humour of Living in great, populous, and consequently, unhealthy Towns, have brought forth a Class and set of Distempers, with Atrocious and frightful Symptoms scarce known to our Ancestors, and never rising to such fatal Heights, nor afflicting such Numbers in any other known Nation. These Nervous Disorders being computed to make almost one third of the Complaints of the People of Condition in England (*EM*, p. i)

The civilized lifestyle of Cheyne's patients, be they of the aristocracy or from lower down the social ranks (but not too low), was making them ill: Britain was too successful. This illness, however, was the price to pay for that high-living lifestyle. Cheyne could provide the cure, but cure required a certain resistance to that lifestyle, and to an extent the lifestyle of the upper and middling orders was inevitable and only to be mitigated, rather than removed, in some idealistic return to primitive living *à la* Rousseau.

Cheyne also presented the English Malady as a disease cluster that did not stretch to insanity: a different thing altogether according to his distinctions. He confessed to his friend and patient Samuel Richardson that he had edited his own brush with madness out of the 'Case of the Author' in *The English Malady*, but 'for the Sake of my Profession and Business lest Patients ever after should have concluded me really Mad, which I was but a little Way from being, only my Senses and Sensibility were rather too acute and on the Stretch'.[23] Here Cheyne's personal mythology required misinformation – in making this separation between refined suffering and madness crystal clear in the public forum at least, Cheyne legitimized the illness for his intended audience and made it positively fashionable. The nerves became fashionable also because the physiological explanation had a social hierarchy built into it: 'The Works of the Imagination and Memory, of Study, Thinking, and Reflecting, from whatever source the Principle on which they depend springs, must necessarily require bodily Organs. Some have their Organs finer, quicker, more agile and sensible, and perhaps more numerous than others'.[24] It is no surprise to find that 'Some' were the upper orders, and that they had finer nerves, a finer accompanying sensibility, and therefore were superior to the lower orders, or at least inferior only in their lack of robustness for dealing with manual, mechanical tasks that did not require their direct involvement in any case. There were different sorts of 'thinkers': 'those who are quick prompt and passionate; are all of weak Nerves; have a Degree of Sensibility; are Quick Thinkers, feel Pleasure and pain the more readily and are of the most lively Imagination' (*EM*, p. 105). 'Slow Thinkers' and 'No Thinkers' (p. 182) were the lower orders, and such orders were decreed by God. Cheyne concluded that:

> There are as many and as different Degrees of Sensibility or of Feeling as Degrees of Intelligence and Perception in human Creatures; and the Principle of both may perhaps be one and the same. One shall suffer more from the Prick of a Pin, or Needle, from their extreme Sensibility, than others from being run thro' the Body; and the first sort seem to be the Class of these Quick Thinkers I have formerly mentioned; and as none have it in their Option to choose for themselves their own particular Frame of Mind, nor Constitution of body; so none can choose his own Degree of Sensibility. That is given him by the author of his Nature, and is already determined, and both are various as the Faces and Forms of mankind are (*EM*, pp. 366–367).

The labourer in the field was not suffering from 'extreme Sensibility', and nor was he a 'Quick Thinker'. His rougher nerves were suited to his environment and occupation, as ordained by God.

The same went for women of the lower orders, but the question of gender was an important one. The new kind of man emerging from this rearranged physiological class order (albeit justifying largely existing notions of class but with enhanced room for the middling sort) could be seen as effeminate if wrongly framed. 'Pillo-Tisanus' invoked a Scriblerian metaphor later to be used by Pope in his attack on Lord Hervey ('Amphibious thing!') in his *Epistle to Dr Arbuthnot* when he accused Cheyne of being of 'that species of Physicians call'd Men Midwives; a sort of amphibious Animals ... or, more properly speaking ... Hermaphrodites of Physick; at least 'till arrived to those years, when they commence Old Women'.[25] Women were seen as possessing super-thin nerves and a sensibility even greater than the men, and were certainly an audience for Cheyne's flattering portrait of nervous disorders, however painful it might be to suffer them. The very language used around sensibility in the *English Malady* was feminized, as Roy Porter has argued.[26]

It was a fine line between a man of feeling and a woman of feeling, so Cheyne's trick partly lay in deploying the notion of the man of feeling as a man of genius: there was already a tradition of melancholy being associated with special talents, but now Cheyne overlaid it with the new vocabulary of the nerves and sensibility. The refined nervous system necessary for experiencing heightened sympathy and emotion was also needed for superior intelligence, that of the 'Quick thinkers' (in the 'Case of the Author', pp. 339–340, Cheyne identifies himself as one such!). Cheyne had explored this idea in his *Essay of Health*, including in his assessments of the literati with whom he mingled socially as well as treated. Poets were a perfect example of the connection of the nerves to literary creativity:

> Those who have a very springy, lively, and elastic Fibres have the quickest Sensations, a weaker Impulse producing a stronger Sensation in them. These generally excel in the Animal Faculty of Imagination. Hence the Poet, – *Genus*

irritable Vatum. And therefore, your Men of Imagination are generally given to sensual Pleasure, because the Objects of the Sense yield them a more delicate Touch, and a livelier Sensation than they do others. (*EH*, p. 144–145)

Cheyne, as we know from his correspondence, considered his Hypped friend and patient Samuel Richardson, novelist and publisher, to be another example of a man of superior sensibility and talents afflicted with hypochondria, which at this time was a word not burdened with the meaning and stigma it has now. Hypochondria stemmed from the area of the body of the same name in the upper lateral region of the abdomen, and was not yet regarded as false suffering. This was not to say that suspicions were not raised about the fashionability and fakery associated with nervous conditions, but that hypochondria held no special distinction above, for example, the cognate conditions of the vapours or the spleen. It is crucial to note that superior sensibility was not reserved for the aristocracy, but could also be a gift from God to the industrious middling sort, a group that included many of the literati (such as Richardson and Alexander Pope), and women from that segment of society as well. Sensibility involved a certain amount of class accommodation, and that worked for Cheyne himself (a mere medic) as well as his readers and patients.

One subtlety of this rank-based concept of nerves was its power to move outside the aristocracy and into the middling orders, such that those of lower birth could access it, not least because it was ordained by God. Samuel Johnson warned his friend, biographer and sufferer of the 'black dog', James Boswell, of the dangers of such misinformation:

> you are always complaining of your own melancholy, and I conclude from those complaints that you are fond of it. No man talks of that which he is desirous to conceal, and every man desires to conceal that of which he is ashamed. Do not pretend to deny it ... make it an invariable and obligatory law to yourself, never to mention your own mental diseases.[27]

Although Johnson squashed his friend's enjoyment of his condition, enabled and encouraged by Cheyne's writings, nevertheless he himself was a beneficiary of this myth of fashionable melancholy – there is no more famous depressive genius in the century than Johnson himself, as immortalised especially in Boswell's biography.[28]

So – Cheyne had put several elements of an attractive package in place for his readers, including his charismatic style, and then combined them with his pièce de résistance, the 'Case of the Author'. 'Case' was a pun on 'body' as well as the medical narrative, and Cheyne's use of his own nervous breakdown, which famously included him ballooning to 32 stone in weight, and subsequent recovery, attracted widespread attention. He pretended to apologise for this generic innovation, telling his 'polite and delicate readers' that his 'low tattle' and 'indecent and shocking egotism', of which he was 'heartily ashamed', were prompted by 'sneers of my Regimen, Case, and Sentiments' (*EM*, p. 362). It is clear, however, that this sop to 'Truth' spoke to a deeper truth in which he shared nervous suffering with his patients and readers, again more akin to the puritan biography, although here without the focus on matters spiritual. This appeal to fellow feeling in the most literal of senses was tremendously successful, not least because, according to David Shuttleton, as Cheyne portrayed them, one's nervous illnesses required 'an ever-vigilant, appealingly indulgent, self-analysis'.[29] As a genre, the medical case study provided the veneer of scientific veracity, but also a human narrative that, in Cheyne's instance, could provide what we now call an 'overcoming narrative' of disability. In one sense, such narratives are a convenient mythology, but in another they provided medical information that could be tremendously helpful to a wider readership of fellow sufferers, however specious the rank-based nerve theory behind the 'Case of the Author'.[30]

Cheyne's account of his own case was both an intimate connection with his fellow valetudinarians, a personal connection through the print medium in a way that had been impossible before popular vernacular medical texts began to appear in force in the eighteenth century, but also a spectacular staging of his own body and mind in the most widely circulated and public of media at the time. Using his own burgeoning celebrity as a Bath and London society doctor, Cheyne upped the ante by publishing himself as a case study, one from which all his readers could learn by example. If Cheyne could cure himself via his ascetic regimen, then so could his reader.

Conclusion

In this chapter we have followed Cheyne's paradoxical progress as demythologiser of arcane medical obfuscation and yet self-mythologiser extraordinaire through from his early career as a budding medic, possibly heading towards academe with a narrow coterie audience of medics, to the high point of his popularity in Bath and London society and abroad, with the publication of the *English Malady* in 1733. A complex mix of factors contributed towards his largely successful self-mythology, including his writing in English rather than Latin, the expansion of the print market, the importance of genre and marketing, his ability as a literary stylist, the nerve medicine and concomitant culture of sensibility that underpinned the fashionability of the English Malady, the quasi-religious simplicity of the milk-and-seed diet set against a burgeoning consumer culture, and the crucial fact of his self-fashioning as both doctor and patient, scientist and fellow sufferer. One must also attribute this success partly to the paradoxically dialogic nature of self-fashioning – Cheyne's bookseller, for example, steering him towards more accessible generic titles, and even the sniping critics themselves, amplifying his reputation even as they sought to destroy it.

Finally, although there is a great deal more work to do on this topic with other writing doctors and health-related workers, Cheyne's self-mythologisation crucially enabled his readers and patients to do the same. If he could self-fashion as a person of feeling, of refined sensibility, intelligence and morality, so could they – male and female alike. The core mythology (and, we must observe, misinformation to modern eyes) of rank-based sensibility in the medical and intellectual senses was a game-changer both for Cheyne and his audience, including literary writers like his friend, publisher and fellow Hypo, Samuel Richardson. If Cheyne 'never wrote a Book in my Life but that I had a Fit of Illness after', as he states in the epigraph, this was, paradoxically, a sign of his talent and, by implication, that of his readers. His great achievement was to extend that very mythology of self-fashioning via sensibility to the other, to his literary audience, while at the same time providing medical information based on a healthy regimen of exercise and diet that, even today, seems eminently healthy in the round.

Notes

1 George Cheyne, *The Letters of George Cheyne to Samuel Richardson*, ed. and published by Charles F. Mullett (Columbia, MO: University of Missouri Press, 1942), letter XLIII, p. 69.
2 Katherine Richards, 'Medical Celebrity in Eighteenth-Century Britain', PhD thesis, West Virginia University (2018), p. 39.
3 Although wider in the sense that the European elite communicated in Latin – Cheyne's popular *Essay of Health*, for example, was translated into Latin by the Revd. John Robertson MD as *Tractatus de Infirmorum Sanitate Tuenda Vitaque Producenda*, 1725. For more on the shift from English to Latin, see Audrey Eccles, 'The Reading Public, The Medical Profession, and the use of English for Medical Books in the 16th and 17th Centuries', *Neuphilologische Mitteilungen* 75:1 (1974): 143–156; K. F. Russell, 'A Check List of Medical Books Published in English before 1600', *Bulletin of the History of Medicine* 21 (1947): 922–958.
4 Robert Hale, letter to Dr. Charlett, Bodleian Library, Oxford, Ballard MSS 24, f.149.
5 George Cheyne, *An Essay of Health and Long Life* (London: printed for George Strahan and J. Leake, Bath, 1724), p. 31. From this point references to this text will appear in text abbreviated in parentheses as follows '(*EH*, p. xxx)'.

6 *EH*. See Mervyn Susser and Zena Stein, 'Germ Theory, Infection, and Bacteriology', in *Eras in Epidemiology: The Evolution of Ideas* (Oxford: Oxford University Press, 2009), pp. 107–122, DOI:10.1093/acprof:oso/97801 95300666.003.0010.
7 See John Armstrong's *'The Art of Preserving Health': Eighteenth-Century Sensibility in Practice*, ed. Adam Budd (Farnham: Ashgate, 2011).
8 This is John Martyn, although David Shuttleton wonders tentatively whether it is Henry Fielding. See David Shuttleton, '"My Own Crazy Carcase": The Life and Works of Dr George Cheyne (1672–1743)', PhD thesis, University of Edinburgh (1993), p. 137. For Martyn see Bertrand A. Goldgar, 'Pope and the *Grub-Street Journal*', *Modern Philology*, 74:4 (1977): 366–380 (at 373).
9 Ian Hacking, 'Kinds of People: Moving Targets: British Academy Lecture', in P. J. Marshall (ed.), *Proceedings of the British Academy*, Volume 151: *2006 Lectures (1)* (Oxford: British Academy, 2007), pp. 285–318, at p. 299.
10 Stuart Tave, *The Amiable Humorist: A Study in the Comic Theory and Criticism of the Early Eighteenth and Early Nineteenth Centuries* (Chicago, IL: University of Chicago Press, 1960), p. 155.
11 Joseph Spence, *Observations, Anecdotes and Characters of Books and Men Collected from Conversation*, ed. James M. Osborn, 2 vols (Oxford: Oxford University Press, 1966), vol. 1, p. 350.
12 Sir William Temple, *Miscellanea*, 3 vols (1680, 1692 and 1702), vol. 3, p. 289f.
13 Cheyne, *Essay of Health*, NLS, Acc. 9345.
14 Pope to Hugh Bethel, 12 July (1724?), *The Correspondence of Alexander Pope*, ed. George Sherburn, 5 vols (Oxford: Clarendon, 1956), vol. 2, p. 178.
15 Shuttleton, 'My Own Crazy Carcase', p. 136; George Rousseau, 'Science Books and their Readers', in Isabel Rivers (ed.), *Books and their Readers in the Eighteenth-Century* (Leicester: Leicester University Press, 1982), pp. 197–255, at p. 214. See Ginnie Smith, '"Prescribing the Rules of Health": Self Help and Advice in the Late Eighteenth Century', in Roy Porter (ed.), *Patients and Practitioners: Lay Perceptions of Medicine in Pre-Industrial Society* (Cambridge: Cambridge University Press, 1985), pp. 249–282.
16 Rousseau, 'Science Books and their Readers', p. 214; David Shuttleton, '"Pamela's Library": Samuel Richardson and Dr. Cheyne's "Universal Cure"', *Eighteenth-Century Life* 23:1 (1999): 60–80.
17 Earl of Ilchester, *Lord Hervey and his Friends: 1726–38* (London: Murray, 1950), pp. 151–152.
18 George Lyttelton, Letter to Pope December 1734, *Correspondence of Alexander Pope*, vol. 3, p. 47.
19 Hester Lynch Thrale, *Thraliana; The Diary of [...] Mrs Piozzi*, ed. K. C. Balderston, 2 vols (Oxford: Clarendon, 1942), vol. 2, p. 778.
20 George Cheyne (1733), *The English Malady: or. a Treatise of Nervous Diseases of all Kinds: as Spleen, Vapours, Lowness of Spirits, Hypochondriacal and Hysterical Distempers [...] with the Author's Own Case at Large*, ed. Roy Porter (London: Routledge, 1991).

21 See Roger Smith, *The Fontana History of the Human Sciences* (London: Fontana, 1997), p. 121.
22 Cheyne also saw the need to impress his professional competence upon his patients, prospective or actual, as Steven Shapin has pointed out in his 'Trusting George Cheyne: Scientific Expertise, Common Sense, and Moral Authority in Early Eighteenth-Century Dietetic Medicine', *Bulletin of the History of Medicine* 77:2 (2003): 263–297, doi:10.1353/bhm.2003.0091. For more on the dual perspective Cheyne inculcated of his identity as both patient and physician, see Paul W. Child, '"The Case of the Author": George Cheyne's Providential Medical Autobiography', *AnaChronisT* 11 (2005): 70–84.
23 Charles F. Mullett (ed.), *The Letters of Dr George Cheyne to Samuel Richardson (1733–1743)* (Columbia, MO: University of Missouri Studies, 1943), xviii, letter LXI, from Bath, 22 May 1742, p. 94.
24 Cheyne, *English Malady*, p. 53.
25 *An Epistle to G—ge Ch—ne M.D. F.R.S. upon his Essay of Health* (J. Roberts, 1725?).
26 Roy Porter (ed.), 'Introduction', in Cheyne, *English Malady*, p. xli; see also Anita Guerrini, *Obesity and Depression in the Enlightenment: The Life and Times of George Cheyne* (Norman, OK: University of Oklahoma Press, 2000), p. 147.
27 James Boswell (1799), *The Life of Samuel Johnson, LL.D*, 4 vols, 3rd edn (London: Charles Dilly), vol. 3, p. 450.
28 See Allan Ingram, *Boswell's Creative Gloom* (London: Macmillan, 1982).
29 Shuttleton, 'My Own Crazy Carcase', p. 178.
30 See D. Christopher Gabbard, '"The Compleat, Common Form": Disability and the Literature of the British Enlightenment', in Clark Lawlor and Andrew Mangham (eds), *Literature and Medicine: The Eighteenth Century* (Cambridge: Cambridge University Press, 2021), pp. 219–241.

4

Studying in solitude: demythologising the masculine medical monopoly with Jane Barker's Galesia and Tobias Smollett's Sagely

Laurence Sullivan

> Here the good and charitable Ladies have Directions given them how to cure Diseases of most Kinds, without much more Expence than their Diet will be of: They are here instructed in what they are generally found to be delighted with, I mean, in being serviceable to their Neighbours: Their Reputation will grow to equal that of a Physician, and, wherever they have the Opportunity given them, will act their Part as well.[1]

After penning a series of medical treatises, the physician Edward Strother (1675–1737) published his first book of popular medicine aimed at a readership of women, particularly those involved in household management. *The Family Companion of Health* (1729) combines elements of both regimen and medical receipt book, genres which had been gaining popularity since the early sixteenth century, to educate its reader on preserving the health of the human body. The volume appears to have enjoyed moderate success, running through three editions – including one published posthumously in 1750 – perhaps due in part to the tantalising promise that, on digesting the information contained within, its readers' medical practice and reputation would rival that of a physician.

Certainly the text touches on medical subjects encompassed within a university education – an option unavailable to women at the time – covering the mechanics of the human body, the circulatory system and other elements of anatomy. Yet despite the lofty promise of his preface, Strother suggests that his primary purpose for writing the book is so that women might 'give Relief to their Menials, without the Assistance of an Apothecary or Physician', thereby limiting their potential patients to domestic servants already within their employment.[2] Offering women the opportunity to elevate their practice to the level of a professional physician, but only within the strict confines of the domestic sphere, speaks to a wider prejudice which had persisted from previous centuries.

Naturally, women who possessed knowledge of the human body and what medicines were effective for healing it could find their services in demand, but such logic also implies a familiarity with drugs which could just as easily do deliberate harm. Throughout the preceding two centuries this duality was laid bare and such thinking would entrench itself in rural parts of Great Britain, leading John M. Riddle to note the extent to which women healers who operated outside the domestic sphere could fall victim to medical misinformation:

> 'Wise women,' sorceresses, midwives, and witches were separate categories in the sixteenth and seventeenth centuries, but people, peasants and officials alike, often conflated them as all made of the same cloth. Women who knew the herbs of healing were candidates for accusations of sorcery and witchcraft. Those who practiced midwifery were especially vulnerable because they knew the poisons that controlled fertility and could cause harm.[3]

Little effort was made to disentangle the terms which defined a woman healer's practice, or the source of their medical knowledge, enabling praise for their healing prowess to be conflated with fear at the realisation that those same skills could be put to nefarious use. Women healers within rural communities were left with few means to combat these enduring myths, as without external qualification to attest to their skill and in possession of knowledge often passed through successive generations – thereby lacking an impartial regulator to assess it – they were dependent on good reputation within their community as proof of ability. Vulnerable to malicious misinformation spread by word of mouth, women healers could only rely on success – or at least maintaining a reputation for success – in order to continue practising medicine. This pressure to maintain both their utility and good social relations within a community ensured that an inherent tension would exist between a woman healer's social standing and her skill. In order to unravel the extent to which these tensions persisted into the eighteenth century, and identify how they might be overcome, this chapter will examine two semi-autobiographical works from the first half of the century.

Jane Barker's *A Patch-Work Screen for the Ladies* (1723) is a novel woven together with poems reworked from the author's previous collection *Poetical Recreations* (1688). The story centres on Galesia, a young woman gifted in the medical sciences and with ambitions of being recognised for those abilities. Yet she is only able to achieve the professional status she desires – the very reputation Strother promises awaits his women readers – on paper, passing off her prescriptions as the work of a male physician. Realising the limiting nature that adopting a false identity would pose for achieving wider acclaim, Galesia – and by extension, Barker – instead seeks to fashion a professional identity which exists beyond the page and embraces the qualities traditionally associated with her gender. Fighting in their own field those physicians who disdained her, and challenging the prejudices of would-be patients bemused by her unusual level of knowledge, Galesia carves out a space for herself in defiance of the myths that surrounded women in medicine.

Tobias Smollett's eponymous hero in *The Adventures of Roderick Random* (1748) experiences first-hand the skill of a self-taught but shunned healer, when he is entrusted to the care of a reputed witch. Seen through the eyes of a skilled ship surgeon – a background Random shares with his author – Smollett's narrative reveals to the reader how a woman healer's reputation does not necessarily reflect reality. Of course, as O. M. Brack reminds us, we must be cautious about identifying any of Smollett's characters too closely with the author himself, pointing to 'the most extreme cases of "inverted autobiography" [which] have centred on the identification of Roderick Random with the youthful Smollett and Matthew Bramble with the elder'.[4] Nonetheless, even in a letter where Smollett dismisses the connection between himself and Random – dated 8 May 1763 to a Richard Smith – the author still openly acknowledges and accepts a few key similarities:

> The only Similitude between the Circumstances of my own Fortune and those I have attributed to Roderick Random consists of my being born of a reputable Family in Scotland, in my being bred a Surgeon, and having served as a Surgeon's mate on board a man of war during the Expedition to Cathagene.[5]

The latter two of these connections, where Smollett acknowledges his education and background as a surgeon as having informed the content of the novel and character of Random, are especially important when we consider how he chooses to represent medical practice of all kinds in the text, both positive and negative. Caring and compassionate, the 'witch's' healing abilities and humility stand in stark contrast to many of the other medical practitioners Random meets during his travels, calling into question the quality of professional qualifications and the reputational benefits they confer.

Read together, both texts demonstrate how a desire to pursue medical practice could push women socially to the peripheries of society, but that it was also this same space, perhaps paradoxically, which offered the most intellectual freedom. Thus able to study those areas of medicine considered previously socially taboo, the significance of their skills in preserving the health of their communities could eventually outweigh the anxiety caused by their failure to conform to societal expectation. At this pivotal point, the study of advanced medicine – and a desire to practise it beyond the boundaries of the domestic sphere – could transmute from a source of social anxiety and suspicion to become instead a socially lubricating medium.

A Patch-Work Screen for the Ladies

The opening scenes of Jane Barker's 1723 novel centre on its protagonist, Galesia, and her older brother's shared love of learning, with the former recounting the days spent studying medicine under the latter's tutelage at the family's country home. This initial instruction she received would have rivalled that of a university education, given her brother trained previously at Oxford, Paris and Leyden – three of the great centres of medical learning in western Europe.[6] Her studies are cut short, however, and her happiness along with them, around the age of twenty when her brother unexpectedly passes away, a fate which, as Jane Spencer points out, is linked closely with her author's own.[7]

Galesia's foundations are then shaken for a second time following the death of her father, when both she and her mother are chased by creditors and hounded by hostile neighbours, causing them to sell off their country estate and move to the unfamiliar city of London in order to escape the growing threat. Finding herself transplanted from the countryside and into the bustling capital, Galesia expresses the extent to which she feels like an outsider in this new environment:

> I lost my self and my Time; and what the World there calls Diversion, to me was Confusion. The Park, Plays, and Operas, were to me but as so much Time thrown away. I was a Stranger to every-body, and their Way of Living; and, I believe, my stiff Air and awkard [sic] Mien, made every-body wish to remain a Stranger to me.[8]

Galesia's otherness grows only more profound with each passing paragraph, but despite her acute feelings of loneliness and the emphasis on physical solitude apparent in Barker's similes, we know that Galesia actually shares this fate with her mother with whom she lives: 'my Mother and I remain'd at Quiet, we not thinking of any-body; nor any-body thinking of us: And thus we liv'd alone (at least in our Actions) in the midst of Multitudes'.[9] In the last of these descriptions we are provided with a key detail, as though it is clear that wider society does not spare a thought for either Galesia or her mother, nor does either woman make a conscious effort to think about anyone but themselves. Their isolation, therefore, is self-imposed.

The apparent reason for this social inertia is that such isolation offers Galesia the opportunity to further her study of medicine, that process begun by her brother's tutoring when the two were younger. Paradoxically, however, it is this same robust knowledge of medicine – which has been allowed to progress precisely because of Galesia's social isolation – that enables her to find her place socially within the great, bustling city of London:

> At home, at our own Lodging, there was as little Quiet, between the Noise of the Street, our own House, with Lodgers, Visiters [sic], Messages, Howd'ye's, Billets, and a Thousand other Impertinencies; which, perhaps, the Beau World wou'd think Diversion, but to my dull Capacity were mere Confusion. Besides which, several People came to me for Advice in divers sorts of Maladies, and having tolerable good Luck, I began to be pretty much known.[10]

The passage opens with a crowded list that evokes noise and chaos, capturing succinctly the sensory overload such stimuli offer to someone wholly unused to the sheer pace of the city. In stark contrast, Barker's following sentence – with its focus on Galesia's newfound role as a provider of medical advice – is measured, calm and ordered. Through her knowledge of medical science Galesia has found a way to make sense of the city; she has stumbled upon purpose and meaning within a community she previously found both baffling and forbidding. Yet still she sets her sights higher.

Medicine has not only provided Galesia with the confidence and sense of self-worth necessary to integrate herself into a society she initially found overwhelming; it also enables her to challenge the gendered status quo in her willingness to consider her own medical practice on a level with male physicians. Yet despite this growing self-confidence, Galesia still views her blossoming reputation as being enabled by 'tolerable good luck', with the implication that she believes, modestly, that her skill alone would have failed without fortune's favour. This ambivalent relationship with her own success begins to shift into a more positive mode as her medical skills come to be recognised by professional apothecaries:

> I was got to such a Pitch of helping the Sick, that I wrote my *Bills* in *Latin*, with the same manner of *Cyphers* and *Directions* as Doctors do; which Bills and Recipes the Apothecaries fil'd amongst those of the Doctors.[11]

Galesia imitates the professional discourse of practising physicians and is wholly successful in the endeavour, effectively challenging them in their own field but in a covert fashion. She is writing in 'ciphers', a complicated form of abbreviated Latin used between physicians and apothecaries to facilitate the fulfilment of prescriptions. This accomplishment demonstrates that she has a working knowledge of subject-specific Latin, the materia medica and, by extension, the power of individual medications and how they function in combination. Although it is unclear if the apothecaries who file her bills are aware of their true source or not, both Galesia and her patients benefit from this unusual form of misinformation. Her bills have been interpreted as the work of a true professional and treated in the same manner as any male physician, with the result that her patients are provided with quality healthcare and the means to access their prescriptions. As multiple apothecaries have responded to her work in the same fashion, these individual acts of misinformation coalesce into a wider mythology, with the implication that repeated (mis)filings have effectively enabled Galesia to become – that most fabled of professionals – a female physician. This sentiment is expressed explicitly in 'On the Apothecaries Filing My Receipts Amongst the Doctors', one of the many poems that punctuate Barker's narrative but one which first appeared in her collection *Poetical Recreations* (1688). Appearing in this new context, the poem's theme shifts its focus subtly from its author and onto her character, associating the voice with Galesia directly. Thus able to show cause and effect holistically in the narrative through its novelistic format, Barker develops something of a vicarious relationship with Galesia as we see the accomplishments chronicled in the original poem, previously confined only to the internal logic of that text, begin to manifest in the wider context of the story here as we witness first-hand Galesia's success both before and after the poem's insertion:

> I hope I shan't be blam'd, if I am proud
> To be admitted in this learned Croud.[12]

The couplet captures how Galesia's initial ambivalence towards her own success, once tempered by her inclusion of the qualifying 'tolerable good luck', has now been displaced by pride. Certainly her bills sit alongside those of professional physicians, but if she has been accepted within 'this learned croud' in any greater sense, then she has seemingly only achieved this status in secret. In response to this limiting factor, she sets her sights on actively surpassing male practitioners, not by imitating them as she has done previously, but by capitalising on the very otherness that prevents her from being openly acknowledged as part of their community. As a core part of this process, Galesia credits her intrinsically feminine qualities – emblemised by her soft hands – as being in part responsible for overcoming a disease where the raw power of male physicians failed:

> As *Saul* 'mongst Prophets turn'd a Prophet too.
> The *Sturdy Gout*, which all Male-Power withstands,
> Is overcome by my soft Female Hands.
> Not Deb'rah, Judith, or Semiramis,
> Cou'd boast of Conquest half so great as this;
> More than they slew, I save, in this Disease.[13]

Like a surgical tool, the softness of the female hands implies finesse and delicacy, accompanied by a tender approach to the patient as opposed to the brute force offered by male physicians – their inability to act with sensitivity being inextricably tied to their gender and therefore endemic to the sex. Yet the use of 'tender' here is not to imply 'tentative': the three historical figures Galesia – and by extension, Barker – lists were all women who 'acted decisively and forcefully' in a military context.[14] By offering a fresh perspective with the accompanying skills unique to what her gender can offer, Galesia is able to approach the figurative battlefield and apply the arsenal of materia medica in a novel way – routing gout through subtle strategy and not overwhelming firepower.

Despite Galesia's multiple instances of self-praise, Barker limits the reader's perspective of the narrative to just her recounting of the story, making us question her definition of success in 'slaying' gout and whether that necessarily equates to gaining acclaim for her accomplishment. Following the logic, Kathryn R. King problematises Galesia's point of view further, arguing that any success the healer might have had with her cure cannot – due to the limited nature of her narrative – rise above the levels of the self-congratulatory:

> Galesia's boast of the triumph of her 'soft female Hands' over 'all Male-Power' is, at best, a fantasy of female power ... If literary authority involves the ability to be seen and to be heard in the realm of public discourse, then Galesia's authority is strictly limited: it enacts 'before a Looking-glass'.[15]

There is certainly truth in this statement. The volume of Galesia's voice within public discourse – when viewed purely though terms of literary authority – is limited. Yet the actions that have formed the basis of that narrative, namely her treating patients and curing those afflicted with gout, will have had a direct effect on their perception of her as a healer – a word-of-mouth reputation which exists independently of her literary authority. Moreover, the process of self-fashioning is not tied intrinsically to the extent of a work's eventual readership: whether the end product is read by only one person or one hundred thousand, the conscious choices involved in an author representing themselves in a certain way remain constant. Of course, the success of self-fashioning is dependent on whether the wider public choose to accept the narrative as it is presented, which is in part informed by the number of people it reaches; but the impetus behind initially pushing that narrative remains unchanged. Galesia, and by extension, Barker, is forced to practise medicine behind the cover of an ambiguous identity which implicitly erases those feminine qualities she wishes to celebrate. Through the power of the written word, Galesia and her creator are able to commit to paper a powerful counter-narrative which demonstrates that women can prove just as effective as men – if not even more so – in the field of medicine, despite the many patriarchal barriers which prevent the possibility of open comparison. Irrespective of the work's eventual reach, the poetical praise Galesia offers her cure for the gout gives voice to a desire to write her own medical contributions, and those of women like her, back into history – the significance of which is only heightened when we consider the extent to which her experiences are entwined with those of her creator.

This palimpsest of authorial identity beneath Barker's writing is laid bare in Jane Spencer's seminal 1983 article. In this essay, Spencer argues that 'Jane Barker's work is especially pertinent to the question of the woman writer's self-definition because it appears to be largely autobiographical', and more recent studies are beginning to uncover the extent to which that statement holds true.[16] Blurring the lines between fictional and lived experience, Kathryn R. King has found evidence that Galesia's poetic praise for her medical conquest over gout may have had grounding in Barker's own life. King cites a 1685 advertisement for 'Dr. Barkers Famous Gout Plaister' which appears at the bottom of a list of recent publications printed by the publisher Benjamin Crayle, stating that the medicament is available for purchase from his establishment.[17] The connection is certainly tantalising given Crayle published Barker's *Poetical Recreations* in 1688, though potentially without her consent, and the two do appear to have known each other personally.[18] Moreover, the self-elevation that may appear in this advertisement from laywoman to the rank of doctor is consistent with Barker's pride at being 'admitted to this learned croud', especially as gout is conspicuously named as the specific ailment whose defeat at her hands 'makes me a fam'd Physician grow'. Moreover, Barker demonstrates through her poetry that she was in possession of the knowledge to create such a medicament for public consumption, for as Carol Shiner Wilson outlines:

> although it was common for seventeenth-century women to be knowledgeable about herbal medicine, it was rare for women to have the knowledge of current medical theories such as Harvey's circulation of blood. Barker incorporates her learned medical knowledge in 'Anatomy' and the apothecaries poem.[19]

Indeed, the poem 'Anatomy' references the anatomists Caspar Bartholin the Younger (1655–1738), Thomas Willis (1621–75) and William Harvey by name, before touching on their contributions to the science – and what Galesia, and therefore Barker, have gleaned from each of them – in verse.[20] Yet the connection between Galesia's knowledge of the science and its significant figures is made more explicit earlier in the text when she informs the reader that her brother:

> assisted me in *Anatomy* and *Simpling*, in which we took many a pleasing Walk, and gather'd many Patterns of different Plants, in order to make a large natural Herbal. I made such Progress in *Anatomy*, as to understand *Harvey's* Circulation of the Blood, and *Lower's* Motion of the Heart.[21]

Thus in possession of anatomical knowledge usually the reserve of men, Barker was well placed to find a treatment effective against gout, for as David Waldstreicher notes, though 'the causes of gout remained obscure in the late eighteenth century, yet the disease had been identified as somehow circulatory and related to diet'.[22] Being well acquainted with Harvey's circulation of the blood and armed with an extensive knowledge of the materia medica herself, Barker would certainly be able to create a novel remedy to counter the gout, one based on the cutting-edge science of the day. In the same way, Galesia uses her knowledge, which rivals that of medical men – as exemplified by the debates with her brother and their collaborative creation of the herbal – to forge a reputation for herself and support her household financially. As much benefit as this knowledge has brought her, it required Galesia to initially resist pressures to conform to social expectation – had she not pushed past these pressures to eventually flourish on her own terms, then she may have languished in the shadowy spaces between social strata:

> My Time and Thoughts were taken up in *Harvey*, *Willis*, and such-like Authors, which my Brother help'd me to understand and relish, which otherwise might have seemed harsh or insipid: And these serv'd to make me unfit Company for every body; for the Unlearned fear'd, and the Learn'd scorn'd my Conversation; at least, I fancy'd so: A Learned Woman, being at best but like a Forc'd-Plant, that never has its due or proper Relish, but is wither'd by the first Blast that Envy or Tribulation blows over her Endeavours. Whereas every Thing, in its proper Place and Season, is graceful, beneficial, and pleasant.[23]

Galesia perceives that her social isolation is initially compounded by her extensive medical knowledge, finding herself in a liminal space where the learned seem to treat her with scorn or outright envy, while the unlearned fear either their own ignorance being exposed, or her familiarity with the human body being used for nefarious purposes. Yet the former camp's apparent scorn is ineffectual, as it does not prevent Galesia curing a disease they collectively could not, while the latter group's fear is understandable but misplaced, born of the socially abnormal nature of a woman being in possession of such specialised medical knowledge, usually the reserve of university-educated men. Although Galesia is ultimately unable to win over the medical men who simply envy her success, and who benefit from ensuring the public remain misinformed about a woman's potential to practise medicine successfully, she is still able to find her 'Place and Season' without their approval by putting her theoretical knowledge into tangible practice and using it to help the people around her. In this way, her knowledge is no longer confined to the medical abstractions of bookish theory – given voice only through impotent academic debate with her brother; instead, she uses it to heal members of her community, the material benefits of which they can observe, admire and applaud. Fear and consternation on the part of her peers is then displaced by approbation and appreciation for her services, and so the intellectual autonomy that her self-imposed isolation provided proves to be the catalyst for her social integration. It is only by standing out and against the social status quo that Galesia is able truly to fit in.

In effect, Galesia has gained autonomy through her mastery of the medical arts, able as she is to support her household financially from the profits of her work. We learn that such an accomplishment is only possible because she has shunned the usual path to stability for women of the eighteenth century – the state of matrimony – when the infidelity of a failed love interest proves to be the catalyst for her cultivating a love of learning:

> False *Strephon* too, I almost now cou'd bless,
> Whose Crimes conduc'd to this my Happiness.
> Had he been true, I'd have liv'd in *sottish Ease*,
> Ne'er study'd ought, but how to *love* and *please*;
> No other *Flame*, my *Virgin Breast* had fir'd,
> But *Love* and *Life* together had *expir'd*.[24]

Had her lover proved constant, she would have lived a life of idleness 'in sottish ease'; instead, his rejection has created the best of all possible worlds, one in which she is able to indulge her passion for studying medicine and, in so doing, reclaim her autonomy. This twenty-line interlude then concludes with a couplet that encapsulates a major theme of the poem: that such relationships serve to distract and dull the industrious mind into contemplating instead only 'how to *love* and *please*'. Women, in short, are prevented from reaching their full potential by the bonds of matrimony, with romance standing as the ultimate distraction from a life of academic accomplishment.

> But I've digress'd too far; so must return,
> To make the *Medick-Art* my whole Concern.[25]

The above couplet physically separates the romantic sentiments from the surrounding ones celebrating medical achievement, figuratively preventing its unwelcome distractions from bleeding into the rest of the poem and literally drawing a line underneath it – just as Galesia has done in her own mind. This preferencing of an already unusual form of study for a woman – anatomical medicine – above finding a romantic partner only adds to Galesia's otherness, for as Jennifer Golightly outlines:

> because the family and the home were so important thematically to fiction in general and to women's fiction in particular, it is difficult to talk coherently about any other aspect of this writing without including a discussion of

the domestic sphere ... to be feminine was, in large measure, to be a wife, a mother, the manager of a household.²⁶

Galesia not only rejects these societal norms of femininity, but also does so in favour of pursuing areas of study outside the realms of what was considered appropriate for women at the time. Her discussion of the domestic sphere amounts to a one-line wholesale rejection of it, before returning to her true passion of medicine. Indeed, when her mother later revives the issue, invoking the spectre of living in an 'uncouth kind of *Solitude*' which her daughter 'too much delighted in', she then goes on to list the same defining features of femininity as those highlighted by Golightly:

> I should be glad, said she, you would avoid, by becoming a good Mistress of a Family; and imploy your Parts in being an obedient Wife, a discreet Governess of your Children and Servants; a friendly Assistant to your Neighbours, Friends, and Acquaintance: This being the Business for which you came into the World.²⁷

Galesia understands and accepts the existence of these societal norms, conceding to herself that 'These were Truths which Reason would not permit me to oppose; but my Reflections on *Bosvil's* Baseness, gave me a secret Disgust against Matrimony'.²⁸ Her study of medicine, and its necessary rejection of those very 'Truths' which would usually govern a woman's place in society, enables Galesia to forge a future for herself outside the scope of her mother's received wisdom, and the entrenched nature of those traditional gender roles which it represents. Instead of operating within the social status quo as a wife, mother, or devoting herself to the management of her household – the roles which both her mother and Golightly identify – Galesia carves out a space for herself as healer, chemist and chief earner for a household consisting solely of women. Moreover, Galesia does not sacrifice her femininity by not embracing the role of wife or mother, for she imbues her work with those qualities, which in turn enable her to provide for her household and so prove she can fulfil the last of Golightly's roles alongside her passion. Of course, Barker was not alone in using the written word to challenge the traditional roles imposed on women, as Elizabeth Kraft demonstrates when she writes that:

> for Aphra Behn, Delarivier Manley, and Eliza Haywood in particular the fundamental obstacle to female happiness was the institution of marriage. Writing at a time when thinkers of both sexes were examining anew all preconceived notions they had inherited from church and state, these women wrote about what they knew best from the position they inhabited in their own place and time.²⁹

The narrative that marriage presented a barrier to intellectual and creative development for women, a state – like that which Barker describes – of complacency and existing only for the comfort of their spouse, would be explored throughout the century. The fact that these women challenged the social status of marriage in an open arena – the literary marketplace – speaks to a growing confidence in the capacity for women to exist independently of a male partner and prove successful in their own right. However, unlike the other women writers listed, Barker subverts social convention from a unique angle by using her medical knowledge to challenge directly a profession dominated by men. Informed by her own medical background and through the voice of Galesia, Barker shows that women are not only able to carry out their medical practice as competently as their male counterparts, but by actively subverting the gender norm, they can also surpass them.

The Adventures of Roderick Random

In chapter thirty-seven of Smollett's first novel, Random and his fellow crewmates are forced to abandon ship just off the shore of Sussex. Angered by the constant mismanagement of the voyage that led to this situation, Random challenges the captain to a duel the moment they reach dry land, but is then betrayed by the rest of the crew and bludgeoned around the back of the head with the butt-end of a pistol. Robbed of his valuables and severely wounded, he is able to crawl into a barn and, after a brief respite, then makes his way to a nearby cottage to seek help. Unfortunately, rather than receiving the help he hoped for, Random is refused entrance before falling into an even worse state:

> About this time I fainted with the fatigue I had undergone, and afterwards understood that I was bandied from door to door through a whole village, no body having humanity enough to administer the least relief to me, until an old woman, who was suspected of witchcraft by the neighbourhood, hearing of my distress, received me into her house, and having dressed my wounds, brought me to myself with cordials of her own preparing.[30]

Before we meet this mysterious character who becomes Random's saviour, we are first introduced to her in chapter thirty-eight's summary, with Random informing the reader that he will be 'succoured by a reputed witch' by the chapter's conclusion.[31] Despite initially remaining nameless, it is the old woman's reputation for witchcraft which stands as the primary trait – both in the chapter summary and in the body of the story itself – and that which defines her. The reader is encouraged, along with Random himself, to make value judgements of her character based on the collective assessment of the village residents, who then quickly reveal themselves to be thoroughly uncharitable people. So endemic is the lack of mercy in this village that one of its primary denizens includes a parson who – failing to display an ounce of Christian charity – 'fell into a mighty passion, and threatened to excommunicate him who sent as well as those who brought me [Random], unless they would move me immediately to another place'.[32] Yet despite all the forgoing, it is only this one ostracised and undervalued member of the community who sees fit to dress Random's wounds and 'succour' him with medicinal cordials of her own preparation.

Random is clearly struck by the old woman's medical abilities, apparently finding no need to redress his wounds from this point onwards, and also openly admitting that her cordials 'brought him to himself' after such a traumatic head injury. Moreover, the old woman provides more than just first aid to Random as she continues to ensure his full recovery, leaving him to comment that: 'I was treated with great care and tenderness by this grave matron, who, after I had recovered some strength, desired to know the particulars of my last disaster'.[33] Smollett elects that Random should refer to the woman reverently as a 'grave matron', with the result that – based seemingly on the strength of her medical practice alone – Random's opinion of his host graduates from the purely descriptive 'old woman' to this more honorific title. Although we later learn that 'Betty' is the woman's given name, in the following chapter it is revealed that her surname is Sagely, providing further indication that Smollett intended her to be read as an archetypal wisewoman.[34] Yet as had been the case for centuries, myths surrounding the source of wisewomen's healing powers ensured that operating as one came with the inherent risk of being branded a witch.[35] Sagely is no exception, having already fallen victim to such misinformation, confiding in Random the status she currently holds among members of her own community:

> I must inform you of the character I bear among my neighbours—My conversation being different from that of the inhabitants of my village, my recluse way of life, my skill in curing distempers, which I acquired from books since I settled here, and lastly, my age, have made the common people look upon me as something preternatural, and I am actually this hour believed to be a witch.[36]

Sagely's confession is revealing in two key ways. First, we learn that she has acquired her knowledge 'from books', making her both an autodidact and thereby evidence for the efficacy of this alternative to a university-led medical education. Moreover, we are told that it is specifically her 'skill in curing distempers' which is the subject of suspicion among her community, not the source of that knowledge. Although apparently not a factor in the villagers' distrust, Smollett still has Sagely highlight to Random how she has gained her skills, suggesting this fact is intended to be important to her personally. Unlike much of Smollett's work, the statement cannot be read comically and lacks any satirical barb, as the success of Sagely's skill is made apparent to the reader through Random himself, providing an implicit endorsement regarding the potential for this form of medical education for the rural healer.

Second, Sagely points to her age as forming another major factor in her being perceived as a witch in the popular imagination. Like Tabitha Bramble of Smollett's *The Expedition of Humphry Clinker* (1771), Sagely's age and gender are tied intrinsically, though implicitly, to her being deemed socially undesirable within her community. On this point, Jolene Zigarovich observes that 'one of the mainstays of the eighteenth-century narrative plot is marriage, and often accompanying it is the theme that women seeking autonomy experience tragic ends'.[37] This is true on two accounts for Sagely, for the irony is that she once married, but the conditions surrounding her engagement caused her to be ostracised by her own family for marrying beneath her station in life:

> I received a letter from my father, importing, that since I had acted so undutifully and meanly as to marry a beggar, without his privity or consent, to the disgrace of his family, as well as the disappointment of his hopes, he renounced me to the miserable fate I had entailed upon myself, and charged me never to set foot within his doors again. – This rigid sentence was confirmed by my mother, who, in a postscript, gave me to understand that her sentiments were exactly conformable to those of my father, and that I might save myself the trouble of making any applications, for her resolutions were unalterable.[38]

Despite the unequivocal rejection from both her parents, Sagely lives happily together with her husband. After his untimely death, however, she briefly takes up residence with a close friend, but then also outlives them. After losing those closest to her, Sagely is spurred into choosing her 'recluse way of life' and indulging her interest in 'curing distempers', which she has taught herself through reading books. Significantly, the situation Random finds Sagely living in is a conscious choice on her part; she has chosen to take up residence on the outskirts of the village and has done nothing to dispel the rumours surrounding her practice of witchcraft. In fact, she knows the primary source of the rumours and the means to remedy the misinformation, but again elects not to take action:

> the parson of the parish, whose acquaintance I have not been at much pains to cultivate, taking umbrage at my supposed disrespect, has contributed not a little towards the confirmation of this opinion, by dropping certain hints to

my prejudice, among the vulgar, who are also very much scandalised at my entertaining this poor tabby cat with the collar about her neck, which was a favourite of my deceased companion.[39]

The Church, here personified by a hypocritical parson and his regressive congregation, acts as a stifling force on Sagely's intellectual curiosity. Blinkered in their beliefs and unwilling to countenance the benefits her knowledge might bring, the majority of the community instead seek to limit her influence, leaving Sagely with only Narcissa and her eccentric aunt as the sole source for cultured company. The parson perpetuates the myths about Sagely's use of malevolent magic that ensure she would not be welcomed back into society, and though she is aware that paying him necessary deference would ease her return to the fold, she elects not to as she views his flock as 'vulgar' and retrograde. Instead, she capitalises on the intellectual freedom that social exclusion can provide. By explicitly refusing to conform to social expectation, Sagely is able to spend her hours studying medicine and experimenting with cordials. In essence, Betty Sagely is complicit in the continuation of her own myth, preferring a life of seclusion over wider social acceptance. Selectively keeping company with the intellectual Narcissa and her family, and writing to Random throughout the rest of his adventures, she eventually rejects the opportunity to live with them both, citing a desire to instead continue living 'peacefully' in her 'solitary widowhood'.[40]

This lifestyle itself manifests as an ironic vicious circle: apparently at first forced upon Sagely by the suspicions of her community, then exacerbated by her study of medicine, which in turn was only possible because of the time and intellectual freedom afforded by her isolation. Smollett presents to the reader the untapped potential which exists within social outcasts – epitomised here by the sharp mind of an aged woman – providing medical care of such quality that even a professional ship surgeon makes repeated praise of her skill. Smollett was in possession of the medical knowledge necessary to show either a character performing correctly any number of health-related tasks, or to heighten their failure through comic deflation. Yet here the narrator himself is a qualified ship surgeon, able to assess the quality of the treatment he receives first-hand and so enabling the endorsement of Sagely's skill to carry increased significance. Random shows the reader that her autodidactic medical education has proved effective, and unlike the community which surrounds her who refuse to engage, he approaches her practice without any accompanying prejudice associated with her age or gender.

Of course, Sagely is not the only medical practitioner who appears alongside Random in the novel. There are a whole host of professional male practitioners who fall victim to Smollett's sharp satirical sting, in stark contrast to Sagely's treatment, as Wendy Moore outlines:

> Smollett ridiculed blundering physicians and lampooned the corrupt Company of Barber-Surgeons with an incisive eye for detail and a cutting wit. Smollett's eponymous hero quakes before a 'dozen grim faces' when he takes his oral examination at Barber-Surgeons Hall. He flounders desperately as one examiner asks how he would treat a man 'with his head shot off' and another inquires how he would help a patient with a 'plethoric habit'. As the examiners squabble over fine points of surgery and anatomy, Roderick escapes with his prized certificate.[41]

Although Smollett fills this scene with satirical barbs and the comic deflation of the barber-surgeons' supercilious self-image, within the world of the text they still stand as a legitimate medical authority – acting as the gatekeepers to Random being able to practise surgery professionally within the navy, despite their obvious ineptitude. Already in possession of surgical skills and a knowledge of pharmacy, Random must still pass this arbitrary exam in order to be conferred with a modicum of the panel's authority – eventually leading him to the low rank of surgeon's third mate aboard the *Thunder*.[42] With their focus on debating the minutiae of lofty medical theories and patently absurd clinical cases, the panel of barber-surgeons' impracticality stands in stark contrast to the straightforward speed, proficiency and medical efficacy with which both Random and the reputed 'witch' operate.

There is a disconnect in the story between low-ranking medics who operate in the field, such as the skilful Random and Mr Thompson, and those in positions of higher authority like Mr Mackshane, who simply dismisses ailing sailors as liars.[43] The myth of authority being connected intrinsically to competency is dispelled by Smollett, with genuine aptitude usually being the reserve of the most undervalued medics. Smollett has shown his reader first-hand the skill with which Random operates as a ship surgeon; he is not like some of his contemporaries who sit on the examination panel idly debating medical theory but never putting any of it into practice. By extension, Random's endorsement of Sagely's capabilities lends her legitimacy because both their curative skills are witnessed empirically by the reader, as opposed to being dependant on titles that merely project a – potentially unearned – sense of medical authority that stands in as shorthand proof of ability. Irrespective of gender, it is the healers who are most often overlooked in Smollett's stories that may, in fact, be the very people keeping society healthy and functional.

Conclusion

The eighteenth century was an age of anxiety when it came to the issue of medical authority and who was equipped to confer it. A hierarchy which differentiated between physicians, surgeons and apothecaries ensured that a practitioner's job title would continue to be associated with their level of skill in the public consciousness, assumptions which would lead to fierce interprofessional rivalry.[44] Yet the exceptional abilities exhibited by Galesia and Sagely – characters who represent women whose skills were easily able to rival those of practising male physicians – went entirely unfactored into that professional framework. Moreover, to reach this level of study both characters needed to live part of their lives in relative seclusion – with Galesia even rejecting the societal pressures of marriage – in order to elevate their practice to include areas like anatomy, themselves treated as taboo subjects for women. Yet despite their laudable skills, both characters still operate from within their homes, peddling near-professional medicine from within the social restrictions of a domestic environment. As Barker's poetry makes so achingly apparent, similar contributions by real women went largely unrecognised in their own time – and the issue has only compounded since.

Either unwilling to be, or simply no longer, supported by a male spouse, the medical knowledge and skills these characters possess provide them with a key function within their fictional communities – countering the risk of being perceived merely as a burden. Yet developing these skills in the first place required a genuine passion for studying the medical sciences, as opposed to being motivated by a potential to profit financially in the future, as without an objective qualification there would be no guarantee that their practice would ever be accepted. Unable to study at university or acquire a degree, women had no immediate access to the academic culture of medicine which had long emphasised theoretical knowledge. Ordinarily locked out from lofty academic debates, the kind exemplified by Smollett's ineffectual board of surgeons, women like Galesia and Sagely were left to focus on the practicalities of medicine and applying themselves where they were needed most.

Yet it remained in the interest of the patriarchal medical establishment to perpetuate the myths of women practitioners' inevitable incompetency, gatekeeping education and professional titles to suppress – if not crush outright – the potential competition. Women could only combat this misinformation by proving the efficacy of their practice on those who would afford them the opportunity. So although both Galesia and Sagely may be safely ignored for a time by their respective communities – in line with what the medical establishment would desire – sickness and disease remain two of life's certainties and there necessarily comes a point when their skills will be required and their service in demand. This is where medicine, with its core aim of ensuring the lasting health of its practitioners and their patients, provides a way for women who fail to conform to the status quo to prevent their own ostracisation. Personal sacrifices and risks would remain a constant for any woman wishing to take up the practice of medicine outside the walls of their own home during the eighteenth century, but those willing to devote their time to advanced study – in spite of the social stigma – could see themselves become a central part of their communities as a direct result of their dedication and in defiance of the myths which had endured from previous centuries.

Notes

1. Edward Strother, *The Family Companion for Health* (London: Fayram, 1729), n.p.
2. Ibid.
3. John M. Riddle, *Eve's Herbs: A History of Contraception and Abortion in the West* (Cambridge, MA: Harvard University Press, 1997), p. 137.
4. O.M. Brack, Jr, 'Smollett and the Authorship of "Memoirs of a Lady of Quality"', in O.M. Brack, Jr. (ed.), *Tobias Smollett, Scotland's First Novelist* (Newark, DE: University of Delaware Press, 2007), pp. 35–73, at p. 35.
5. Tobias Smollett, *The Letters of Tobias Smollett*, ed. Lewis M. Knapp (Oxford: Clarendon Press, 1970), p. 112.
6. Jane Barker, *A Patch-Work Screen for the Ladies* (London: Curll, 1723), p. 2.
7. Ibid., p. 27; Jane Spencer, 'Creating the Woman Writer: The Autobiographical Works of Jane Barker', *Tulsa Studies in Women's Literature* 2:2 (1983): 165–181 (at 166).
8. Barker, *Patch-Work Screen*, pp. 42–43.
9. Ibid., p. 50.
10. Ibid., p. 55.
11. Ibid., p. 56.
12. Ibid., p. 56.
13. Ibid., p. 57.
14. Carol Shiner Wilson (ed.), *The Galesia Trilogy and Selected Manuscript Poems of Jane Barker* (Oxford: Oxford University press, 1997), p. 117.
15. Kathryn R. King, 'Galesia, Jane Barker, and a Coming to Authorship', in Carol J. Singley and Susan Elizabeth Sweeney (eds), *Anxious Power: Reading, Writing, and Ambivalence in Narrative by Women* (New York: State University of New York Press, 1993), pp. 91–104, at p. 95.
16. Spencer, 'Creating the Woman Writer', p. 166.
17. Kathryn R. King, 'Jane Barker, *Poetical Recreations*, and the Sociable Text', *ELH* 61:3 (1994): 551–570 (at 569).
18. Ibid., pp. 557, 559.
19. Wilson, *Galesia Trilogy*, p. xxiv.

20 NB A longer, alternative version of this poem appeared previously in *Poetical Recreations* as 'A Farewell to POETRY, WITH A Long Digression on ANATOMY'.
21 Barker, *Patch-Work Screen*, p. 10.
22 David Waldstreicher, 'The Long Arm of Benjamin Franklin', in Katherine Ott, David Serlin and Stephen Mihm (eds), *Artificial Parts, Practical Lives: Modern Histories of Prosthetics* (New York: New York University Press, 2002), pp. 300–326, at p. 300.
23 Barker, *Patch-Work Screen*, p. 11.
24 Ibid., p. 57.
25 Ibid., p. 58.
26 Jennifer Golightly, *The Family, Marriage, and Radicalism in British Women's Novels of the 1790s: Public Affection and Private Affliction* (Lewisburg, PA: Bucknell University Press, 2012), p. 24.
27 Barker, *Patch-Work Screen*, pp. 79–80.
28 Ibid., p. 80.
29 Elizabeth Kraft, *Women Novelists and the Ethics of Desire, 1684–1814: In the Voice of Our Biblical Mothers* (Aldershot: Ashgate, 2008), p. 33.
30 Tobias Smollett, *The Adventures of Roderick Random*, 2 vols (London: J. Osborn, 1748), vol. 2, p. 11.
31 Ibid., vol. 2, p. iii.
32 Ibid., vol. 2, p. 11.
33 Ibid.
34 Ibid., vol. 2, pp. 13, 19.
35 Leigh Whaley, *Women and the Practice of Medical Care in Early Modern Europe, 1400–1800* (London: Palgrave MacMillan, 2011), p. 5.
36 Smollett, *Roderick Random*, vol. 2, p. 14.
37 Jolene Zigarovich, *Sex and Death in Eighteenth-Century Literature* (Abingdon: Routledge, 2013), p. 12.
38 Smollett, *Roderick Random*, vol. 2, pp. 12–13.
39 Ibid., vol. 2, pp. 14–15.
40 Ibid., vol. 2, p. 344.
41 Wendy Moore, 'The Adventures of Roderick Random', in *British Medical Journal*, 343:d5718 [online], updated 14 September 2011 [cited 27 September 2021], available at https://www.bmj.com/content/343/bmj.d5718, last accessed 19 October 2023.
42 Smollett, *Roderick Random*, vol. 1, pp. 42, 243.
43 Ibid., vol. 1, pp. 248–249.
44 Maureen McNeil, *Under the Banner of Science: Erasmus Darwin and his Age* (Manchester: Manchester University Press, 1987), p. 126.

5

'Take physic, Pomp': imagining dog doctors in eighteenth-century Britain

Stephanie Howard-Smith

> Now round his grave, ye Mastiffs, scowl,
> And let the staunchest Blood-hound howl;
> And Oh! thou faithful Spaniel, tear
> The weeds that grow his tomb-stone near
> …
> Drive from the spot each puppy swift,
> Who here presumes a leg to lift;
> For here – Oh! let your growls arise –
> Your friend, your great Physician lies!

So concludes William Meyler's 1792 epitaph on the 'Celebrated Canine Doctor' of Bath, James Whittick.[1] The dog doctor was in some ways a new actor in the eighteenth-century medical marketplace, and his novel specialism provided easy fodder for comic writers. Behind such jokes, however, the dog doctor's presence in literature demonstrates a sincere interest in how owners saw fit to deal with their sick pets, as well as a greater societal unease with the place of companion animals in elite British society. Unlike Whittick (as described in the poem) and his living peers, the fictional dog doctor generally only had a single set of human/canine clients: wealthy women and their little companion dogs. Over the last two hundred years, the eighteenth-century fantasy of the wealthy woman's dog doctor (presented at best as an obsequious parasite and at worst a conman) has given way to a fresh myth – that dogs received no specialist healthcare until the Victorian, Edwardian or even post-war periods.

The dog doctor's limited archival presence means that any study of the dog doctor's practice must contend with his representation in Georgian literature. This is partly because the activities of fictional dog doctors offer some indication of their services, clients and occupational backgrounds, which were rarely recorded elsewhere. Far more importantly, however, it is because the dog doctor was inextricable from his representation in literature, in which he was almost without exception presented as a quack out to exploit what Laura Brown terms the 'immoderate love' of female owners.[2]

Dog doctors in eighteenth-century Britain

This chapter takes as its focus the construction of the dog doctor in eighteenth-century British culture, beginning by situating the dog doctor's canine patients in their social and cultural contexts. Through considering some of the ways the dog doctor insinuated himself in eighteenth-century culture, while exploring his appearances in lapdog satires of the late eighteenth century, I argue that he inevitably appears as an accessory in the act of challenging established hierarchies of both species and sex.

Workers, companions and commodities: eighteenth-century dogs and the birth of the canine service economy

The current consensus on chronologies of veterinary history seems often to be based on a misunderstanding of the role dogs played in eighteenth-century society. Animal health scholar Joanna Swabe claims that 'historically speaking, the diseases and afflictions of dogs and cats received very limited veterinary attention' because of their limited worth to humans:

> In centuries past, dogs and cats simply did not warrant the therapeutic attentions of medical science; whilst useful creatures – for protection, pest control and companionship – they were essentially of little economic value and easily replaceable.[3]

Likewise, in his study of the eighteenth-century farrier, Michael MacKay says of veterinary care for companion species, that while 'dogs and cats caught the eye of sentimentalists, they were far less valuable and required much less care than the horse'.[4] However, the dog doctor's skill and expertise were in demand from a range of dog owners and guardians, not only 'sentimentalists'. Such statements fail to account for the importance of the dog as a source of labour and as an object of affection in eighteenth-century Britain. Both urban and rural economies relied on canine labour in the form of home and business security, shepherding and vermin control. Dogs were also essential in many sports and pastimes across the social spectrum, from dog fighting to patrician fox hunting, shooting and hare coursing. However, dogs also had value beyond their skills in the yard, farm or field. Sentimentality was itself a powerful emotional register. It was crucial to both the popularity and the popular perception of dog ownership in the eighteenth century – and therefore to the dog doctor's practice and its representation in literary culture.

Although people have kept dogs as companions for thousands of years, historians of human–animal relations identify the eighteenth century as the point at which pet keeping first became a 'widespread phenomenon' in Britain. Ingrid Tague argues that the period saw 'growing acceptance of pet keeping' as a form of leisure, alongside an increased emphasis on practicing kindness to animals. Yet, as Tague also notes, pet ownership also attracted a great deal of criticism, much of it concentrated on companion dogs in general and lapdogs in particular. Although almost always presented as a feminine phenomenon, men owned lapdogs too, and male lapdog owners were often charged with effeminacy.[5] The material comfort in which some dogs lived – especially when compared to humans – was the focus of much of this criticism. Although only the very luckiest animals might have their own specially made dog bed, the dogs of Britain's elite had access to their own cushions, luxury leather collars, bowls, clothes and a relatively rich diet. Dog ownership was slowly creating its own material culture; again, while keen hunters spent considerable amounts of money on building kennels and supporting their packs and the men who cared for them, writers and artists tended to target the material comforts with which women provided their lapdogs.[6] To some, the dog doctor was yet another indication of the privileges enjoyed by companion dogs – privileges not afforded to all people – and as a result, a cultural history of the dog doctor is inseparable from that of the Georgian lapdog.

Defining the dog doctor

It is obvious that much of the eighteenth-century literature featuring the ministrations of dog doctors – which was often satirical in intent – was not intended to accurately represent their working practices. Almost all writing about the dog doctor has him summoned to heal a companion animal by its female owner. Such companion dogs could only represent a relatively small proportion of dogs in the eighteenth century, yet dog doctors were employed by a wide range of people living in Georgian and Victorian Britain to minister to the health of a similarly wide range of dogs.[7] Stewards on country estates would be expected to discuss the dog doctor's diagnosis of a sickly spaniel or hunting hound in correspondence with their master.[8] Crucially, the dog doctor's services included one of the few practices believed to protect against canine madness. Until the early nineteenth century, owners of both 'genteel' dogs and common curs would have their dogs 'wormed' – a preventative operation in which the frenulum of the tongue is removed. Worming was reputed to make the animal resistant to contracting (and therefore, transmitting) canine madness, the condition that could present as hydrophobia in humans, now understood as *rabies lyssavirus*.[9] Dog doctoring could be serious business.

This is not to say that dog doctors did not treat the beloved companions of female pet owners. Although writers (of both fiction and non-fiction) generally presented them as untrustworthy conmen, as in George Coleraine Hanger's 1814 recollections of the 'Queen's dog physician', who is paid generously for providing a non-service and 'goes away contented, laughing in his sleeve at her ladyship', letters and diaries by canine caregivers provide a counterpoint to the stereotype.[10] Mary Coke's journals, for instance, record her reliance on the authority of the local dog doctor, and in her correspondence Hester Piozzi likewise praised the 'great deal of good' the medicines prescribed by Streatham dog doctor William Shirley did to her 'poor little Flo'.[11] Indeed, some dog doctors cannily tailored their services to the demands of wealthy female dog owners. In late-eighteenth century London, specialist canine businesses effectively operated as a one-stop shop for dog owners (much like the French *tondeurs de chien*, who clipped fur and performed operations). Richard Endersby sold dogs from his shop on Oxford Street, but the adverts he placed in newspapers note that dogs were 'bled, physick'd and clipt' there too.[12] Perhaps this explains the immaculately groomed lapdog atop a cushion on the trade cards advertising the business of late eighteenth-century London's celebrity dog doctor, John Norborn (Figure 5.1). Although Norborn treated men's sporting dogs too, he advertised his business in a manner which confirmed the cultural stereotype that

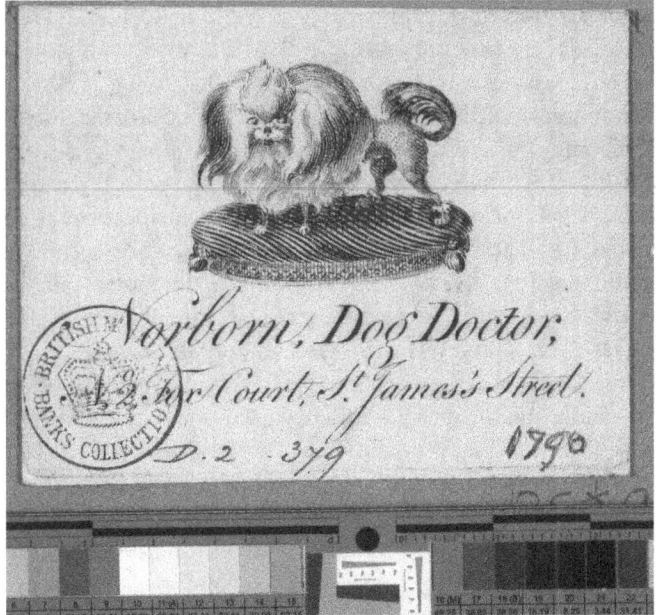

Figure 5.1 Trade card of John Norborn (*c.*1790), British Museum (D,2.379).
© The Trustees of the British Museum. All rights reserved.

dog doctors chiefly administered to the pets of wealthy women. The adverts he took out in newspapers also coded his prospective clientele as elite and female while emphasising his polite respectability, directing 'Ladies, &c. having dogs laboring under the severest disorders' to apply to 'the Doctor'.[13]

The practitioners whom dog owners called upon in times of crisis came from a range of backgrounds. As with Lady Tempest, fictional owner of Pompey the Little, the wealthiest dog lovers might seek the services of a physician or surgeon. Farriers – and from the 1790s onward, veterinary surgeons – generally practised on horses and livestock, but sometimes also applied their expertise to ill dogs. The farrier himself, however, was only one rung up from the dog doctor as a maligned animal healthcare practitioner and was frequently presented as illiterate and ignorant. But whereas the farrier's reputation has since been rehabilitated or re-evaluated in contemporary scholarship, no such attempt has been made for the dog doctor.[14] The dog doctor was at the bottom of a hierarchy which stretched across human and animal medical care. His place in order is reflected by Captain Crowe in Tobias Smollett's *Launcelot Greaves*; when criticising the provincial surgeon-midwife Mr Fillet for his overenthusiastic blood-letting, Crowe denigrates him as 'that there surgeon, or apothecary, or farrier, or dog-doctor, or whatsoever he may be', listing the medical trades in hierarchical order of descending respectability.[15]

The archetypical canine healthcare specialist 'dog doctors' were primarily engaged in trades or occupations that had little to do with the health of humans or animals, but had simultaneously developed a reputation for healing sick animals within their community. Dog doctoring was the main source of income only for a certain few. Unlike human practitioners represented in literature, the question of professionalism or irregularity was absent – there was no such thing as a qualified education or licence in canine healthcare. There were no apprenticeships, universities or colleges to educate prospective dog doctors on the particulars of canine healthcare as there were for farriers, surgeons, medical students and – from 1791 onwards – veterinary surgeons, who were mainly instructed in the anatomy and healthcare of horses. Perhaps because of this, canine healthcare practice was not as rigidly stratified as its human (or equine) equivalent.[16] The label was likewise deployed haphazardly. For instance, in a 1785 medical treatise Robert Hamilton described his fellow physician Robert James (inventor of James's Fever Powder) as a 'professed Dog Doctor', and an Ipswich gaoler who wormed dogs on the side was also pronounced 'a considerable Dog Doctor' himself.[17] Many practitioners may not have self-identified as dog doctors at all – in Frances Burney's 1782 novel *Cecilia*, Mr Morrice attempts to convince Cecilia to enlist the services of a 'most excellent dog-doctor, as we call him'.[18] It seems probable that healers who dabbled in curing dogs often rejected this term, given its widespread usage as an insult. Although the *Oxford English Dictionary* records the first instance of the phrase 'dog doctor' in Tobias Smollett's 1771 picaresque novel *Humphry Clinker*, the dog doctor was by no means a product of the second half of the eighteenth century. As early as 1710, a Whig MP was using the term to disparage the clergyman Henry Sacheverell, a Doctor of Divinity.[19]

The dog doctor's predecessor, the dog-leech, had also been frequently invoked as a slur since the early seventeenth century. In Jacobean and Caroline theatre the insult is usually directed at practitioners of human medicine: in Jonson's *The Alchemist* ('Out, you dog-leach,/ The vomit of all prisons'); in Fletcher's *The Mad Lover* ('Surgeon, syringe,/ dog-leach'); and in Machin and Markham's *The Dumb Knight* ('A very mountebank of wench-flesh, an empiric,/ A dog-leech for the putrified sores/ Of these lust-canker'd great ones'). In John Ford's *The Lover's Melancholy*, Rhetias despairs of 'empirics, that will undertake all cures, yet know not the causes of any disease! Dog leeches!'[20] The dog-leech's work almost always appears in the abstract, and the term is an insult directed at the lowest order of human practitioners.

A history of the literary dog doctor

The outline of the fictional eighteenth-century dog doctor had begun to emerge in the days of the dog-leech. In Thomas Nabbes's 1638 comedy *The Bride*, Mrs Ferret recommends the skill of her neighbour who cured her dog's mange and thus gained a reputation as 'an excellent dog-leech'. Like later fictional clients of dog doctors, Mrs Ferret is a wealthy woman with compromised human relationships (she henpecks her justice husband). Most importantly, her dog's name, Shock – a stock name for a lapdog with a 'shock' of white hair and also the name of a variety of bichon-type dogs – marks him out a lapdog, and therefore a luxury and high-status companion animal.[21] Mrs Ferret's ownership of and attention to the well-being of such a pet is a further mark against her character.

Although lapdogs had appeared in misogynistic satires on women and femininity prior to the mid-eighteenth century, the lapdog trope was reinvigorated by the 1751 publication of Francis Coventry's *The History of Pompey the Little*.[22] Coventry's work follows the circulation of Pompey, the lapdog, through English society, in which he plays various roles, including that of a much-loved companion, a fashion accessory and even a guide dog. The novel was extremely popular. Such was the ubiquity of *Pompey the Little* that in 1801 (half a century after its initial publication), the *Morning Chronicle* reported a Marylebone dog doctor had put up a 'whimsical' business sign. Over his door was not only his name, but a portrait of a 'lady's lap-dog' and the words 'Pompey the Little': 'Under it, by way of motto, stands the quotation from Lear, "Take physic, Pomp"' – a witticism which relied as much upon public knowledge of Coventry's canine hero as it did the work of Shakespeare.[23] Satires of lapdog ownership seem to increase both in number and invective following the publication of Coventry's novel, which obviously struck a chord with its readers (and inspired other writers to pen similar satirical criticisms of women and their pets). Likewise, dog doctors did not emerge as a secondary target of satires against lapdog-owning women until after the publication of *Pompey the Little*, although they had been practising for decades.

Pompey the Little codified some of the main beats of the anti-lapdog satire: an erotic element to the relationship between lapdog and female owner; a disparity between the ways a mistress treats her pet and the people who are dependent on her care or attention (be they spouses, children, servants – or even enslaved workers); an almost obsessive focus on the well-being of their pets; the provision of luxury goods and services for dogs. Unsurprisingly, this included employing medical practitioners to heal the dog. Although the specialist dog doctor does not make an appearance in *Pompey the Little*, when its canine protagonist becomes fatally ill towards the end of the book, his owner, Lady Tempest, 'spared no Expence for his Recovery, and had him attended by the most eminent Physicians of London'.[24] The dog doctor and his clients were the next logical targets for satirists who criticised lapdog ownership in the second half of the eighteenth century.

From the mid-1750s onwards, perhaps partly because *Pompey the Little* had laid the groundwork for further anti-lapdog satires, dog doctors became increasingly common in satirical fiction. Among the earliest imaginings of the dog doctor is the following report published in September 1755 in the *Derby Mercury*:

> Last Saturday a favourite Dog belonging to a Lady near Grosvenor-Square was put into a Coffin, and being carried by her two Chairmen on a Horse, was interred between Primrose-Hill and Hampstead. The Footmen walked before, and the Dog Doctor, who had attended him all the preceding Night, behind.

The article was almost certainly copied from a London paper, given that the next day it was printed in the *Oxford Journal*.[25] The original report could be based in truth, but its sensational claims may be inspired by Eliza Haywood's fiction *The Invisible Spy*, which was published the previous year (but dated 1755) and describes a similar funerary procession.[26] Regardless of whether the initial report had any basis in reality, it caught the imagination of readers. A few weeks later, it appeared in the *Caledonian Mercury*. Some of the specifics had been changed – Grosvenor Square swapped to Upper Brook Street, for instance. This new version also reported that 'for [*sic*] or five of her Servants are going to the Salt-water to be dipped', a popular cure for the bite of a mad dog – implying the dog was a victim of hydrophobia who had attacked people before its death.[27] These fictional reports established the basis of the dog doctor as a stock character in late eighteenth-century and early nineteenth-century satire: its main target was almost always a wealthy woman. Her dog doctor was a willing actor and a beneficiary in a charade ridiculous to outside observers and driven by what was considered to be an improper and irrationally strong attachment to an animal.

The dog doctor and gendered medical satire

Not even established works were safe from the spectre of the greedy dog doctor. The theatricals staged at the Austrian ambassador's home in Twickenham in January 1802 included a performance of Moliere's classic farce, *Le Medicin malgre lui*. However, the amateur dramatists had deemed it necessary to censor some of the play for an audience of 'chaste ears', adding instead a brand new scene. In it, a small child, played by the ambassador's youngest daughter, seeks the doctor's advice about 'her favourite Bijou'. Bijou, to Sganarelle's surprise, is no jewel, but the name of her little dog. He 'affects great surprise at being taken for a dog-doctor' but is predictably unwilling 'to let any thing escape his rapacity', and takes the girl's payment before inventing a cure.[28]

However, unlike Sgnarelle in the adapted play, the dog doctor as imagined in eighteenth-century literature was generally a secondary target compared to the woman who employed him. As sensibility gained cultural traction from the 1760s onwards, the lapdog became increasingly deployed as a mark against the humanity or true sensibility of their women owners. In 'Suffering Things: Lapdogs, Slaves, and Counter-Sensibility', Markman Ellis explores the role of 'counter-sensibility' in the reactions of female characters to the suffering of their companion dogs. Ellis argues that lapdogs, 'recipients of misdirected sentimental feelings, inordinate caresses, excessive affection and grief', act as emblems of 'the malevolent, spiteful, and hypocritical quality of their female owners, who demonstrate an "unfeeling" nature' for other people. Here, counter-sensibility operates in the 'disparity between absent feeling' for suffering people and 'excessive feeling' for sick or injured lapdogs.[29] Summoning a dog doctor was the perfect indicator of a character's tendency towards this counter-sensibility; few other acts can suggest such a level of emotional or financial investment in a dog's well-being.

In this light paying for specialist canine healthcare was not simply folly or even a waste of money, but evidence of a more troubling phenomenon. In 1774, the *Morning Post* presented what it reported to be a bill for £4 8s. 6d. from a dog doctor named Richard Hendersby (probably a reference to the aforementioned Richard Endersby). Perhaps the bill was a fictionalised joke, as some readers might consider the alleged complaints of the dogs (e.g. 'curing two other greyhounds of a cough') to be trivial. Hendersby, however, was not really the focus of the article; its targets were fashionable female dog owners who were happy to pay for such services, doting on their canine companions while ignoring the plight of vulnerable humans:

> the following bill, furnished by a dog doctor to one of these adorers of dogs, will, it is to be hoped, awake them from that kind of idolatry, bring them to a sense of feeling for their fellow creatures in distress, and also expose an insult upon common sense permitted to these, as well as other quack doctors.[30]

Writers continued to present the inequality between women's lapdogs and humans as the rationale behind their attacks on the dog doctor and their clients into the nineteenth century. In his account describing the Queen's dog physician, published forty years after Hendersby's 'bill', George Coleraine Hanger not only compared the lapdog's overly rich diet to that of impoverished children, but bluntly declares that 'I think it scandalous to give dogs what a human being would be grateful to receive'.[31] Female pet owners stood accused of upsetting the natural order by promoting their dogs' welfare above that of people.

The perceived absurdity of healthcare for dogs was also highlighted by the nature of fictional canine complaints and cures, which often leant towards the trivial or the disgusting. This was the case from the start of the dog healer's appearances in eighteenth-century literature. In 'Memoirs of P. P.: Clerk of this Parish', a Scriblerian parody of religious autobiographies attributed to Alexander Pope and John Gay, the narrator (while discussing his so-called 'twofold Profession' as a cobbler-cum-barber), details the 'Chirurgery ... I practiced in the Worming of Dogs'. Among the highlights of P. P.'s illustrious career is the occasion in which he was 'was sought unto to geld the Lady Frances her Spaniel, which was wont to go astray. He was called *Toby*, that is to say, *Tobias*'.[32] P. P.'s obsequious joy and self-importance in performing tasks for the local clergy and gentry – in this case a very undignified one – is part of the piece's satirical barb. More notably, in Tobias Smollett's *Humphry Clinker* (1771), Chowder, the canine companion of middle-aged spinster aunt Tabitha Bramble, is involved in an 'accident' during her family's stay at Bath: 'A famous dog-doctor was sent for, and undertook to cure the patient, provided he might carry him home to his own house; but his mistress would not part with him out of her own sight – She ordered the cook to warm cloths, which she applied to his bowels with her own hand'.[33] Again, the dog doctor is almost incidental here – the narrator (Bramble's niece), and Smollett by extension, are far more interested in her overreaction than they are the dog doctor. (Similarly, Tabitha's anecdote about Chowder's laxatives in her very first letter says more about her obsession with the dog's health than it does the animal's bowels.[34]) Of course, later in the novel Tabitha abandons Chowder when she finally finds a human suitor, and it becomes clear that he was just a proxy for her misdirected affection.

At least, however, Chowder's problems are not necessarily of Tabitha Bramble's making. This is not true of many of the fictional dog doctor's clients. Often, the animal is only suffering from an ailment directly caused by the affection of his/her indulgent (female) owner. Meyler's epitaph on Whittick noted that he favoured starvation when a 'fair' client's 'darling of her heart/ Was pamper'd, and oppress'd with pain' – the dog's pain arises as a consequence of pampering.[35] As a result, the dog doctor's treatment often took the form of neglecting an animal suffering from abuse accidentally inflicted by a well-meaning owner. For instance, in John Wolcot's (AKA Peter Pindar) 1794 poem 'The Lady's Lapdog, and the Coachman', the reader is introduced to the titular canine: 'Fat was our CHLOE – like a ball of grease;/ So round, a foot-ball quite, and fair her fleece'. The dog refuses to eat any other food aside from 'nice *tid-bits*', and only then with much solicitation from her owner. She is treated by the owner's coachman, Jehu, who refuses to offer Chloe anything other than the food scraps which made up a typical Georgian dog's diet – offal, stale bread and cheese rinds. A battle of the wills follows, and Wolcot imagines a dialogue between dog and man (e.g. '"Well, Chloe, can you take your liver?" – "No / No thank ye, Jehu"'). Eventually, the hungry dog relents and happily eats anything Jehu offers. On her return Chloe's owner – not suspecting the 'rough mode of cure' which could cost Jehu his job – is delighted, praising the coachman's skill: 'Then into Jehu's hand she slips a guinea / And Jehu's thought a very fine physician'.[36]

A similar story is found in other texts in which dog doctors appear. In John Thomas Smith's memoir, he recollects living next door to the London dog doctor Norborn and overhearing between the exasperated dog doctor's wife and a respectable client:

'What! but is your bitch ill again? I am sure we brought it about – it was fed upon nothing but bread and milk.'

'Bread and milk!' exclaimed Mrs. Nollekens; 'why we give it some of the best bits of our yard-dog's paunches.'

'Bless you, good woman! then it will never be well: the Doctor can do nothing for it, that I can tell you.'[37]

Successive generations of writers also were drawn to the story of the sly dog doctor and the overly trusting, overly fond owner (although Jehu's stale bread came to be replaced by industrially manufactured kibble), even as specialist canine healthcare became increasingly acceptable.[38] (In nineteenth- and twentieth-century variations of this story, including that told by the vet James Herriot, the practitioner sequesters the dog's usual luxurious fare for himself.)[39] Restricted diets were almost certainly a common practice, and were probably necessary for many dogs fed rich foods. During a stay in Moscow in 1807, the Irish diarist Martha Wilmot's dog Themise was forbidden meat and instead prescribed a diet of milk, bread and water by a 'famous Dog Doctor'.[40] Starvation diets were recommended by veterinarians in the United States well into the twentieth century, and canine obesity presents a serious animal welfare issue today.[41] Of course, in the first half of the eighteenth century, George Cheyne promoted the health benefits of a not dissimilar diet for humans.[42] However, focusing on overfed dogs (rather than any other complaints treated by dog doctors, such as mange, broken legs or fits) also enabled criticism of this mode of pet keeping more generally, and therefore of female dog owners. The immoderate fondness that drove a woman to overfeed her dog was the same fondness that led her to employ a dog doctor.

The fictional dog doctor's practice represented an upset of the social order, as women chose to concentrate their financial resources and affection on a 'useless' animal. This was compounded by the class dynamics of such interactions. The fictional dog doctor is generally depicted as socially inferior to his clients, and writers reinforce this difference. In Smith's memoirs, for instance, the wife of John Norborn (named as Mrs Norman) has a propensity for malapropisms (e.g. 'You don't know the *disponsibility* I am in'). Her client, Mary Nollekens, the wife of a famous sculptor, even upbraids the dog doctor's wife for her vulgar mode of address ('Is that the way to speak to a lady?'). However, the dog doctor has the power in these interactions, and Nollekens' posturing is of little interest to Mrs Norman – when her client entreats her to come downstairs to talk, she responds by reeling off a list of the A-list canine patients she is currently busy looking after.[43] The human physician summoned by dog owners to revive an ailing pet remained a staple of satirical literature even after the rise of the specialist dog doctor. This physician-cum-dog doctor shares more in common with the stock drawing-room physician than he does other fictional dog doctors, and adheres to the same tropes;

he is argumentative and has a strong sense of self-importance (albeit punctured by the fact he is employed to heal a small fluffy dog and not a hypochondriac human).[44] In a 1789 comic-erotic poem written by the Bath physician Anthony Fothergill, 'On the Premature Death of Cloe Snappum', after the titular lapdog is crushed between her mistress's thighs while her owner has an orgasmic spasm, 'two doctors held a learn'd debate/ On Cloe's case – alas, too late!'[45] Like other physicians in satire, most notably Pompey's London professionals, whose intervention unfortunately 'rather hastened than delayed his Exit', the moonlighting doctors invariably seem to be of little help to their patients.[46] This development, of course, is also common in satires on doctors and their human patients. A 1784 elegy on the death of Bungy, the Newfoundland dog of Charles Robinson, Canterbury's recorder, claims that doctors and dog doctors alike disagreed on his treatment, their haphazard application of different cures increasing his pain and hastening his death.[47] In many ways, writing about dog doctors also conformed to the conventions of medical satire more generally – the (dog) doctor consistently takes advantage of his wealthy clients' neuroses and gullibility.

Physicians were usually keen to avoid comparison with dog doctors. Hester Piozzi reported in her correspondence that her physician friend, Dr George Smith Gibbes, was 'agonised' by the nature of his representation as 'Dr Faddle' in an 1807 satire of Bath society, in which his alter ego is summoned to attend a lapdog suffering from cholic. Faddle prepares to throw every treatment at the animal ('a purge and a blister, a bleeding and clyster, will again set all to rights'), but the 'suffering angel' dies in front of him.[48] Physicians themselves could be particularly scathing about dog doctors. James Whittick first rose to local prominence in 1786 when the physician and poet Dr Henry Harington published a satirical broadside taking the form of a mock Latin 'diploma' supposedly awarded to Whittick, 'the celebrated *Canine Professor of Physic*' of Bath. Whittick's place of residence, Guinea Lane, is noted to be 'very aptly named', suggesting that Harington considered Whittick's interest in canine healthcare to be fundamentally pecuniary in nature. Harington's cynical attitude to Whittick's abilities and motivations may perhaps also be evident in his listing dog killing as one of the main duties of the dog doctor.[49] Harington's satire on the real Whittick aligns here with depictions of fictional and fictionalised dog doctors who are consistently shown to value the worth of dogs and the utility of canine healthcare wildly differently from their clients. After his patient dies, Faddle reveals a seething hatred of the animal: ('Gad so the nasty little son of a bitch is really gone, I believe').[50]

The visual culture of dog doctoring

As a cultural construction, the dog doctor was for the most part a literary phenomenon. While the multitalented *tondeurs de chien* (dog barbers) routinely attracted the interest of French artists, the dog doctor made little impact on English visual satire. Indeed, the *tondeur de chien* appeared more frequently than his cross-channel counterpart in the work of British cartoonists. He appears as a skinny and dishevelled figure grasping an unwilling canine patient in Henry William Bunbury's *View of the Pont Neuf at Paris*, later copied in detail in at least two other English prints (Figures 5.2 and 5.3). Such cartoons cast the dog barber as inherently French, and specifically Parisian, and perhaps therefore implicitly effeminate, or at least contrary to the ideals of hearty English masculinity. The print produced by James Bretherton after Bunbury was even subtitled 'La Francia'.[51]

Thomas Rowlandson, who copied Bunbury's *Pont Neuf* himself, also turned his attention to English cobblers whose signs tell the viewer they also work as a dog doctor or dog wormer and cat gelder.[52] In one watercolour (Figure 5.4), the cobbler Thomas Stichwell appears as a balding middle-aged man intent on his work. A female customer sits beside him while he works on a shoe while his wife, unimpressed by the attention he is receiving from a buxom young woman, leans out of the window above his shopfront. (Rowlandson was repeatedly drawn to cobblers and their marital (dis)harmonies.[53])

It is hard to know what to what degree Stichwell's side-job informs Rowlandson's depiction of the cobbler. The dogs loitering in front of his shop front seem almost incidental, paying no attention to him at all. It is unclear whether one of the dogs belongs to either one of the women, although they appear to be wearing collars. The dogs are clearly healthy animals and not in obvious need of dog doctoring. Whereas the dog doctor is typically presented as exploiting women's over-affection for their pets, here the women may be willing to exploit their pets to engage with the muscly cobbler-cum-dog doctor as an object of sexual desire. The act of being able to touch a customer's feet seems to offer intimacy itself, as suggested by the 1784 etching *Wit's Last Stake*, where the cobbler-cum-dog gelder seems to relish the opportunity to work on the Duchess of Devonshire's shoes.[54] Whether Thomas Stichwell actively courts such attention from his admirers is up to the interpretation of the viewer. The dogs may echo the human interaction in the print – the larger dog, nonplussed by the attentions of the irritating smaller terrier, mirroring the apparently untempted Stichwell.

There appears to be relatively little comment on dog doctoring here – nor a satire on pet keeping or pet owners as there is in many of Rowlandson's

Dog doctors in eighteenth-century Britain 109

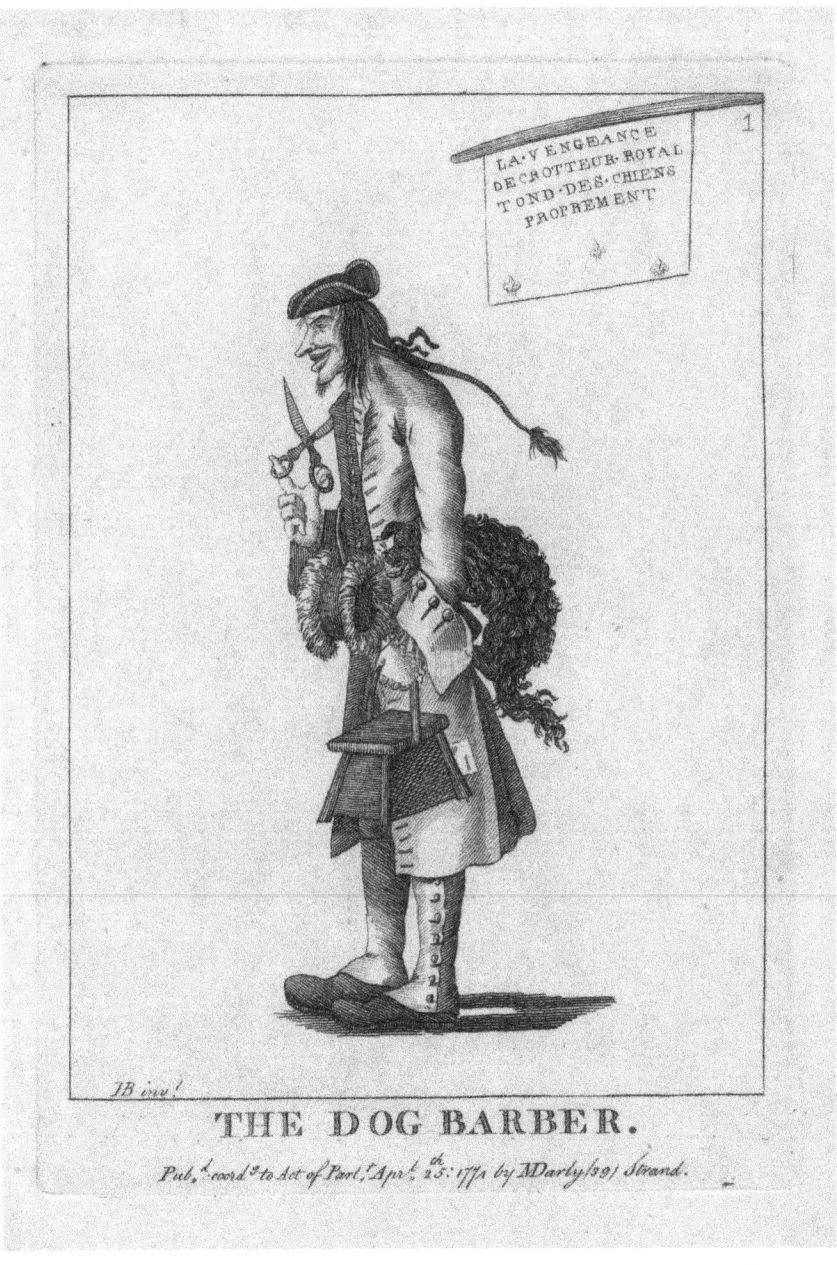

Figure 5.2 After Henry William Bunbury, *The Dog Barber* (1771), etching, 22.4 × 13.8 cm, Metropolitan Museum of Art, New York, The Elisha Whittelsey Collection, The Elisha Whittelsey Fund, 2011.

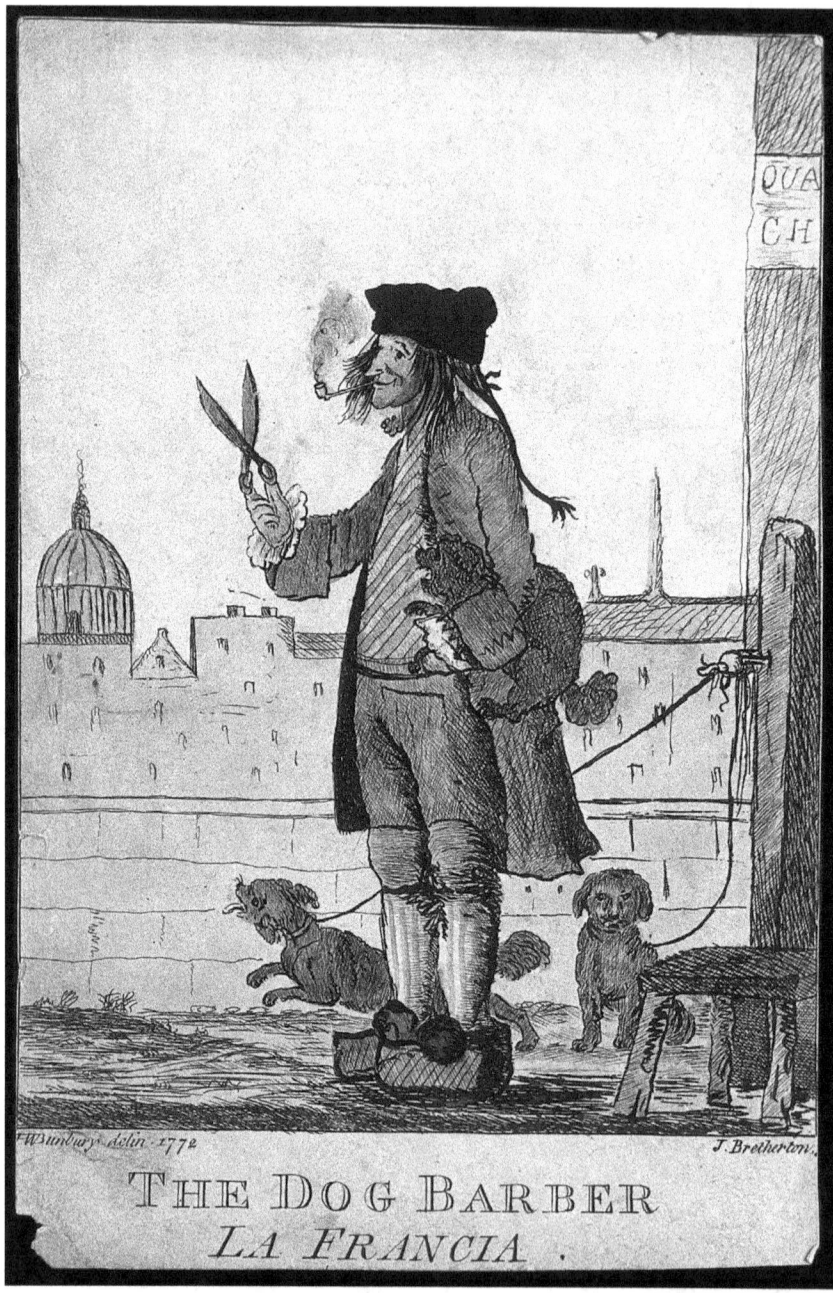

Figure 5.3 James Bretherton after Henry William Bunbury, *The Dog Barber. La Francia* (1772), coloured etching, 24 × 15.8 cm, Wellcome Collection. Public Domain.

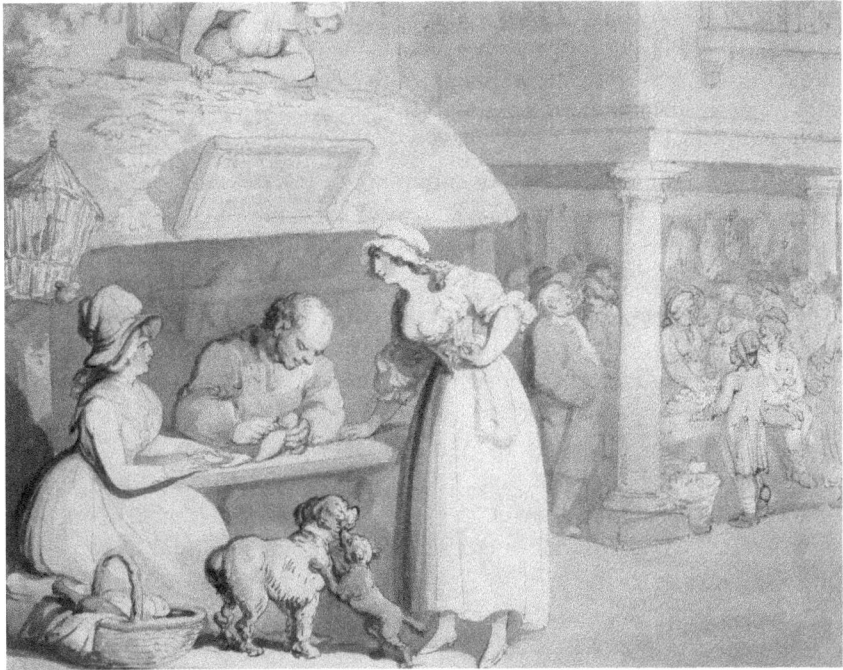

Figure 5.4 Thomas Rowlandson, *Tommy Stichwell, Cobbler and Dog-Doctor* (late 18th – early 19th century), pen, ink and watercolour over pencil, 24 × 30.25 cm, Lot 85, Old Masters, British & European Paintings, Wednesday 6 March 2019, Woolley & Wallis, p. 32. © Woolley & Wallis Salisbury Salesrooms.

other prints and in most literature in which the dog doctor makes an appearance. Indeed, another preparation of the same scene removes the angry wife and identifies the cobbler (now Timothy Botch) as a part-time porter rather than a dog doctor.[55]

Conclusion

In 1803, the veterinary surgeon (and former army surgeon) Delabere Blaine complained that 'the very term dog doctor conveys an idea remote from gentility: but it is not the unworthiness of the pursuit, but the kind of persons who have hitherto followed it, that has made it so'.[56] Blaine's disparaging of his unqualified counterparts was certainly intended to set himself apart from his competitors, but these prejudices were reflective of the period and replicated in its novels and satirical poetry. Such beliefs were, he predicted, hard to change. The term 'dog doctor' was employed as an insult against veterinarians dealing with canine health throughout the Victorian period and well into the mid-twentieth century.[57] Veterinary surgeons working in small animal practice were dogged by suggestions that their 'speciality was effete and trivial'.[58] Even in 1921, veterinarians warned their peers who practised on dogs that their work 'often aids the rotten sentiments of a useless section of community who are unfit to be fathers or mothers'.[59] This assumption can be traced back to the eighteenth century and to the depiction of dog doctors in Georgian literature as reliant upon the patronage of wealthy mistresses who doted on their little dogs at a time when pet keeping was routinely presented as the sole province of histrionic women who had strong attachments to their dogs out of proportion with societal expectations, and who did not fulfil their obligations to their families or society in general. The literary dog doctor helped to seal the reputation of the dog doctor as an ignorant opportunist – someone with little interest in the well-being of dogs and a strong desire to take advantage of their owners. Of course, if owners genuinely suspected that the dog doctor's services were of such little use, they would not have employed them – unless, of course, being seen to employ a figure to attend to the health of one's pet was considered as a commendable impulse in itself, which, as this chapter has established, it was not.

The representation of dog doctors in Georgian literary culture was driven by a societal discomfort at the ever-rising status of companion dogs in British homes. It was this trend that ushered in (among other things) the development of a cottage industry in canine healthcare. The dog doctor emerged before pet care became a mass 'commercial enterprise' – that would come later, in the Victorian period – and as a result his presence appeared particularly symptomatic of the confused priorities of wealthy dog owners of the day.[60] The fictional canine health practitioner (be he a physician, surgeon, specialist dog doctor or otherwise) serves as an indicator of the pet's financial and emotional value to his mistress – satires on the dog doctor were almost always necessarily satires of a certain kind of elite femininity. Just as the employment of canine-specialist vets in Edwardian London later served to challenge the 'veterinary establishment's view that dogs were "unworthy" patients', the employment of dog doctors by the owners of pets challenged an established hierarchy which placed dogs below other 'useful' animals and, of course, well below humans.[61] This demand for specialist canine healthcare made evident the inequality between the human poor and the canine rich. In this context, when the role of the dog remained largely contested, imagining the dog doctor and his services presented an opportunity to mediate the changing status of companion dogs within society and to criticise the women who supposedly enabled such a shift in the status quo.

Notes

1. William Meyler, 'Epitaph on the Celebrated Canine Doctor, Whittick', in *Poetical Amusement on the Journey of Life; Consisting of Various Pieces in Verse: Serious, Theatric, Epigrammatic and Miscellaneous* (Bath: Meyler, 1806), pp. 150–152.
2. I have used male pronouns throughout this chapter when discussing the dog doctor as the dog doctor was exclusively configured as a man in eighteenth-century Britain. Laura Brown, *Homeless Dogs and Melancholy Apes: Humans and Other Animals in the Modern Literary Imagination* (Ithaca, NY: Cornell University Press, 2010), pp. 65–89.
3. Joanna Swabe, 'Veterinary Dilemmas: Ambiguity and Ambivalence in Human–Animal Interaction', in A. L. Poderscek, E. S. Paul and J. A. Serpell (eds), *Companion Animals and Us* (Cambridge: Cambridge University Press, 2000), pp. 292–311 (at p. 294).
4. Michael Hubbard MacKay, 'The Rise of a Medical Specialty: The Medicalisation of Elite Equine Care c.1680–c.1800', PhD Thesis, University of York (2009), pp. 12, 336, available at http://etheses.whiterose.ac.uk/14229/1/625453.pdf, last accessed 10 April 2020.
5. Ingrid Tague, *Animal Companions: Pets and Social Change in Eighteenth-Century Britain* (University Park, PA: Pennsylvania State University, 2015), pp. 2, 228–229, 106–108, 125–127. Tague herself briefly discusses dog doctors in *Animal Companions* (pp. 38–40).
6. Stephanie Howard-Smith, 'In the Dog House: British Canines at Home, 1688–1832', *Home Cultures* 18:2 (2021): 129–149, available at https://doi.org/10.1080/17406315.2021.1963610, last accessed 19 October 2023.
7. For an analysis of the working practices of eighteenth-century dog doctors, see Stephanie Howard-Smith, 'The First Dog Doctors: Canine Healthcare Practitioners in the Eighteenth-Century Medical Marketplace', Social History of Medicine (forthcoming at the time of writing).
8. Joan Wake and Deborah Champion Webster (eds), *The Letters of Daniel Eaton to the Third Earl of Cardigan, 1725–1732* (Kettering: Northamptonshire Record Society, 1971), pp. 66–73.
9. Robert James, *A Treatise on Canine Madness* (London: Newberry, 1765), p. 203.
10. George Hanger, *To All Sportsmen, Farmers, and Gamekeepers* (London: Stockdale, 1814), pp. 66–67.
11. Mary Coke, *The Letters and Journals of Lady Mary Coke*, ed. James Archibald Home, 4 vols (Edinburgh: David Douglas, 1896), vol. 4, p. 444; Edward A. Bloom and Lillian Bloom (eds), *The Piozzi Letters: The Correspondence of Hester Lynch Piozzi 1784–1821*, 6 vols (Newark, DE: University of Delaware Press, 1989), vol. II: *1792–1798*, p. 139.
12. *Public Advertiser* (17 May 1784), p. 4.
13. *Morning Herald* (9 April 1788), p. 2.
14. MacKay, 'The Rise of a Medical Specialty', pp. 81–82. See also Joan Lane, 'Farriers in Georgian England', in A. R. Michell (ed.), *The Advancement of*

15. Tobias Smollett, *The Adventures of Sir Launcelot Greaves*, 2 vols (London: Coote, 1762), vol. 1, p. 25.
16. Roy Porter, *Disease, Medicine and Society in England, 1550–1860* (Cambridge: Cambridge University Press, 1995), pp. 11–12.
17. Robert Hamilton, *Remarks on the Means of Obviating the Fatal Effects of the Bite of a Mad Dog* (Ipswich: Shave and Jackson, 1785), pp. 135–145.
18. Frances Burney, *Cecilia, or Memoirs of an Heiress*, 5 vols (London: Payne and Cadell, 1782), vol. 4, p. 156.
19. '"dog", n.1.: C1. a. (a) dog doctor n.' *OED Online*, available at www.oed.com/view/Entry/56405, last accessed 2 May 2019. Cropley to Stanhope, 23 April 1710, Stanhope MSS 34/16, Kent Record Office, quoted in Clayton Roberts, 'The Fall of the Godolphin Ministry', *Journal of British Studies* 22:1 (1982): 71–93, available at http://www.jstor.com/stable/175657, last accessed 28 February 2023.
20. Ben Jonson, *The Alchemist* (London: Burre, 1612); Gervase Markham, *The Dumbe Knight* (London: Bache, 1608); John Fletcher, *The Mad Lover*, in *Comedies and Tragedies written by Francis Beaumont and John Fletcher* (London: Robinson and Moseley, 1647); John Ford, *The Lover's Melancholy* (London: Seile, 1629).
21. Thomas Nabbes, *The Bride* (London: Blaikelocke, 1640), vols. 1 and 4.
22. See Brown, *Homeless Dogs and Melancholy Apes* and Jodi L. Wyett, 'The Lap of Luxury: Lapdogs, Literature, and Social Meaning in the "Long" Eighteenth Century', *Lit: Literature Interpretation Theory* 10:4 (1999): 275–301.
23. *Morning Chronicle* (29 September 1801), p. 3.
24. Francis Coventry, *The History of Pompey the Little* (London: Cooper, 1751), p. 265.
25. *Derby Mercury* (14 September 1755), p. 3; *Oxford Journal* (15 September 1753), p. 1.
26. Eliza Haywood, *The Invisible Spy*, 4 vols (London: Gardner, 1755), vol. 1, p. 27.
27. *Caledonian Mercury* (1 October 1753), p. 3.
28. *Morning Chronicle* (12 January 1802), p. 3.
29. Markman Ellis, 'Suffering Things: Lapdogs, Slaves and Counter-Sensibility', in Mark Blackwell (ed.), *The Secret Life of Things: Animals, Objects, and It-Narratives in Eighteenth-Century England* (Lewisburg, PA: Bucknell University Press, 2007), pp. 93–113 (pp. 100–102).
30. *Morning Post* (12 January 1774), p. 2.
31. Hanger, *To All Sportsmen*, p. 66.
32. Alexander Pope and John Gay, 'Memoirs of P. P.: Clerk of this Parish', in *Miscellanies*, 3 vols (London: Motte, 1727), vol. 2, pp. 268–284 (at pp. 275–276).
33. Tobias Smollett, *The Expedition of Humphry Clinker*, 2 vols (London: Johnston, 1771), vol. 1, pp. 119–120.

34 Ibid., vol. 1, p. 4.
35 Meyler, 'Epitaph on the Celebrated Canine Doctor', p. 151.
36 John Wolcot [Peter Pindar], 'The Lady's Lap-Dog, and the Coachman', *Pindariana; Or Peter's Portfolion* (London: T. Salisbury, 1794), pp. 66–70.
37 John Thomas Smith, *Nollekens and His Times: Comprehending a Life of that Celebrated Sculptor; and Memoirs of Several Contemporary Artists, from the Time of Roubiliac, Hogarth, and Reynolds, to that of Fuseli, Flaxman, and Blake*, ed. Wilfred Whitten, 2 vols, 2nd edn (London: Lane, 1829), vol. 1, pp. 135–137.
38 John George Wood, *Petland Revisited* (London: Longmans & Co., 1884), pp. 117–119.
39 Henry Sutherland Edwards, *Malvina*, 3 vols (London: Hurst and Blackett, 1871), vol. 1, pp. 139–142; James Herriot, *If Only They Could Talk* (London: Joseph, 1970).
40 Edith Helen Vane-Tempest-Stewart and H. M. Hyde (eds.), *The Russian Journals of Martha and Catherine Wilmot, 1803–1808* (London: Macmillan, 1935), pp. 294–296.
41 Susan D. Jones, *Valuing Animals: Veterinarians and their Patients in Modern America* (Baltimore, MD: Johns Hopkins University Press, 2003), p. 122; C. Pegram, E. Raffan, E. White, A. H. Ashworth, D. C. Brodbelt, D. B. Church and D. G. O'Neill, 'Frequency, Breed Predisposition and Demographic Risk Factors for Overweight Status in Dogs in the UK', *Journal of Small Animal Practice* 62:7 (2021): 521–530.
42 Carol Houlihan Flynn, *The Body in Swift and Defoe* (Cambridge: Cambridge University Press, 1990).
43 Smith, *Nollekens and His Times*, vol. 1, p. 136.
44 Genice Ngg, 'The Changing Face of Quack Doctors: Satirizing Mountebanks and Physicians in Seventeenth- and Eighteenth-Century England', in S. M. Hilger (ed.), *New Directions in Literature and Medicine Studies* (Basingstoke: Palgrave Macmillan, 2017), pp. 333–356 (pp. 348–350).
45 Anthony Fothergill, 'On the Premature Death of Cloe Snappum, a Lady's Favourite', *An Asylum for Fugitive Pieces, in Prose and Verse, Not in Any Other Collection: With Several Other Pieces Never before Published*, 3 vols (London: Debrett, 1789), vol. 3, p. 249.
46 Coventry, *Pompey the Little*, p. 265.
47 T. W., 'Elegy on the Death of Bungy', *Gentleman's Magazine* (August 1784), p. 614.
48 Richard Warner [Peter Paul Pallet], *Bath Characters: Or, Sketches from Life* (London: Wilkie and Robinson, 1807), pp. 16–17.
49 Henry Harington, 'The Following Diploma Lately Obtained by the Celebrated Canine Professor of Physic in this City' [broadside] (Bath, 1786). I am grateful to Gill Lynch for her translation of the Latin portion of the diploma.
50 Warner, *Bath Characters*, p. 17.
51 After Henry William Bunbury, *View on the Pont Neuf at Paris* (1771), etching, 25.1 × 37.7 cm, British Museum; After Henry William Bunbury, *The Dog Barber* (1771), etching, 22.4 × 13.8 cm, Metropolitan Museum of Art; James

Bretherton after Henry William Bunbury, *The Dog Barber. La Francia* (1772), coloured etching 24 × 15.8 cm, Wellcome Collection.

52 Thomas Rowlandson, *Tommy Stichwell, Cobbler and Dog-Doctor* (c.1789), pen, ink and watercolour over pencil, 24 × 30.25 cm, Lot 85, Old Masters, British & European Paintings, Wednesday 6 March 2019, Woolley & Wallis, p. 32; Thomas Rowlandson, *The Cobbler: Tom Stichwell Dog Wormer And Cat Gelder* (1789), watercolour, 27.9 × 35.6 cm, Paul Mellon Photographic Archive (PA-F02122-0003).

53 Thomas Rowlandson, *The Coblers Cure for a Scolding Wife* (1809), hand-coloured etching, 36.9 × 26.5 cm, Royal Collection Trust (RCIN 810778).

54 Thomas Rowlandson, *Wit's Last Stake, or the Cobbling Voters and Abject Canvassers* (1784), hand-coloured etching, 26.3 × 36.2 cm, Metropolitan Museum of Art (59.533.62).

55 Martin Birnbaum, *Jacovleff and Other Artists: Alexandre Jacovleff, William Blake and Other Illustrators of Dante, Thomas Rowlandson, Aubrey Beardsley, Marcus Behmer, Arthur Rackham, Hermann Struck, Anne Goldthwaite* (New York: Struck, 1946), p. 117.

56 Delabere Pritchett Blaine, *A Domestic Treatise on the Diseases of Horses and Dogs* (London: Boosey, 1803), p. 142.

57 Andrew Gardiner, 'The "Dangerous" Women of Animal Welfare: How British Veterinary Medicine Went to the Dogs', *Social History of Medicine* 23:3 (2014), 466–487 (at 467–468). Neil Pemberton and Michael Worboys, *Mad Dogs and Englishmen: Rabies in Britain, 1830–2000* (Basingstoke: Palgrave, 2007), pp. 197–198.

58 Gardiner, 'The "Dangerous" Women of Animal Welfare', p. 485.

59 Alison Mary Skipper, 'Form, Function and Fashion: Health, Disease and British Pedigree Dog Breeding During the Long Twentieth Century', PhD Thesis, King's College London (2021), p. 174.

60 Sarah Amato, *Beastly Possessions: Animals in Victorian Consumer Culture* (Toronto: University of Toronto Press, 2015), pp. 41–48.

61 Alison Skipper, 'The "Dog Doctors" of Edwardian London: Elite Canine Veterinary Care in the Early Twentieth Century', *Social History of Medicine* 33:4 (2020): 1233–1258 (at 1257), available at https://doi.org/10.1093/shm/hkz049, last accessed 28 February 2023.

6

'A man of common understanding': venereal disease, myth and reading as a protective practice in eighteenth-century Britain

Declan Kavanagh

In eighteenth-century writing on the *lues venerea*, or venereal disease, authors frequently present the debilitating effects of the ailment in a way that clearly foregrounds how gonorrhoea and the pox intersect with formative ideas about what it means to be a white and male Briton. Venereal disease was rampant in the period and the prolific nature of treatises on the subject attests to the fact that the disease was still something of a mystery. As Noelle Gallagher notes in her study, *Itch, Clap, Pox* (2018):

> at the same time that venereal disease remained shrouded in mystery, it also seemed to be worryingly *present*; many eighteenth-century commentators warned that the disease was already rampant and continuing to spread, and although no reliable data on infection rates exist for this period, medical historians have speculated that syphilis in particular had reached epidemic proportions by the 1700s.[1]

The discourse on venereal disease, written across numerous treatises and dissertations throughout the period, worked to focalise questions of male sexual desire and agency. In this chapter, I explore the medical writing on venereal disease alongside the prose fiction of Tobias Smollett and the life writing of James Boswell in order to showcase how writing about sexual infection in this period provided a canvas upon which questions of male ability and debility were writ large. Reading medical observations on the disease reveals how men were sometimes encouraged not to fear medical knowledge but to become men of common understanding; to be, in other words, agents of their own self-recovery. While writers like Smollett used the novel form to model men's mastery of their own sexual health, private diary accounts like Boswell's instead foreground his distrust of medical intervention in the wake of his infection, before detailing the anxieties that underpinned the distemper's cure.

Indeed, the literature on venereal disease, as represented in publications like Daniel Turner's *Syphilis: A Practical Dissertation on the Venereal Disease* (1717),[2] brings to the fore considerations of disability, not only in the context of the debilitating effects of venereal disease itself, but also in discussions of its possible cures. As Turner cautions, ability – here coded as 'age' and 'strength' – should be a key determinant when preparing a cure for the patient as 'after a sufficient Quantity either of the internal or external Medicine before used, let the Turpeth Mineral but with due Regard to the Age and Strength of your Patient, in the Quantity or Dose'.[3] The 'Turpeth Mineral' dosage, namely the amount of the powder given containing a mercuric sulphate, is applied in direct proportion here to the perceived infirmity or otherwise of the patient in question. Turner also alludes to the paradoxical way in which the materials of an apothecary's dispensing closet can have adverse effects once handled by the dispenser: 'When I consider how prejudicial the said Mineral, their Foundation, is daily found, more especially to the nervous System, of all the Mechanicks occupy'd about the same: Not to mention the dismal Havock it makes among the Miners, it is very rare to find a working Painter, more particularly the Grinders of their Whites; the Gilders; nay some of the Plumbers, and also Glasiers, without Paralysis or Tremor'.[4] In a sentence that links men from an array of occupations, Turner marks out the hazardous ramifications of sustained close contact with mercuric sulphate. Not only apothecaries, but also painters, grinders, miners, plumbers and glaziers, all risk suffering from trembling and palsy. In this way, Turner demonstrates how reading his *Practical Dissertation* amounts to a protective practice for his readers. By presenting his readers with the dangers of mercuric sulphate, Turner offers knowledge that will help these men to avoid its debilitating impact.

As Turner's *A Practical Dissertation on Venereal Disease* shows, debility is interwoven into the fabric of the discourse on venereal disease, not only in the discourse's account of the ravages of the disease, but also in its consideration of the harmful nature of the very materials that are often used to 'cure' it. Moreover, as Turner reminds his reader, if the preparation of the 'cure' can lead to debility for a number of men, then the task of securing treatment for the infected man also has the potential to be socially ruinous. Addressing doctors but also, by extension, surgeons and apothecaries, Turner remarks: 'I would exhort each of you, that in this particular Part of your Profession, you are truly to every one, that under such Predicament, puts, as I may say, his Life, or which is almost the same to a modest Man, his reputation, in your Hands'.[5] Here Turner employs the trope of the doctor's hands, recurrent in various accounts of the disease, to signal the disproportionate power of the apothecary, or the physician, who administers treatment to a man with a venereal distemper and, in doing so, also firmly grips the man's reputation. As I will explore later on when discussing Boswell's *London Journal* (1762–63), the return to the image of the doctor's hands in passages such as these communicates the coded threat of an effeminising subjection for the man seeking out a cure. Not only is the afflicted man at the mercy of a physician in terms of the duration and cost of his treatment, he is also at the mercy of his practitioner when it comes to the health of his own reputation. Writing on venereal disease and its possible cures, as Turner's dissertation on syphilis reveals, was as much about these diseases as it was about prompting male readers to carefully think through the complex negotiations of masculinity that could potentially arise when grappling with venereal diseases.[6]

The fraught question of how men could navigate their own social and financial ruin when seeking treatment for venereal disease served to frame publications on the topic decades after Turner's *A Practical Dissertation on Venereal Disease* appeared. In a much later publication entitled *Observations Concerning the Prevention and Cure of the Venereal Disease* (1796), William Buchan frames his intervention as providing a substitute for the physician's knowledge 'where he cannot be had'. As the following excerpt bears out, Buchan is keen to outline the relationship between reading and practice in upholding the myth of masculine invulnerability. Reading his *Observations* will help men to avoid 'becoming the prey of ignorance and avarice'; reading then, as a protective practice, will secure one's reputation and the myth of male invulnerability that reputation maintains:

> It is easy to say that every man afflicted with the venereal disease, ought to have recourse to the best advice; but how is he to obtain it? The best advice is not easily purchased. Besides, men afflicted with the venereal disease are often in situations where no medical assistance of any kind can be had. These are the men for whom the following observations were thrown together. They are not designed to supersede the physician, but, in some measure, to supply his place where he cannot be had; and to prevent those who are not able to employ him, from becoming the prey of ignorance and avarice.[7]

In the opening pages of his *Observations*, Buchan markets his book to the reader by setting out the predicament in which men find themselves when experiencing the onset of the first symptoms of a sexually acquired infection. Buchan is clear that men are often in situations in which 'no medical assistance of any kind can be had'. While pointing out that his *Observations* are not meant to negate a physician's medical knowledge, Buchan clarifies that the text is intended as a resource for those who lack easy access to such care and, more pointedly, as a preventative measure for men who would become the 'prey of ignorance and avarice'. The perils attending managing sexual health then are twofold in so much as men might find themselves without any access to 'advice' or they might unwittingly become the victim of a practitioner's exploitative guidance. On the latter point, Buchan is keen to outline the specific issues surrounding physicians and their treatment of venereal diseases:

> It is a just observation, that there is a greater difference between a good physician and a bad one, than between a good physician and none. When I say a bad one, I mean the self-created doctor, who, while he knows nothing, undertakes everything. A man of common understanding, with the assistance of books, will conduct his own cure better than many of those who make a trade of curring the lues venerea. Nor is it a matter of small importance for a man to know when he is properly treated. It is on the ignorance of the patient that the Charlatan presumes. He knows there is no danger of detection while the patient is taught to dread, even the least dip, in medical knowledge.[8]

In this brief passage, Buchan sets up a binary between the 'self-created doctor' who 'knows nothing [but] undertakes everything' and the 'man of common understanding' who 'with the assistance of books, will conduct his own cure better than many of those who make a trade of curring [sic] the lues venerea'. Men, the reader is told, 'should at least have as much information about this malady as to know when he has got it'.[9] Rather than being completely ignorant, Buchan points out that ordinary men already possess intimate knowledge about their own health. Within the vein of Enlightenment empiricism broadly conceived, Buchan criticises 'the speculative physician [who] may amuse himself with plausible theories, and even believe that he can cure all diseases by his favourite system' but who 'when he comes to real practice, he will find that his art can only be learned at the patient's bed-side'.[10]

Knowledge, like an infection, is 'acquired'. In his criticism of the speculative physician, Buchan further emphasises the value of the common man's personal knowledge and the textual knowledge that he can glean through independent book learning. As Buchan further explains:

> The knowledge of all diseases is acquired, like that of men, by observation. Reading, no doubt, has its use, but it will never make a physician, any more than it will make a mechanic, or a complete seaman. I would rather trust myself in the hands of an experienced nurse, than of a theoretical physician.[11]

The 'speculative physician', versed in theory but with little or no practical experience, is dismissed here in favour of 'the hands of an experienced nurse'. Here, once again, the metaphor of the hands returns, although in the guise of the presumably female nurse's more practical experience. Buchan's message is a carefully crafted one that suggests that men should find a balance between theoretical and practical approaches to the treatment of venereal complaints. More implicitly, the discussion in this part of *Observations* works to centre authority on venereal treatment away from 'self-created' doctors. It is unclear whether or not Buchan is solely targeting physicians, or also taking aim at apothecaries who primarily 'treat' venereal disease, but the implication is that the trade in venereal disease treatment is populated by duplicitous practitioners who profit from ignorant men who fear 'even the least dip, in medical knowledge'. Medical 'Charlatan[s]' can dispense unsound advice and administer placebo nostrums because the 'common man' neglects, out of fear, to take books like Buchan's into *his own hands*. Independent book learning is foregrounded here in Buchan's *Observations* as a protective practice, which literate lay men can engage in to protect themselves against the costly misinformation – both reputational and physical – supplied by quacks.

To avoid being 'under the hands' of an exploitative doctor, surgeon or apothecary, Buchan encourages his invariably male reader to 'use their own understanding' in 'matters that concern their own health'.[12] For one man to be 'under the hands' of another man suggests the potential relinquishing of power from one man to another. Buchan suggests here how exercising one's own understanding can help to retain men's agency in personal health matters. Explaining the intended reach of his *Observations*, he asserts that:

> It is far from my intention to write a complete treatise on the venereal disease. This has been very fully accomplished by others; neither would it suit the nature of my performance, which only aims at exhibiting such a view of that malady as will enable any person of common sense to know when he has caught the infection; and, at the same time, to suggest the proper means for preventing its progress, or removing it in the early stages.[13]

The man of 'common sense', Buchan argues, can not only learn to identify when he has been infected with the pox or gonorrhoea, but he can also learn 'the proper means for preventing its progress, or removing it in the early stages'. Over the course of his lengthy *Observations*, Buchan advises in detail how men might best privately 'cure' their chancres, chordees, bougies, gleets, phymosis and venereal ulcers. In the following passage, Buchan deftly guides his reader through the process of self-curing a running venereal infection by preparing a solution and injecting it by syringe into the urethra:

> As soon as the running appears, and there is no inflammation, stricture, or swelling of the parts to forbid it, my practice is immediately to use an astringent injection. Of these there is great variety. What I prefer is the white vitriol dissolved in water: This may be used in various proportions, from half a dram of vitriol to a whole dram, to the pint of water: But, for the conveniency of my patients, I generally give it in the following manner: That they may not have trouble in preparing the medicine, I dissolve an ounce of white vitriol in four ounces of water, and desire the patient to put a teaspoonful of it to a common sized tea-cupful of water. Of this he is to throw up two or three small syringefuls, five or six times a day, keeping in the injection for some time by grasping the fore-part of the penis with his hand. This operation is easier performed than described, and can be better done by the patient himself than by any one else.[14]

The preparation of an astringent injection is carefully demystified here as Buchan explains how to prepare the treatment before putting 'a teaspoonful of it to a common sized tea-cupful of water'. As the solution is made using objects that are readily available in the domestic setting, such as 'a common sized' teacup, Buchan foregrounds for his reader how a cure can be self-administered in private and with some ease using common household objects. The 'tea-cup' also symbolises the fashionable practice of polite conversation over a cup of tea or a dish of coffee. Here Buchan, in, perhaps, a calculated way, gestures towards the impolite gossip that the infected man might excite in publicly seeking out the services of a quack. Buchan's *Observations* reminds men that administering a cure in private will protect their reputational health as well as their physical condition; reading here amounts to a protective practice, which upholds the myth of male impenetrability.

Moreover, in describing the injection, Buchan lingers on the disconcerting intimacy of the prolonged and frequent touch that is required to administer the cure. Not only is it the man's genitalia that is touched but the most sensitive part of his genitalia – 'the fore-part of the penis' – that must be 'grasp[ed]'by the 'hand' in order to inject the solution into the urethra a number of times a day. In this passage, the image of the doctor's hands is invoked only to be immediately expelled by Buchan's assertion that 'This operation is easier performed than described, and can be better done by the patient himself than by any one else'. What would ordinarily be an intrusive and emasculating procedure under the hands of a doctor, is instead framed as a simple operation that is best done by the hands of the patient himself. Buchan's *Observations* firmly invests the man who suffers from venereal disease with agency in his own sexual health. Dispelling fears about being subjected to financial, physical and reputational damage under the hands of a doctor that we find in texts like Daniel Turner's *A Practical Dissertation on Venereal Disease*, Buchan imagines a 'man of common sense' who, gleaning instruction from the pages of his *Observations*, can learn to identify an infection early, formulate a cure and administer it all within the privacy of his own lodgings. Undergirding Buchan's writing is a view of men as being autonomous, sovereign and able subjects. Whereas earlier treatises like Turner's communicated the close relationship between debility and venereal infection, even to the point of describing how possible cures could be debilitating in and of themselves, Buchan's intervention, much like the medical self-instruction presented in his earlier *Domestic Medicine* (1769),[15] is keen to stress how men might be empowered to protect themselves from medical misinformation and to privately overcome such infection and, by extension, the chronic debility and reputational ruin that it engenders.

Roderick Random and the sentimentality of sexual health

The kind of male agency that William Buchan peddles in his *Observations* has an earlier, albeit overlooked, cultural life in the form of the novel. In *Roderick Random*, Tobias Smollett offers his reader a central protagonist – Roderick Random – who models agency over his own sexual health and the health of others, particularly women, by taking venereal matters literally into his own hands. If by the close of the eighteenth century, medical authors like William Buchan were promoting men's sexual agency over the financial, reputational and bodily ruination frequently wrought by venereal disease, then earlier in the period, novelists like Tobias Smollett were ventilating questions of men's understanding of medical knowledge and sexual health in their own writing. The question of embodiment is central to Smollett's prose fiction. As Aileen Douglas argues in *Uneasy Sensations: Smollett and the Body* (1995), Smollett in '*Roderick Random* makes the definition of the human body an issue, insists that the body is not naturally social, and says that even strong relationships are often impaired by our unstable physicality'.[16] As a non-practising physician turned novelist, Smollett exploits the body in his fiction as a palimpsest for cultural and political conflict while also demonstrating, through characters like Roderick Random, how male embodiment is always already enmeshed in social perceptions of men's physical ability: to be legible as a man is to be able-bodied. In my reading of the novel, I show how Roderick's relationship with Nancy Williams, a sex worker who is destitute and suffering from a raging venereal distemper, instances a crucial moment in the novel in which a shared recognition of mutual corporeal instability works, not to impair a relationship, but to strengthen it. In encountering Miss Williams, Roderick's behaviour examples a practice of care towards her – and towards himself – that enacts the kind of agency over one's sexual and reputational health that Buchan champions in his *Observations* (1796) and in his earlier *Domestic Medicine* (1769). This oft overlooked moment in *Roderick Random* utilises the sentimental mode to model an ethics of care in relation to sexual health, which narrativises male agency over the debilitating effects of venereal maladies.

Roderick examples Buchan's later 'man of common understanding' in so much as his eight-month apprenticeship with Mr Lavement, a Huguenot apothecary, affords him ample opportunity to grow in 'industry and knowledge',[17] while also, crucially, observing the deceptive nature of Lavement's commercial trade in venereal treatments:

> He had a great deal of business; but as he was mostly employ'd among his fellow refugees, his profits were small. – However, his expence for medicines was not great, he being the most expert man at a succedaneum, of any

apothecary in London, so that I have been sometimes amaz'd to see him without the least hesitation, make up a physician's prescription, though he had not in his shop one medicine mention'd in it.[18]

Roderick's observation of Lavement's dealings chimes somewhat with Buchan's later assertion in his *Observations* that many quick apothecary 'cures' merely heal a venereal sore while 'the poison has been taken into system, it is only *shutting the door while the thief is in the house*'.[19] Lavement's 'cures' for venereal disease are ineffective because they are inauthentically composed. Buchan is keen to stress how most apothecary remedies are indeed inauthentic as they effect only cosmetic changes. Moreover, Smollett's depiction of Mr Lavement, and later support for Miss Williams, resonates with Buchan's warnings against the reputational and physical harm bound up with apothecaries who proffer venereal cures. In many ways, Roderick's education during his journeymanship also, by extension, offers an education to Smollett's male reader on the hazards of investing in apothecary treatments. Reflecting on Lavement's venereal disease treatment, Roderick relates that:

> there was one for the venereal disease, that brought him a good deal of money; and this he conceal'd so artfully from me, that I could never learn its composition: But during the eight months I stay'd in his service, he was so unfortunate in the use of it, that three parts in four of those who took it, were fain to confirm the cure with a salivation under the direction of another doctor.[20]

Roderick's interest in Lavement's undisclosed composition for his venereal disease treatment is purely a monetary one as, through careful observation, Roderick has ascertained that the treatment does not work; it has failed to stop the distemper running its course and statistically 'three parts in four' of the men who seek it out end up with a confirmed pox and must therefore undergo another treatment under the hands of yet another practitioner. The 'industry and knowledge' that Roderick gains is bound up with the dual realisation that men seeking venereal treatments can be entirely exploited for financial gain and that in matters of venereal treatment it is ultimately better to take matters into one's own hands.

When Roderick is forced out of Lavement's service by the conspiratorial machinations of Squire Gawky and the apothecary's daughter, he somewhat ironically discovers that he himself has contracted a venereal distemper:

> Thus I found myself, by the iniquity of mankind, in a much more deplorable condition than ever: for though I had been formerly as poor, my reputation was without blemish, and my health unimpaired till now; – but at present my good name was lost, my money gone, my friends were alienated, my body infected by a distemper contracted in the course of an amour.[21]

Tarnished by the slander of his former co-inhabitants, without employment, and now in the full grip of venereal infection, Roderick's predicament instances the kind of moment in Smollett's prose fiction in which, as Aileen Douglas argues, the definition of the human body is problematised. Friendless, without financial support, and suffering from a venereal distemper, Roderick, and by extension Smollett's reader, is prompted to confront the stark limitations of male reputational prestige in a world in which the body is vulnerable and wholly subject to debilitating infection. Curiously, Smollett does not allow the reader to zone in on Roderick's newfound vulnerability as it is at this precise moment in the novel that Miss Williams's own suffering gets foregrounded. Any possible sympathy that the reader might have for Roderick's own miserable condition is quickly transposed onto the character of Miss Williams as Roderick's hopeless passivity gets exchanged for decisive action as he responds to Miss Williams's infirmity by running downstairs and dispatching his landlady 'to a chymist's shop for some cinnamon-water' for the patient.[22] We are told that Nancy Williams had 'put herself into the hands of an advertising doctor, who having fleeced her of all the money she had, or could procure, left her three days ago in a worse condition than that in which he found her; – that except the cloaths on her back, she had pawned or sold every thing that belonged to her, to satisfy that rapacious quack'.[23] The ruin of venereal disease is sentimentalised by Smollett as through Miss Williams an injured femininity, rather than a pugnacious masculinity, becomes the signifier of the disease.

Assuming the role of apothecary, Roderick proposes to Williams 'that she should lodge in the same room ... which would save some money; and assured her I would myself undertake her cure as well as my own, during which she should partake of all the conveniences I could afford to myself'.[24] Through a sentimentalised fictive account of a sex worker suffering from venereal disease, Smollett showcases an ethics of care between Roderick and his patient, Miss Williams, which allows Roderick to exercise agency over his own sexual health while also treating a less fortunate case than his own. Roderick's infection and the threat that it poses to his own reputational and physical health gets subsumed here into his charitable administration of a cure for his 'careful nurse'[25] and, simultaneously, for himself. Roderick as nurse to Nancy Williams might suggest his emasculation only for the fact that, in this instance, such action exchanges his own vulnerability for practical assertion. Roderick and Nancy lodge in two separate dwellings while undergoing treatment (a situation that contradicts Roderick's proposal that they will lodge in the same room), and the two-month long regime is interrupted at one point by Nancy's arrest and wrongful transportation to Marshalsea. Smollett's account of this arrangement between Roderick and Nancy is taken up by Nancy's telling of her own chequered past; there is no information given about the kind of treatment that Roderick is administering. On one level, Nancy's venereal disease treatment and recovery works as a plot device to allow her to voice her own history on her own terms. In doing so, she reveals how her 'nocturnal adventures' led to her becoming 'infected with the disease', while later, she surmises that 'the most fashionable woman of the town is as liable to contagion'.[26] Yet, however sympathetic the reader might be to Miss Williams's plight, her reformation in the 'homely garb of a country wench'[27] can only ever be plausible if she is fully cured of her venereal distemper. Though we are not given details about how Roderick effects his cure, we can conjecture that the use of water, readily available in the lodging, is likely involved. As Annika Mann notes, Tobias Smollett 'published only one medical text in his lifetime', namely his *Essay on the External Use of Water*, which 'advocates bathing in pure rather than mineral water to purge the body of waste matter'.[28] In his *Essay*, Smollett alludes to venereal disease twice. Firstly, he evokes venereal chancres when he mentions the usefulness of water in wounds that have 'become *fistulous*, from the nature of their situation, such as those in the Urethra', and secondly, when he lists 'venereal Distemper' as one of the ailments that is eased by a 'warm Bath'.[29] Whether or not Roderick cures himself and Nancy by the external use of water (he requests cinnamon water initially), we are nonetheless told that he 'attended her with such care and success, that in less than two months, her health, as well as my own, was perfectly re-established'.[30] Undergirding this vignette, in which Nancy Williams voices her history, is the quieter performance of Roderick not only listening in sympathy – within an ethics of care – but also actively modelling for the reader an example of a man using his own book learning and common sense to intervene in, and prevent, the socially ruinous and physically debilitating effects of venereal disease. Smollett's portrayal of Roderick instances how reading and observation can both be protective practices in curing Miss Williams, while his charitable action upholds the myth of male invulnerability and strong social prestige.

James Boswell's *London Journal* as illness narrative

If Smollett's *Roderick Random* promotes agency in the face of debilitating venereal disease, then non-fictive eighteenth-century accounts, such as James Boswell's diary entries on his gonorrhoea infection, foreground crisis rather than cure. Such crisis invites a reading of the *London Journal* (1762–63) as an illness narrative which involves thinking about his anxious account of gonorrhoea infection as multifaceted; Boswell, in his own account, is less a man of 'common understanding' in Buchan's terms, and more like a man plagued with anxiety about the financial damages that attend infection. Scholarly writing about Boswell's melancholy, or anxiety, is not new. Allan Ingram's *Boswell's Creative Gloom: A Study of Imagery and Melancholy in the Writings of James Boswell* (1982) was ground-breaking in its book-length focus on melancholia and in exploring how 'Boswell uses imagery ... in order to project himself onto the world, but he also uses it to look inwards and to attempt to achieve a greater understanding of himself'.[31] However, approaching his life writing as an illness narrative does signal a departure, because it dispenses with moralistic views of his life as being characterised by failed self-regulations and troubling excesses, while also moving away from diagnosis or medicalisation as an analytic outcome. Boswell has been variously read as an alcoholic, as a hypochondriac and as a sex addict. Lennard J. Davis reads him as an obsessive; for Davis, Boswell's writing partakes in 'a defining moment, beginning in the middle of the eighteenth century in England and France' 'when obsession becomes itself something so problematic that people begin to write about it, study it, turn it into a medical problem, and then try to cure it'.[32] In my reading of the *London Journal*, I show how Boswell orientates his writing towards the realisation of his own health – a mental and physical health that is premised on able-bodied and hetero-compulsory norms.

As Stella Bolaki notes in *Illness as Many Narratives* (2016), an illness narrative is defined as 'illness stories or narratives [which give] expression to the subjective or lived experience of a particular disease or condition, which is distinct from the clinical definition of disease understood as an organic dysfunction within biomedicine'.[33] In his *Journal*, Boswell gives textual expression to his experiences of illness, both physical and mental, in ways that exceed period-specific medical definition. Of course, some of his conditions are more readily assimilated into disease narratives than others. Boswell's contraction of gonorrhoea is a case in point. However, while the infection itself is described in terms of a 'distemper', or disease, with physical symptoms, 'a little heat in the members of my body sacred to Cupid', it is, at first, described in terms that relate to Boswell's subjective anxiety-ridden experience of the disease, when he narrates how he 'began to feel an unaccountable alarm of unexpected evil'.[34]

More precisely, Boswell's monitoring of his sexually transmitted disease through his journal writing exceeds the disease's own narrative parameters. His distemper has an affective reach that moves beyond the bodily discomfort it engenders. When his infection is confirmed it is by his doctor-friend, Douglas, who tells Boswell that he has an 'evident infection and that the woman who gave it [to him] could not but know of it'.[35] Boswell's account of the diagnosis exemplifies an illness narrative for the direct way that it separates out the clinical experience of the disease from the subjective one. In his journal entry, Boswell figuratively splits his doctor Douglas from his friend Douglas when he writes:

> And here let me make a just and true observation, which is that the same man as a friend and as a surgeon exhibits two very opposite characters. Douglas as a friend is most kind, most anxious for my interest, made me live ten days in his house, and suggested every plan of economy. But Douglas as a surgeon will be as ready to keep me long under his hands, and as desirous to lay hold of my money, as any man. In short, his views alter quite. I have to do not with him but his profession.[36]

What is most apparent is that Boswell distrusts not his friend, but his friend's *profession* and the misinformation that the profession peddles. He does not believe that his doctor will prioritise his health above his own monetary interests. From this point on in the *Journal*, Boswell makes clear the divide between his own experience of his illness and the surgeon's diagnosis of his distemper; his illness, and, by extension, his own reputation, must be managed away from the medical profession, which he perceives distorts truth for its own financial gain.

Others have argued that Boswell's journal writing exposes cycles of failed self-regulation. As Susan Manning notes, '[his] Journals are the long record of his unsuccessful struggle to subject the vagaries of his own character to a "long habit of philosophical discipline," to *impose* unity and regularity on the wayward motions of his mind'.[37] Manning's Boswell consistently sets himself up for failure; he is the author of his own malaise, investing himself in the Enlightenment's pervasive ethical project of self-improvement, only to realise, and then textually record, his inability to be *disciplined*. According to Manning, 'we read Boswell for the naked candour with which his writing identifies, subscribes to, and repeatedly fails to enact, this power of choice and enlightened self-interest over behaviour'.[38] Manning moralises when she isolates 'the least edifying "pleasures of Boswell"', namely 'the melancholy cycle of his repeated "lapses" into drunkenness and verbal and sexual incontinence, ... which the journals attempt to write out of the existence of the "composed" character'.[39] If we as readers take pleasure in Boswell's 'impermissible "pleasures"', Manning assures that such pleasure is at the level of structure and style, not spectacle; readerly pleasure is derived not from our enjoyment of Boswell's inebriations and sexual improprieties but instead from the ways in which Boswell attempts to 'expunge' these episodes from his text.[40] Within the very rhythm of Boswellian prose is a paradoxical impulse to record the facts of one's deviation as a means of effacing such deviation.

Diagnosing Boswell as a depressive addict – addicted to sex and to alcohol – Manning argues that his records of depression, drunkenness and debauchery feature in his narrative as 'vessels with holes through which meaning has leaked away'; the documentation of such leakage serves to recuperate, if only in narrative, that which is materially unrecuperable: the condition of idleness, drunken debaucheries and the fleeting pleasures of casual sex. Following Manning, it might be tempting to consider Boswell's self-documenting of melancholia as forming a textual space in which meaning has 'leaked away'.[41] My reading refutes the idea that Boswell's writing on his pleasures and his melancholia signifies his attempt to write away, or write out, such deviation. Far from being textual black holes, devoid of meaning, such accounts emerge as being productive of the very kind of reputational and myth-making strategies that shore up Boswell's identity as a white, bourgeois and able-bodied man in 1760s Britain.

The distinction between Manning's reading of Boswell's writing and my own centres on the difference between *oscillation* and *orientation*. Whereas Manning sees Boswell as addictively swinging between sin and reformation, pleasure and abstinence, noting how every 'failure leads only to a further reiteration of the same attempt',[42] we might instead focus on how, in writing his *London Journal*, Boswell *orientates* himself in private self-narration to offload and protect himself from reputational damage. It is tempting to focus, as Manning does, on the pendulum dynamic of the *London Journal*; however, such a focus obscures the steadying orientation that underwrites all textual oscillation. As Sara Ahmed notes, in her book *Queer Phenomenology* (2006), 'compulsory heterosexuality operates as a straightening device, which rereads signs of queer desire as deviations from the straight line'.[43] Ahmed's comment on compulsory straightness reminds us that orientation produces its own kinks: namely, for Boswell, an adherence to those parallel straight lines of compulsory heterosexuality and public sociability and able-bodiedness traced in his *London Journal*. While Boswell's writerly voice swings between anxiety and calm, he remains orientated toward his own contentment. Such moments of ease have been curiously left out of readings of the anxious Boswell. For example, we can see this in his journal entry on 12 December 1762 in which he recounts having his 'feet washed with milk-warm water' and going to bed 'to sleep soft and contented'.[44] Having his feet washed was one of Boswell's favourite pastimes; the sensuality that this experience involves, I think, is beautifully evoked by the detail that the water is 'milk-warm'. The orientation away from melancholy toward mirth, is also an orientation towards able-bodiedness in so much as heightened states of acute anxiety incapacitate him. On 11 December 1762, he writes:

> The truth is with regard to me, about the age of seventeen I had a very severe illness. I became very melancholy. I imagined that I was never to get rid of it. I gave myself up as devoted to misery. I entertained a most gloomy and odd way of thinking. I was much hurt at being good for nothing in life. ... Many a struggle was in my mind between melancholy and mirth.[45]

In this candid admission, Boswell locates his self-recognition of his mental illness as occurring during his adolescence. When such melancholy inevitably returns to overwhelm in adulthood, Boswell narrates it in terms of his ability, not debility:

> Tuesday 4 January: 'I thought my slender diet weakened me. I resolved to live hearty and be stout. This afternoon I became very low-spirited. I sat in close. I hated all things. I almost hated London. O miserable absurdity! I could see nothing in a good light. I just submitted and hoped to get the better of this.'[46]

In this written account, his melancholy is contained in the past; it is temporally secure, but it is still productive of meaning. This account is not a vessel, which *leaks meaning*; rather it is a biographical orientation point that holds significance as an indication of that which can be overcome. Although the passage reveals his submission to melancholy, the final line reorientates Boswell, and his reader, to face a future when he hopes 'to [have got] the better of this'. Whatever the discernible black spots, whatever the kinks in the line, Boswell's orientation is always towards ability, or, in his own words, 'to live hearty and be stout'.

Yet, Boswell's strategy to 'get the better of this [melancholia]' is not only tied to able-bodiedness but also to homosocial reputation and to his own conceptions of manliness. Boswell conceives of his melancholia in terms of his own masculinity and the masculinities of other men. He writes about how his friend, Erskine, 'goes upon system, which is just to keep himself as easy and happy as he can, and to make the best of everything'.[47] On his friendship with Erskine, he writes: 'Being with Erskine gives me a simplicity of sentiment and makes me very easy as to what men in general make such a work about'.[48] Yet when other male friends, like James Macdonald, learn of Boswell's submission to Erskine's affective 'system', they question it as an effective choice for any man:

> When [Macdonald] heard Erskine's sentiments (which, by the by, are much my own, and which I mentioned just to see what he would say), he was perfectly stunned. 'Why', says he, 'he must not be a man.'[49]

Boswell, too, accepts that Erskine's indifference is somehow suspect, yet he resolves:

> to have a degree of Erskine's indifference, to make me easy when things go cross; and a degree of Macdonald's eagerness for real life, to make me relish

things when they go well. ... The great art I have to study is to balance those two very different ways of thinking properly.[50]

To be a fashionable man in 1760s Britain is to adhere to homo and hetero sociability, yet Erskine's modelling of self-care emerges as a kink in the straight line, which Boswell resolves to straighten out by reorientating himself toward a balance between Erskine's unmanly inaction and Macdonald's manly action. Boswell must balance the taking of health advice with his own reputation as a man. As with the earlier reading of *Roderick Random*, in health matters reputation matters more.

Boswell's *London Journal* is a particularly useful text for thinking about intersections of illness narrative: namely, experiences of venereal infection and mental health. Sexual intercourse makes him the most anxious, and it is in the arena of sexuality that physical and mental illness intersect for Boswell.[51] He is anxious for his ability to be proven and he is anxious that he will not be able enough to 'act the vigorous part'.[52] His gonorrhoea infection brings the connections between compulsory able-bodiedness and compulsory heterosociability into sharp relief. Boswell's account of his infection with 'Signor Gonorrhoea'[53] demonstrates how sexual infection disorientates trajectories that align with compulsory able-bodiedness and heterosociability; to suffer the distemper, and its treatment in confinement, is to also to suffer deviation, however unwilling, from these injunctions to be seen and to be capable. While scholars have correctly read syphilis and gonorrhoea as fashionable diseases of the rake and his lifestyle, Boswell's private diary account of his distemper reminds us not only of the reputational perils that subtend fashionable infection but also how the mode of cure upsets injunctions to sociability and ability that inform the myth of masculinity.[54] We might in this instance think of Boswell's infected penis as the leaky vessel that goes unacknowledged in Manning's reading. Recovering Boswell's intimate relationship with his own body reveals the illness narratives that orientate his life and his writings.

Detailing his gonorrhoea infection, Boswell describes the leakage as the 'deep-tinged loathsome matter', which 'are the strongest proofs of an infection'.[55] This moment becomes the occasion for Boswell to display the strongest proof of his masculinity and able-bodiedness. Reflecting on his interview with Louisa, the woman he claims infected him, he writes: 'During all this conversation I really behaved with a manly composure and polite dignity that could not fail to inspire an awe, and she was pale as ashes and trembled and faltered'.[56] Far from practising the kind of ethics of care that Roderick exhibits towards Mrs Williams, Boswell's encounter with Louisa amounts to a selfish rejection of the sexual partner; it is not about care but rather about shoring up possible reputational damage in the face of the woman who he believes penetrated him by infecting him. For Boswell, while he does not take matters into his own hands like Roderick, his infection, far from leaking meaning, instead necessitates the reinvestment of meaning as the very discharge of the distemper gets reimagined in his *London Journal* as the sublime textual site upon which to reorientate its author, and his reader, toward reputational and physical protection.

As I have argued in this chapter, across the varied eighteenth-century accounts of venereal disease that emerge in David Turner's and William Buchan's medical literature, Tobias Smollett's fiction and James Boswell's life writing, we are consistently shown how infection and its treatment raises broader concerns for men and women about the class of practitioners who offer medical assistance and about what receiving treatment will realistically mean for one's reputational and physical health. For Smollett, men can master their own sexual health and avoid the ruinous reputational consequences of a doctor who peddles misinformation about the disease and its cure. In all of the cases parsed here, eighteenth-century accounts of venereal disease provide a textual space for men to think through the charged relationship between their own prized virility and potential for debility. As these narrative examples have shown, for a man to be infected with the pox is also somehow to unwittingly confront the demands placed upon the maintenance of masculinity itself. On the one hand, as Boswell bemoans, infection opens up the common man to a world of misinformation, myth and potential reputational ruin, yet as Buchan and Smollett attest, such an infectious world is also one in which reading itself can become a protective practice.

Notes

1 Noelle Gallagher, *Itch, Clap, Pox: Venereal Disease in the Eighteenth-Century Imagination* (New Haven, CT: Yale University Press, 2018), p. 5.
2 All references are to the 1724 edition of Daniel Turner's *Syphilis: A Practical Dissertation on the Venereal Disease* (London: Walthoe, 1724), which was accessed in print at the British Library, London.
3 Turner, *Syphilis*, pp. 1–2.
4 Ibid.
5 Ibid.
6 For primary and secondary materials that address female experiences of venereal disease see: Samuel Solomon, *A Guide to Health, or, Advice to Both Sexes, to Obtain a Radical and Permanent Cure for those Secret Infirmities of Nature which Delicacy often Forbid to Disclose* (London: Printed for the author, [1796?]); Ann Lewis and Markman Ellis (eds), *Prostitution and*

Eighteenth-Century Culture: Sex, Commerce and Morality (London: Pickering and Chatto, 2012).
7   William Buchan, *Observations Concerning the Prevention and Cure of the Venereal Disease. Intended to Guard the Ignorant and Unwary Against the Baneful Effects of that Insidious Malady* (Dublin: Wogan, 1796), pp. 3–4. This edition was accessed in print at the British Library.
8   Ibid.
9   Ibid., p. 4.
10 Ibid., p. 11.
11 Ibid.
12 Ibid., pp. 19–20.
13 Ibid., p. 28.
14 Ibid., p. 41.
15 William Buchan, *Domestic Medicine; or, the Family Physician [...] Chiefly Calculated to Recommend a Proper Attention to Regimen and Simple Medicines* (Edinburgh: Balfour, 1769).
16 Aileen Douglas, *Uneasy Sensations: Smollett and the Body* (Chicago, IL: University of Chicago Press, 1995), p. 56.
17 Tobias Smollett, *The Adventures of Roderick Random*, ed. Paul Gabriel-Boucé (Oxford: Oxford University Press, 1999 [1748]), p. 100.
18 Ibid.
19 Buchan, *Observations*, p. 99.
20 Smollett, *Roderick Random*, p. 100.
21 Ibid., p. 114.
22 Ibid., p. 116.
23 Ibid.
24 Ibid., pp. 116–117.
25 Ibid., p. 117.
26 Ibid., pp. 136, 137.
27 Ibid., p. 138.
28 Annika Mann, *Reading Contagion: The Hazards of Reading in the Age of Print* (Charlottesville, VA: University of Virginia Press, 2018), p. 84.
29 Tobias Smollett, *An Essay on the External Use of Water*, ed. Claude E. Jones (Baltimore, MD: Johns Hopkins University Press, 1935), p. 55.
30 Smollett, *Roderick Random*, p. 138.
31 Allan Ingram, *Boswell's Creative Gloom: A Study of Imagery and Melancholy in the Writings of James Boswell* (London and Basingstoke: Macmillan, 1982), p. iii.
32 Lennard J. Davis, *Obsession: A History* (Chicago, IL and London: University of Chicago Press, 2008), p. 6.
33 Stella Bolaki, *Illness as Many Narratives: Arts, Medicine and Culture* (Edinburgh: Edinburgh University Press, 2016), pp. 3–4.
34 James Boswell, *Boswell's London Journal, 1762–1763*, ed. Frederick A. Pottle (Melbourne: Heinemann, 1950), 18 January 1763, p. 149.
35 Ibid., 20 January 1763, p. 157.

36 Ibid., pp. 157–158.
37 Susan Manning, 'Boswell's Pleasures, the Pleasures of Boswell', *British Journal for Eighteenth-Century Studies* 20:1 (1997): 17–32, at 17.
38 Ibid.
39 Ibid.
40 Ibid., p. 18.
41 Ibid., p. 23.
42 Ibid., p. 25.
43 Sara Ahmed, *Queer Phenomenology: Orientations, Objects, Others* (Durham, NC and London: Duke University Press, 2006), p. 23.
44 Boswell, *London Journal*, p. 81.
45 Ibid., pp. 77–78.
46 Ibid., p. 120.
47 Ibid., 11 December 1762, p. 78.
48 Ibid.
49 Ibid., p. 79.
50 Ibid., 2 January 1763, p. 79.
51 Sex makes Boswell anxious: 'I was a little uneasy at this, though it could not be helped. It kept me longer anxious till my ability was known. I have, together with my vivacity and good-humour, a great anxiety of temper which often renders me uneasy. My grandfather had it in a very strong degree'. Ibid., 7 January 1763, p. 126.
52 Ibid., 2 January 1763, p. 118.
53 Ibid., 19 January 1763, p. 155.
54 For syphilis as a fashionable disease see: Emily Cock, 'The *à la Mode* Disease: Syphilis and Temporality', in Allan Ingram and Leigh Wetherall Dickson (eds), *Disease and Death in Eighteenth-Century Literature and Culture: Fashioning the Unfashionable* (Houndsmill: Palgrave Macmillan, 2016), pp. 57–75.
55 Boswell, *London Journal*, 20 January 1763, p. 156.
56 Ibid., p. 160.

7

Sir Anthony Carlisle's gothic (medical) intervention: carving the criminal body in *The Horrors of Oakendale Abbey*

Bethany Brigham

Until 1832 there was simply no sufficient supply of dead bodies for the teaching and study of human anatomy in England. Debated at popular, medical and parliamentary levels, the anatomy issue was finally addressed by the Anatomy Act, which secured a supply of subjects for dissection, a supply made up of those unfortunate enough to die in a hospital or workhouse and go unclaimed by friends and relatives.[1] As there were few alternatives prior to the 1832 Bill, private anatomy schools and teaching hospitals contended for the anatomical subjects provided by the body snatcher. The sheer extent of the demand for these stolen bodies was documented by the body snatcher Joshua Naples, who in *The Diary of a Resurrectionist, 1811–1812* (1896), recorded the transactional history of the body-trafficking trade. The Royal College of Surgeons published this rare inside perspective of the body-snatching era long after the trade had been eradicated and strategically framed the diary with an account of the period leading up to the anatomy reform assembled by James Blake Bailey, the college's librarian. While Bailey claimed the history was appended to the diary to make it 'more interesting', the publication allowed the college to authoritatively navigate, and subsequently reclaim, the narrative surrounding the Anatomy Act.[2] Indeed, *The Diary of a Resurrectionist* is significant as a medically sanctioned intervention that attempted to reaffirm the necessity of anatomy reform by outlining the myth and misinformation that surrounded the activities of the medical practitioner during the body-snatching era.

Yet, the history constructed by Bailey is itself an interwoven fabric of newspaper articles, committee reports, medical discourse and literature such as the gothic-inflected tales of Samuel Warren's *Passages from the Diary of a Late Physician* (1830–37).[3] An indiscriminate blend of 'fact' and fiction, Bailey's account demonstrates that no comprehensive examination of the anatomy debates can dispense with gothic fiction. Literary scholars have considered the way in which gothic fiction tied anatomy practices to criminality and murder, suggesting that the genre reflected and magnified the public's distrust of medical practice and their fear of body snatching. For example, Tim Marshall places both editions of *Frankenstein* (1818/1831) alongside the anatomy debates in order to suggest that Mary Shelley's novel, which conspicuously features an undead being made up of body-snatched criminals and paupers, 'voices the social perception that it is the surgeons who murder to dissect'.[4] The years immediately preceding the Anatomy Act were certainly coloured by the medical establishment's implication in incidents of 'Burking', a popular phrase that alludes to the infamous spate of murders carried out by William Burke alongside William Hare in 1828. The murders were committed so that the men could sell the bodies of their victims to the Edinburgh anatomists and their actions – along with the 'Burking' carried out by Thomas Williams, John Bishop and James May in London just three years later – propelled the passing of the Anatomy Act.[5] However, Marshall also suggests that by confirming the 'nationwide phobia about "body snatching" possibilities', *Frankenstein* 'assembles the case' to end the horrors of the body-snatching era by legislative means, highlighting gothic fiction's alternate position as a means of intervention that substantiated the medical establishment's anatomy rhetoric.[6] Building on Marshall's claim, this chapter addresses the gothic's role within the anatomy debates by positing 'Mrs Carver's' *The Horrors of Oakendale Abbey* (1797) as a similar means of gothic (medical) intervention that, like *Frankenstein* and *The Diary of a Resurrectionist*, made the case for reform.[7]

First published anonymously by William Lane's Minerva Press, *The Horrors of Oakendale Abbey* was subsequently attached to the author 'Mrs Carver' by the Minerva Library Catalogue of 1814, alongside three other novels: *Elizabeth: A Novel* (1797), *The Legacy: A Novel* (1798) and *The Old Woman* (1800).[8] This particular author is significant, as Don Shelton claims that 'Mrs Carver' was the pseudonym of an established surgeon and anatomist, Sir Anthony Carlisle (1764–1840), a man with a vested interest in the anatomy issue. Little has been done to assess the broader implications of this claim, yet as noted by Shelton, *The Horrors of Oakendale Abbey* is a 'rare and knowledgeable' source on body snatching, veined through with detailed medical knowledge.[9] *The Horrors of Oakendale Abbey* centres on the heroine Laura, who is imprisoned in the abandoned Oakendale Abbey by its aristocratic owner. Hoping to seduce the young orphan, Lord Oakendale believes that the seclusion and horrors of the building will 'sooner dispose a mind, like hers, to coincide with his wishes'.[10] When Laura receives keys to the abbey, she finds the rooms littered with corpses, skeletons and the walking undead, which she assumes are 'artful delusions' laid out by Lord Oakendale (41). However, the Bluebeard's-castle-style format transforms when she discovers that the abbey has been commandeered as a dissection theatre where body snatchers covertly deliver bodies. Grounded in the medical realities of late eighteenth-century England, the 'Carver' novel is therefore a fitting focus for this chapter, as its textual intervention becomes increasingly evident when positioned alongside debates taking place at the time of the novel's conception, and when the medical background of its potential author is taken into account.

The anatomy debates have been rigorously examined by Ruth Richardson in her seminal work *Death, Dissection and the Destitute* (1987), which understandably focuses on the first few decades of the nineteenth century when body snatching and 'Burking' became an undeniably visible feature of English culture as those involved with the anatomy trade increasingly found themselves facing prison sentences, fines and hard labour. However, notable attempts to resolve the anatomy issue and to address body snatching were also made before the turn of the nineteenth century. As stated by Richard Ward, the late eighteenth century represents 'a particular moment when the claims of medical science competed with those of criminal justice in harnessing the power of the criminal corpse'.[11] Those found wanting both morally and judicially could consequently find themselves destined for the anatomist's table, a precedent set by the Murder Act of 1752, which made anatomisation the post-execution punishment for murderers. Throughout the anatomy debates, various alternatives to body snatching were hotly debated, including offering the bodies of prostitutes, suicides or those who came to their death by duelling, prize-fighting, and drunkenness up to the anatomy schools.[12] Such suggestions confirmed the association between anatomy, immorality and criminal punishment; indeed, anatomisation symbolised a social, legal and medical death, making dissection a particularly disturbing prospect for the English public. Despite widespread outrage towards body snatching, popular aversion toward dissection thus slowed the enactment of anatomy legislation long into the nineteenth century, leaving practitioners with little choice but to fight for further criminal bodies at the gallows or pay the increasingly high fees demanded by the 'resurrection men'. However, the late eighteenth century remains significant as a moment when political debates about how to deal with body snatching subsequently informed parliamentary discussions regarding the type of offences that should qualify criminals for the post-execution punishment of dissection.

While many medical practitioners sought to avoid the publicity that would come with legislation and preferred to obtain bodies by 'authorised stealth', when Sir Robert Peel questioned several surgeons about their preferred source of supply for anatomical subjects in 1823, most of the anatomists concurred with the idea of extending dissection to all criminals.[13] Carlisle made his own position in this debate very clear, raising emphatic objections about dissecting the poor who, he claimed, would only come to fear the hospital or workhouse.[14] Carlisle instead suggested that a 'programme of economy' would allow criminal bodies to become a viable solution to the anatomy issue, a view that is certainly relevant to a consideration of *The Horrors of Oakendale Abbey* as gothic (medical) intervention.[15] Joining the themes of body snatching and anatomy with the spectacle of the criminal corpse, 'Mrs Carver' both conspicuously addresses the concerns of late eighteenth-century English society and manipulates gothic convention to meet medical demand. This chapter will therefore position *The Horrors of Oakendale Abbey* within the anatomy debate by positing the Minerva Press novel as a uniquely qualified vehicle for disseminating the anatomy argument of a medical practitioner like Carlisle. I will then examine the ways in which 'Carver' foregrounds the pressing need for reform by constructing popular beliefs surrounding death and anatomy practices as a form of myth and misinformation that facilitated body snatching and that proved a barrier to legislative change. Finally, this chapter will demonstrate that, in *The Horrors of Oakendale Abbey*, 'Carver' posits the criminal body as both central to the advancement of medical knowledge and as a viable alternative to body snatching, thus offering a suitably gothic solution to the 1790s anatomy debate.

Minerva Press and the author-anatomist

Sir Anthony Carlisle took a position as surgeon at Westminster Hospital in 1793, embarking on what would prove to be a successful and varied medical career. An esteemed anatomist and scientist, he was President of the Royal College of Surgeons in 1828 and 1837 and an elected Fellow of the Royal Society.[16] Carlisle was a pioneer of medical advancement: he was the first to make surgical use of the carpenter's saw and he substituted the clumsy and crooked knife generally used in amputations with a thin, straight-edge blade.[17] No stranger to the arts, Carlisle was also a student of the Royal Academy, where he later acted as Professor of Anatomy for sixteen years.[18] His 'sensational lectures were the talk of the town', and one even reportedly brought William Hazlitt to the point of fainting when a human brain and a heart were passed around on dinner plates.[19] A purveyor of gothic showmanship, Carlisle makes a fitting author-anatomist. As noted by Shelton, even the pseudonym 'Mrs Carver' appears to be a playful reference to his position as the carver of bodies.[20]

Over the course of his forty-seven-year career, Carlisle boasted of high-ranking patients such as the Duke of Gloucester and the Prince Regent (later George IV).[21] However, Carlisle's position at Westminster Hospital was voluntary, and he would have certainly welcomed another source of income while building his professional reputation and more lucrative private practice. Robert Southey's correspondence suggests that Carlisle looked beyond the medical establishment for this subsistence. A letter from Southey to Hugh Chudleigh Standert – a surgeon with literary inclinations – states that Carlisle 'introduced me to *The Critical* in 1798, & I wrote some years for it at the low rate of three guineas per sheet'.[22] Southey's reference to writing reviews for *The Critical Review or, Annals of Literature* – first edited by yet another literary surgeon, Tobias Smollett – points to Carlisle's entanglement with the world of low-paid hack writing in the period when the 'Carver' novels were being published. Southey also notably explored the problem of body snatching in his 1797 ballad 'Mary', which tells the tale of the eponymous maid of the inn, who is dared to visit an abbey in the middle of the night where she witnesses 'in the moon-light two ruffians appear / and between them a corpse did they bear'.[23] Mary goes mad after discovering that her lover is one of these body snatchers and the ballad concludes with the image of the lover's gibbet. Sharing the same year of publication and similar gothic mechanisms, Southey's ballad and *The Horrors of Oakendale Abbey* both place considerable emphasis on the post-execution punishment of the body snatcher.

Carlisle was undoubtedly influenced by his literary circle, which included radical figures such as Mary Wollstonecraft, William Godwin and Thomas Holcroft. Indeed, Charles Lamb described Carlisle as 'the best storyteller' he had ever heard, highlighting a literary flair that complemented Carlisle's medical showmanship and love of wordplay.[24] Godwin is well known for using his own fiction as political intervention, as he published his gothic novel *Things as They Are; or, The Adventures of Caleb Williams* (1794) as a supplement to *An Enquiry Concerning Political Justice* (1793). Furthermore, Southey's 'The Surgeon's Warning' (1796) and Holcroft's *Adventures of Hugh Trevor* (1794/1797) both addressed anatomy practices and body snatching, although the former was decidedly more critical of the anatomist than the latter. In *Letters Written in Sweden, Norway and Denmark* (1796), Wollstonecraft even argued that 'a general knowledge of the component parts of the human frame' was necessary for combatting medical quackery and the harmful popular beliefs that arose as a result.[25] The writer was here responding to a public execution in Denmark where 'two persons came to the stake to drink a glass of the criminal's blood', a practice that was widely regarded as an 'infallible cure for the apoplexy'.[26] Wollstonecraft resolutely dismissed such remnants of 'exploded witchcraft' as a source of myth and misinformation.[27] Those closely associated with Carlisle – as well as Mary Shelley – constituted a network of writers that all that took up the concerns of the anatomy debate in the late eighteenth century.

Sitting within a vast and interconnected network of literary interventions, the Minerva Press novel thus demands consideration as the potential vehicle of Carlisle's own gothic intervention. As noted by Elizabeth Neiman, even the conventions shared between Minerva's own network of authors could become an outlet for aesthetic innovation that 'enabled novelists to contribute actively to pressing debates'.[28] Despite its contemporary reputation as 'a factory of cheap, formulaic novels', the Minerva Press offered its writers more than just a quick source of income.[29] The 'Carver' novel was published in a period when the Minerva Press dominated the market, producing texts that were relatively low cost and ever more available through circulating libraries.[30] Challenging a 'false equivalency' between female authorship and female readership, scholars have more recently demonstrated that the Minerva Press catered for a diverse audience made up of men and women from many different walks of life.[31] As an anonymous Minerva Press author, Carlisle could therefore gain access to a wide readership, while protecting his professional standing and avoiding accusations of bias or self-interest.

It is important to note that, as few in the labouring classes earned more than ten shillings a week during the Romantic period, the subscription fees to circulating libraries would largely have excluded the lower classes from the novel's potential readership.[32] Nonetheless, the physical aspects and cost of *The Horrors of Oakendale Abbey* indicate that the text was specifically intended for a middle-class audience. A single-volume novel priced at 4 shillings and 6 pence, *The Horrors of Oakendale Abbey* was substantially cheaper than the latest Walter Scott romance, a comparatively larger text that would have cost around 42 shillings.[33] This novel was also considerably cheaper than the other 'Carver' texts: for example, *Elizabeth* was a three-volume text with each volume costing 3 shillings, making the overall price for the full text 9 shillings.[34] While the author had little say over selling prices, composing a single-volume text promoted greater circulation by making the novel cheaper and therefore more accessible and publishers tended to produce more copies of the first volume of a text than any other, knowing that consumers were unlikely to read beyond the first of a multivolume work.[35] A single-volume Minerva novel like *The Horrors of Oakendale Abbey* could thus convey its central message quickly and concisely, making it an effective means of disseminating information among the middle classes. The Minerva novel then makes a fitting choice for the author-anatomist. It is particularly apt that Lane's Press was named after the Roman goddess Minerva, a patroness of the arts, crafts and trades – including medicine.

Anatomising the 1790s context

In 1795, the *Journal of the House of Commons* suggested that body snatching had become 'so frequent as to diffuse a general uneasiness, especially in the breasts of the middling and lower orders of the community, whose feelings cannot by any argument be reconciled to it'.[36] The *Journal* here reflects on the wide-scale consequences of a particular case of body snatching from February that year, when three men were found moving bodies from a Lambeth burial ground. Further enquiry revealed an elaborate body-snatching scheme had been operating in the area that even supposedly involved eight reputable surgeons. As a result, a general meeting between various London parishes was held at the Crown and Anchor Tavern, where the community's response was recorded:

> In consequence of such discovery, people of all descriptions, ... began like mad people to tear up the ground ... by which a great number of empty coffins were discovered, the corpses having been stolen from them; great distress and agitation of mind was manifest in every one, and some, in a kind of phrensy, ran away with the coffins of their deceased relations; and the generality of the populace were so ripe for mischief, that they attacked a house with stones and brick-bats, upon the bare suspicion that the occupier had been concerned in, or privy to the robbery of the ground, and it was with difficulty they were prevented from demolishing it.[37]

The reaction of the Lambeth parishioners highlights a deep and emotional investment in the burial of their loved ones and the outrage that was felt towards the desecration of graves. While the account describes the parishioners of St Mary's as 'people of all descriptions', suggesting that the case affected all levels of society equally, the *Journal* is right to identify the lower and middling orders as predominantly fearful of body snatching. Few from within these classes would have had access to sophisticated body-snatching deterrents or watchmen, and even fewer were privileged enough to be buried in vaults or inside churches and chapels.[38] Usually buried in open parish churchyards, it was the lower and middling classes that were largely at the mercy of body snatchers.

The record of this particular meeting is significant as it not only details the public's response to body snatching but also encapsulates the suspicions and beliefs that surrounded anatomy practices. Indeed, one member of the meeting reportedly claimed that an 'Articulator' (or dealer in bones), was involved with the body-snatching scheme and made 'the most wanton use of some [bodies] that fall into his hands, substituting human skulls for nail boxes, and having the skeleton of a child, instead of a doll, for his own child to play with'.[39] In a similarly superstitious vein, another claimed the stolen bodies had 'been converted into a substance like Spermaceti, and candles made of it, and that Soap has also been made of the same material'.[40] Southey's 'The Surgeon's Warning' demonstrates that such beliefs were not specific to the Lambeth parishioners but rather reflected a wider perception of medical practitioners. Southey's contemporaneous poem ventriloquizes the words of a dying surgeon, who fears that he will face retribution on the anatomy table when the resurrectionist comes for his body. Echoing the Lambeth Parishioners, Southey's surgeon admits: 'I have made candles of infants fat / The Sextons have been my slaves / I have bottled babes unborn, and dried / Hearts and livers from rifled graves'.[41] His words are saturated with the gothic mythologies of anatomy that clearly took root in the eighteenth century and slowed the progress of reform long into the nineteenth. While broadly acknowledged, the class distinctions apparent in the Lambeth body-snatching case demonstrate that the fears and beliefs of a more specific section of society contended with the demands of the medical establishment.

The same contention is visible in *The Horrors of Oakendale Abbey*, but the emphasis on class distinctions in the novel only bolsters its position as an intervention that mediates the myth and misinformation around medical practice. Indeed, the body snatchers of Oakendale Abbey hide under the cover of 'ghastly visions' and stories of a murdered woman who appears after dark with 'streams of blood running from her throat', blending supernatural superstition with the deviancy associated with anatomy and the body-snatching trade (11–12). However, 'Carver' dismisses both, making it clear that the Abbey was 'the terror of many generations' because the superstitious fears of the local peasantry facilitated the operations of the body-snatching gang (5). While conventional to the gothic romance, it is pertinent that superstition is derided as a symptom specifically of the lower classes, particularly as *The Horrors of Oakendale Abbey* was mainly produced for a middle-class Minerva Press readership. As suggested by Susan Lawrence, in a period when the middle class was seeking to consolidate its social status, those from within the middle class began to distance themselves from superstitions associated with the lower orders.[42] Adopting the more enlightened attitude of the upper classes, Lawrence suggests that the middle class tacitly accepted dissection as an unsavoury but necessary part of medical education.[43] A similar trend is apparent in popular death culture, as while the family and friends of the deceased traditionally retained and watched over the body until the day of burial, those of the middle class began to adopt the upper classes' preference for deferring these funerary services to the undertaker.[44] The 'Carver' novel thus appears as a medically inclined appeal, specifically directed at a middle-class audience that was fearful of the body snatcher, but that was also shifting its attitude towards the corpse.

In her exploration of the gothic corpse within anatomical culture, Laurence Talairach-Vielmas points to the way in which 'Carver' manipulates the gothic form in *The Horrors of Oakendale Abbey* in order to address the concerns of its intended audience. Providing one of the few readings of the 'Carver' novel in relation to Shelton's claim, Talairach-Vielmas suggests that the author revisits the familiar formulas of Clara Reeve and Ann Radcliffe, using medical reality to dismiss the supernatural and highlight the gothic 'as an artificial assemblage of conventional motifs'.[45] Those familiar with Radcliffe's corpus would thus expect 'Carver' to safely dismiss the supernatural with vaguely rational explanations, but the author instead innovatively replaces supernatural terrors with the all-too-real horrors of body snatching. Talairach-Vielmas addresses this element of the novel by suggesting that if Carlisle was indeed the author then he simply capitalised on his medical knowledge and the fear surrounding 'illicit anatomy'.[46] Yet, the figure of the anatomist is conspicuously omitted from *The Horrors of Oakendale Abbey*, while the body snatcher is thrust to the forefront of the narrative, suggesting that the novel capitalises on the horrors of body snatching rather than anatomy. Furthermore, 'Carver's' dismissal of the 'artful delusions' attached to the Abbey offers a metacommentary on the artificiality of gothic convention, while simultaneously applying gothic convention to draw attention to the fallacy of supernatural superstition. This double-edged manipulation of the 'supernatural explained' formula is thus especially fitting in a novel set in 1790s England, published during a period when popular belief slowed the cause of anatomy reform.

The implementation of anatomy legislation in England was indeed sluggish. While the 1788 case of Rex v. Lynn made it an offence to take a body from a churchyard under Common Law, the dead were not legally classed as property, and disinterring a corpse only became a criminal offence if personal items like the shroud were also taken. In 1795, the MP Sir John Frederick attempted to address this loophole when he put forward 'A Bill More Effectually to prevent the Stealing of Dead Bodies', which sought to upgrade body snatching to a felony. Frederick's Bill was certainly a reflection of public opinion, as it was introduced because of a petition from the Lambeth parishioners, 'on behalf of themselves, and the *public in general*', who were 'deeply affected at the very alarming and growing evil of robbing the several church yards, burying grounds, and other places of interment'.[47] The Bill was followed by that of the backbench MP, Richard Jodrell, who suggested in 1796 that dissection should be made a punishment for a wider range of offences, such as burglary or robbery. While both Bills were rejected, Frederick and Jodrell's proposals are significant, particularly when examined as a joint venture. Notably, Jodrell forged the connection between the two Bills when he claimed in Parliament that 'he entertained the upmost horror' towards the stealing of dead bodies and 'lamented the fate' of Frederick's Bill.[48] Indeed, if graverobbing had been upgraded to a felony in 1795, body snatchers themselves could have become newly eligible for the anatomist's table under the terms of Jodrell's Bill just a year later. Such an expansion on the allowances made by the Murder Act would certainly have addressed the anatomy issue by increasing the supply of bodies and potentially eradicating the body-snatching trade.

Frederick and Jodrell's Bills were in fact part of a string of legislative attempts that would have covertly addressed the anatomy supply issue by increasing the severity of criminal punishment. William Wilberforce's 1786 'Dissection of Convicts Bill' was an early version of this legislation that, as noted by Richard Ward, was 'decisively motivated by the needs of medical science'.[49] Urged by his family surgeon William Hey, Wilberforce put the proposed Bill forward in order to draw attention to 'the extreme difficulty that surgeons experienced in procuring bodies for dissections, and the shocking custom of digging them up after burial'.[50] Ward attributes the rejection of this Bill to a feeling in Parliament that murder was the greatest of offences and should be exclusively attached to the severest of punishments.[51] Such a precedent upheld the notion that anatomisation was a moral and judicial punishment, a notion that only bolstered the general antipathy towards dissection and that likely contributed toward the rejection of the 1795 and 1796 Bills. Distinctly propelled by the demands of the medical establishment, the late eighteenth-century Bills were also rejected because the State was clearly aware of the negative perception of anatomy practices and was unwilling to risk coming under public fire by enacting legislation that openly favoured the anatomists. Indeed, in *The Diary of a Resurrectionist*, Bailey notes that the Home Secretary had once told a deputation that 'there was no difficulty in drawing up an effective Bill; the great obstacle was the prejudice of the people'.[52] Yet, the ever more frequent and violent responses to graverobbing, exemplified by the Lambeth body-snatching case, suggests that legislation could be tolerated if it expressly sought to eradicate body snatching and if suitable subjects for dissection could be found. The portrayal of popular superstition as a lower-class fallacy that facilitated body snatching thus foregrounds *The Horrors of Oakendale Abbey* as a highly strategic address, presented at a time when it was necessary, and increasingly possible, to reconcile the middle classes with anatomy practices.

Carving the criminal corpse

In 1794, *The Times* reported that over a hundred bodies, 'some whole, some mangled', were found at a property in the East End of London.[53] According to the article, a full account of the circumstances could not be published because they were 'too horrid to meet the public eye', but the reporter's proclamation that the Archbishop of Canterbury should move Parliament to make it '*death* to rob a churchyard' made the 'shocking brutality' of the substantial body-trafficking operation evident.[54] Highlighting body snatching as an offence deserving of the severest form of punishment, this timely suggestion captures the late eighteenth-century appetite for reform. The article certainly substantiates the claims of Michel Foucault, who in *Discipline and Punish: The Birth of the Prison* (1975) suggests that while 'modern codes' of punishment were established around the end of the eighteenth century, England was particularly loath to see the disappearance of the public execution.[55] Indeed, the number of capital crimes in England grew to over two hundred, and judges felt themselves 'dangerously soft' if they commuted the death sentence; more men and women were in fact hanged as a proportion of the population during the Romantic period than at any other time before or since.[56] While a growing public discourse increasingly denounced the public spectacle of torture as a form of 'Gothic' savagery, post-execution punishment also endured in England as many felt that the fear attached to anatomisation was a more effective deterrent than the gallows itself.[57] Calls for amelioration ultimately prevailed, but the Bills of 1795 and 1796 were undoubtedly the product of a specific moment in English history when the penal system seemed to offer both a viable solution to the anatomy issue and a suitably gothic alternative to body snatching – criminal bodies.

Similarly a product of this particular moment, *The Horrors of Oakendale Abbey* also proves to be centred around the criminal body, as 'Carver' reflects on the logistical problems of anatomy supply and strategically addresses the gothic mythologies that surrounded anatomy practices. This point is most obviously made in the novel when Laura stumbles into a room where she finds the body of a woman hanging against a wall. A cloth covering all but the face, the indecent treatment of this body is clearly intended to shock readers, but the 'ghastly and putrefied appearance of which bespoke her to have been for some time dead', further shows the body to be unfit for dissection (47). In juxtaposition to this dead body, Laura is then terrified by a zombie-like male figure that escapes from the body snatchers' storeroom of bodies. While the woman's 'absolute death' is signalled by her putrefied state, this 'undead' male figure makes for an unsuitable anatomical subject perhaps because he is not dead enough:

> The face was almost quite black; the eyes seemed starting from the head; the mouth was widely extended, and made a kind of hollow guttural sound in attempting to articulate. (47)

The in-between status of this 'undead' being would indeed be problematic. As Ruth Richardson asserts, popular death culture of the period was 'coloured by a prevailing belief in the existence of a strong tie between body and personality/soul for an undefined period of time after death'.[58] Grounded in teachings from the Book of Revelation, beliefs that the body and soul remained united, or could reunite, after death meant that few wanted to risk offering their body up for dissection. In *Letters*, Wollstonecraft demonstrated how such anxieties could shape notions of how the dead should be treated when she responded to a display of embalmed bodies in a church in Norway. Wollstonecraft expressed abhorrence towards the preservation process because it involved a dismantling of the body that will 'remain till the day of judgment, if there is to be such a day; and before that time it will require some trouble to make them fit to appear in the company of angels, without disgracing humanity'.[59] Even while dubious about Judgement Day, Wollstonecraft's thoughts were clearly pervaded by the idea that the body's state when it entered the grave affected its potential resurrection.

The apparent walking corpse in *The Horrors of Oakendale Abbey* thus represents a popular quasi-Christian belief system that, in giving the corpse a supernatural or spiritual element, palpably resisted scientific medicine.[60] Yet 'Carver's' use of the 'supernatural explained' conspicuously casts such beliefs aside. The 'undead' figure in fact reveals himself to be a criminal named Patrick who, taken only half-dead from the gallows, was claimed for dissection by the same resurrection men he used to work for. Patrick's resurrection story therefore addresses specific cultural anxieties that underpinned the anatomy debates, particularly as Patrick's thoughts at the gallows centre on 'the wretched state to which his body would be subjected after he was dead' (159). In response to his fear, a clergyman attempts to impress the criminal's mind with the idea that 'the more immortal and immaterial part of him … could not suffer by the hands of men', challenging a belief that significantly problematised dissection by severing the tie between body and soul in death (159). Notably, 'Carver's' convenient remoulding of contemporary orthodoxy appears to align *The Horrors of Oakendale Abbey* with the views and concerns of its potential author, particularly as in a letter from 1796 Southey claimed that Carlisle often expressed views that were 'atheistical'.[61] Grounding Patrick's revival in the corporeal circumstances of hanging both addresses popular belief systems that medical practitioners had to contend with throughout the anatomy debates and reflects on medical realities of the period.

Many criminals were brought down from the gallows 'half-hanged' as the cessation of heart or brain function proved indeterminate in times of trauma, when the body could shut down and merely assume the appearance of death.⁶² It is thus unsurprising that gothic tales about subjects that return to life on the anatomy table were mythologised in this era. Elizabeth Hurren notes that as the Murder Act required surgeons to anatomise those hanged for murder and anatomists were also supplied with bodies brought from the gallows, 'the dissection room was where the boundaries of life and death might be glimpsed together'.⁶³ However, the medical fascination with galvanism, resuscitation and suspended animation demonstrates that practitioners sought to dismiss the corpse's supernatural associations by resolving the uncertain status of death scientifically.⁶⁴ Carlisle's friend and teacher, the surgeon and anatomist John Hunter, had exactly this ambition when he agreed to attempt to revive Reverend William Dodd, King George III's chaplain who was sentenced to death for committing forgery in 1777.⁶⁵ The self-styled 'Macaroni Parson' was brought down from the gallows after forty minutes and taken to an undertaker's parlour where Hunter tried and failed to bring Dodd back to life.⁶⁶ While giving death a set of fixed biological conditions proved difficult, Patrick's medically explained resurrection in *The Horrors of Oakendale Abbey*, like Dodd's failed resuscitation, challenges the supernatural power of the corpse by at least demonstrating that revival was only possible to those who had not undergone an 'absolute death'.

The close associations between Dodd's execution and that of 'Carver's' Patrick – who is also exposed to the severest penalties of the law for forgery – suggests that the author was familiar enough with the incident to have drawn on it twenty years later, further drawing Carlisle in line with *The Horrors of Oakendale Abbey* as its potential author. Carlisle's name and perspective on the body-snatching issue are essentially stamped on *The Horrors of Oakendale Abbey* as the body snatcher tells Lord Oakendale that his gang frequently procured bodies 'that were hanged at, or near Carlisle' (137).⁶⁷ Highlighting a significant site of execution in the period and also seemingly alluding to the author's own hidden identity, 'Carver' substitutes the insufficient and unsuitable corpses supplied by the body snatcher with the criminal corpse. Indeed, the fear of post-execution punishment expressed by Patrick, who is only too aware of being 'reserved for dissection', points to the anatomisation of criminals – notably executed for crimes other than just murder – as both an effective deterrent and a fitting alternative to body snatching (156). Ironically, as forger and body snatcher, Patrick would have become doubly eligible for the anatomist's table if the proposed legislative changes of 1795 and 1796 had been enacted. Published in the wake of the failure to enact this legislation, and aligning with contemporaneous discussions about the efficacy of capital punishment, *The Horrors of Oakendale Abbey* thus picks up where the parliamentary debates left off:

> Thus was this mystery at once explained, and the ghosts of Oakendale-Abbey were indeed the dead; but brought thither by those unfeeling monsters of society, who make a practice of stealing our friends and relations from the peaceful grave where their ashes, as we suppose, are deposited in rest! (138)

The dead would certainly not return to 'ashes'; they simply would not remain in their graves long enough. This passage is undoubtably a timely jab at the hesitancy of the State as 'Carver' reminds readers that they remained vulnerable to being disinterred by such 'monsters of society'. In *The Horrors of Oakendale Abbey*, the penitent resurrectionist who expected to be 'disjointed by the hell-hounds at Oakendale' ultimately escapes punishment (156). So too with the rest of the body-snatching gang, despite Lord Oakendale's efforts to 'set on foot a prosecution, and an order to apprehend, or cause to be apprehended, those wretches who had, for so many years, been the terror of Oakendale' (139). The reader is told that 'his exertions on this score proved fruitless; the perpetrators of these acts taking care to secure themselves beyond the reach of justice', indicating that the body snatchers would long continue to operate (139–140). As demonstrated by *The Horrors of Oakendale Abbey*, until the enactment of anatomy legislation, it would thus not be ghosts but rather the dead that would remain the persistently haunting problem.

Conclusion

Transforming the generic expectations of the 'supernatural explained', *The Horrors of Oakendale Abbey* proves an innovative means of conveying the needs of the medical practitioner to a popular audience at a particularly pertinent moment in the late eighteenth century. The 'Carver' novel pressed for increasingly necessary legislation by directing the reader's attention towards the gothic horror of body snatching and by addressing the popular beliefs that surrounded anatomy practices. In line with the views of its potential medical author, the 'Carver' novel most noticeably positioned the criminal body as a viable and largely acceptable alternative to body snatching. However, until the 1832 Anatomy Act repealed the conditions of the Murder Act, popular prejudice towards dissection continued to outweigh medical need, leaving the late eighteenth-century anatomy debate unresolved. This lack of resolution is perhaps reflected in the novel's ending which, like the identity of the author, is suitably ambiguous. The narrative closure offered by Laura's reunion with her lover Eugene is conflictingly denied when she is revealed as Lord Oakendale's niece, inheriting both Oakendale Abbey and its body-snatching issue on the death of her newfound uncle. With no recourse to legislation, Laura's 'virtues' alone must dispel 'THE HORRORS OF OAKENDALE-ABBEY' (172).

Whether written by 'Carver' or Carlisle, *The Horrors of Oakendale Abbey* was undoubtedly created to speak to its own contemporary moment and the concerns of its middle-class audience. As the novels produced by the Minerva Press were known for their short shelf lives and were rarely ever reprinted beyond their first editions, *The Horrors of Oakendale Abbey* was not a text written with posterity in mind. However, the novel holds an important place within a distinct network of literary interventions that shaped the public's perception of medical practice during the anatomy debates. While Elizabeth Neiman notes that 'no one single novel transforms the conversation', Minerva's penchant for imitation and its well-known formulas in fact facilitated the 'Carver' novel's potential as gothic (medical) intervention.[68] Indeed, a process of gothic perpetuation, from both within and outside of the Minerva Press network, ensured that *The Horrors of Oakendale Abbey* had a much greater legacy than the author probably intended. Boasting a unique publication history, *The Horrors of Oakendale Abbey* found its way to America where it was republished in serial form in the Philadelphia periodical *The Dessert of the True American* (September–October 1798). The text was again printed as a single volume in 1799 by John Harrison of New York, and a further new edition was printed in Pennsylvania as late as 1812.[69] The literary afterlife of *The Horrors of Oakendale Abbey* therefore encompasses more than the novel's own single publication history and its impact should be considered beyond English shores. Most importantly, while the specific subject matter of *The Horrors of Oakendale Abbey* may be inextricably tied to its own contemporary moment, the text's occupation with mediating the myth and misinformation that surrounds medical practice is a recognisably modern concern.

Acknowledgements

The research presented in this chapter was supported by the Arts and Humanities Research Council. I must also thank the curators at the University of Pennsylvania for allowing me to access the 1797 edition of *The Horrors of Oakendale Abbey*.

Notes

1 See Ruth Richardson, *Death, Dissection and the Destitute* (London: Routledge & Kegan Paul, 1987) and Elizabeth T. Hurren, *Dying for Victorian Medicine:*

English Anatomy and its Trade in the Dead Poor, c.1834–1929 (Basingstoke: Palgrave Macmillan, 2012) for examinations of how sufficient this supply actually was.
2. James Blake Bailey, *The Diary of a Resurrectionist, 1811–1812: To which are Added an Account of the Resurrection Men in London and A Short History of the Passing of the Anatomy Act* (London: Swan Sonnenschein & Co., 1896), p. v.
3. Warren reportedly studied medicine before becoming a lawyer, his *Passages* were printed in serial form in *Blackwood's Edinburgh Magazine*.
4. Tim Marshall, *Murdering to Dissect: Grave-Robbing, Frankenstein and the Anatomy Literature* (Manchester: Manchester University Press, 1995), p. 50.
5. Richardson, *Death, Dissection and the Destitute*, p. xv.
6. Marshall, *Murdering to Dissect*, pp. 11–12.
7. The 1797 edition of this novel is housed in the Singer-Mendenhall Collection, Kislak Centre for Special Collections, PR4452.C58 H6.
8. Dorothy Blakey, *The Minerva Press, 1790–1820* (Oxford and London: Bibliographical Society, 1939), p. 181.
9. Don Shelton, 'Sir Anthony Carlisle and Mrs Carver', *Romantic Textualities: Literature and Print Culture, 1780–1840* 19 (2009): 54–69, at 55.
10. Mrs Carver, *The Horrors of Oakendale Abbey* (London: Minerva Press, 1797), p. 15. The wording of this line differs by edition. In the modern reprint, the line is: 'sooner dispose a mind, like hers, to coincide with his base desires' (Zittaw Press, 2006), p. 40.
11. Richard Ward, 'The Criminal Corpse, Anatomists and the Criminal Law: Parliamentary attempts to Extend the Dissection of Offenders in Late Eighteenth-Century England', *Journal of British Studies* 50:1 (2015): 63–87, at 86.
12. Bailey, *Diary of a Resurrectionist*, p. 31.
13. Richardson, *Death, Dissection and the Destitute*, pp. 162–163.
14. Ibid., p. 164. Carlisle made similar claims in 1834 before the Select Committee on Medical Education.
15. Ibid.
16. R. J. Cole, 'Sir Anthony Carlisle F.R.S.', *Annals of Science* 8:3 (1952): 255–270, at 264–265. While Cole's dates are pulled from the RCS official records, W. F. Bynum claims Carlisle was president in 1829 and 1839; see 'Sir Anthony Carlisle', *Oxford Dictionary of National Biography*, available at https://www.oxforddnb.com/display/10.1093/ref:odnb/9780198614128.001.0001/odnb-9780198614128-e-4687, last accessed 3 November 2023 (para. 2 of 7).
17. Cole, 'Sir Anthony Carlisle', p. 265.
18. Ibid., p. 260.
19. W. T. Whitley, 'Turner as a Lecturer', *Burlington Magazine for Connoisseurs* 22 (February 1913), p. 257.
20. Shelton, 'Anthony Carlisle and Mrs Carver', p. 55.
21. Cole, 'Sir Anthony Carlisle', p. 266.
22. Robert Southey, Letter to Hugh Chudleigh Standert (14 December 1809), *The Collected Letters of Robert Southey: Part One*, available at https://romantic-circles.org, last accessed 17 August 2020 (para. 3 of 5).

23 Robert Southey, 'Mary', *Poems, by Robert Southey* (London: Printed by N. Biggs, for Joseph Cottle, Bristol, and G. G. & J. Robinson, 1797), p. 168, ll. 79–80.
24 Don Shelton, 'Anthony Carlisle and Mary Shelley: Finding Form in a *Frankenstein* Fog', *Athens Journal of Philology* 6:2 (2019): 105–130, at 109–110.
25 Mary Wollstonecraft, *Letters Written in Sweden, Norway and Denmark* (Oxford: Oxford University Press, 2009), p. 105.
26 Ibid.
27 Ibid.
28 Elizabeth Neiman, *Minerva's Gothics: The Politics and Poetics of Romantic Exchange, 1780–1820* (Cardiff: University of Wales, 2019), p. 102.
29 Ibid., p. 1.
30 Ibid., p. 4.
31 E. A. Neiman and C. Morin, 'Re-evaluating the Minerva Press: Introduction', *Romantic Textualities: Literature and Print Culture, 1780–1840* 23 (2020): 11–23, at 13.
32 William St Clair, *The Reading Nation in the Romantic Period* (Cambridge: Cambridge University Press, 2004), p. 195.
33 Blakey, *Minerva Press*, p. 279; price of Scott text from St Clair, *The Reading Nation*, p. 40.
34 Blakey, *Minerva Press*, p. 279.
35 St Clair, *The Reading Nation*, p. 244.
36 'March 30th', *Journal of the House of Commons*, 50 (December 1794–June 1795): 383.
37 Laurence Dopson, 'St Thomas's Parish Vestry Records and a Body-Snatching Incident', *British Medical Journal* 2:4618 (1949): 69.
38 Richardson, *Death, Dissection and the Destitute*, p. 81.
39 Dopson, 'St Thomas's Parish', p. 69.
40 Ibid.
41 Robert Southey, 'The Surgeon's Warning' (1796), *Poems, by Robert Southey*, Vol. II (Bristol: Biggs & Cottle, 1799), p. 165, ll. 33–36.
42 Susan C. Lawrence, 'Anatomy and Address: Creating Medical Gentlemen in Eighteenth-Century London', in Vivian Nutton and Roy Porter (eds), *The History of Medical Education* (Brill: Rodopi, 1995), pp. 199–228, at p. 205.
43 Ibid.
44 Richardson, *Death, Dissection and the Destitute*, pp. 4, 23.
45 Laurence Talairach-Vielmas, *Gothic Remains: Corpses, Terror and Anatomical Culture, 1764–1897* (Cardiff: Cardiff University Press, 2019), p. 41.
46 Ibid., p. 35.
47 'March 30th', *Journal of the House of Commons*, p. 383.
48 'March 11th', in *The Parliamentary Register; or, The History of the Proceedings and Debates of the House of Commons*, Vol. 44 (London: Printed for J. Debrett, Piccadilly, 1796), p. 288.
49 Ward, 'The Criminal Corpse', p. 64.

50 Ibid., p. 70. See also '16th May', *Journal of the House of Commons* 20 (January 1786–July 1786): 227.
51 Ward, 'The Criminal Corpse', pp. 81, 84.
52 Bailey, *Diary of a Resurrectionist*, p. 89.
53 'Ship News', *The Times* (22 March 1794), p. 3.
54 *The Times*, p. 3 (original italicization).
55 Michel Foucault, *Discipline and Punish: The Birth of the Prison* (London: Penguin, 1991), pp. 7, 14.
56 St Clair, *The Reading Nation*, p. 259.
57 Foucault, *Discipline and Punish*, p. 39.
58 Richardson, *Death, Dissection and the Destitute*, p. 7.
59 Wollstonecraft, *Letters*, p. 109.
60 Richardson, *Death, Dissection and the Destitute*, p. 29.
61 Robert Southey, Letter to Grosvenor Charles Bedford (19 August–7 September 1796), *The Collected Letters of Robert Southey: Part One*, available at https://romantic-circles.org, last accessed 21 July 2021 (para. 19 of 24).
62 Elizabeth T. Hurren, *Dissecting the Criminal Corpse: Staging Post-Execution Punishment in Early Modern England* (London: Palgrave Macmillan, 2016), p. 6.
63 Ibid., p. 237.
64 Ibid.
65 Wendy Moore, *The Knife-Man* (London: Bantam Press, 2006), p. 361.
66 Ibid., pp. 361–362, 369. 'Macaroni' refers to someone who exceeds the ordinary bounds of fashion.
67 In the 2006 edition the phrase is 'they frequently procured bodies after word interned at or near Carlisle' (158). The use of this word is hard to determine, however it seems to point to the procurement of bodies stolen after burial rather than taken from the gallows.
68 Neiman, *Minerva's Gothics*, pp. 26–27.
69 Peter Garside, James Raven and Rainer Schowerling, *The English Novel 1770–1829: A Bibliographical Survey of Prose Fiction Published in the British Isles* (Oxford: Oxford University Press, 2000), p. 710.

8

Mislabelling and the medical printer-publisher: demystifying the ephemera of Elizabeth Rane Cox (1765–1841)

Helen Williams

Medical bookselling was, and continues to be, a trade adjacent to, while facilitating, the medical professions. It required working within a network of medical practitioners and authors, and a successful business depended upon keeping up to date with the latest medical innovations, scholarship and celebrities. It was one of the trades in which women could openly participate, bookselling and printing being in this period predominantly family businesses, conducted from the family home, and therefore co-opting the labour of women and children but without them necessarily receiving the credit for that work.[1] While printing and bookselling continue to be the trades most often considered in scholarship exploring eighteenth- and nineteenth-century individuals in the book trades, the recovery of jobbing print work has been much more difficult, and rarely do we get a sense of the entrepreneurs, and especially female entrepreneurs, who carved their own niche in the marketplace.[2] In the early years of the nineteenth century, when medical labelling remained in a state of chaos, Elizabeth Cox née Rane (1765–1841) referred to herself when writing her will in 1840 as a 'Medical Bookseller Labeller &c' by trade.

The discipline of book history since 1980 has had the effect of glorifying the book as object and marginalising the printed matter that necessarily circulated around the codex, creating what Michael Harris has called a 'dialectic of ephemera and books'.[3] Such a dialectic has emerged through a historic – and gendered – reification of Literature with a capital L, which is most often transmitted via the codex, at the expense of other forms in which women may have thrived as authors and producers.[4] The dialectic endures precisely because ephemera is simultaneously promiscuously abundant (too much) and undervalued, disposable, and therefore rare (too little). This chapter follows work undertaken by James Raven and Gillian Russell to rehabilitate the ephemera of the book trades in order to better understand the print cultures of the past and their wider social impacts.[5] In applying the interventions of print and book history, and particularly of the growing discipline of women's book history, to early nineteenth-century medical labels, this chapter argues for a renewed attention to printed ephemera as a means of better understanding the material conditions of medicine, of the singular contribution of one woman to medical history, and of her attempts to overcome barriers to medical knowledge and health in the early nineteenth century.[6] I argue that Elizabeth Cox was central to nineteenth-century medical print culture, significant to both practitioners and patients, but continues to be overlooked today, despite her printing innovations leading to the improvement of dispensing practice in England and overseas and her business producing what has been recognised as 'the most successful booklet of the nineteenth century'.[7]

Accidental poisoning

In 1828, the *London Medical Gazette* reported on the 'State of the Medical Profession in St. Petersburgh', praising the rigour with which apothecaries conducted their work:

> the medical administration is more strict even than in any other part of Europe. Not only must every prescription be signed with the name of the physician whose advice has been taken, but it must also mention the patient for whom it is written, with the day of the month and year. To the medicine a label is affixed, mentioning, besides the date and hour of its delivery, its price, and the name of the 'Aptekare' and his shop.[8]

The article was an excerpt from Augustus Bozzi Granville's *St. Petersburgh: A Journal of Travels to and from that Capital* (1828), amplifying Granville's representation of the Russian pharmaceutical professional for the *Gazette's* London practitioners. The success of the 'Aptekare', or pharmacist, consisted of the strictness with which they sealed each medicine and then labelled it with a string of standard requirements. In contrast with Russia, at this time in England there were no official requirements for medical labelling, and limited means of identifying medicines and their ingredients.[9] As Stuart Anderson has demonstrated, it was not until the 1840s that public concern about access to poisons emerged,[10] though Granville's description of St Petersburg indicates a cultural moment of concern around a decade earlier. Borrowing from Granville, the article concluded: 'Did such regulations exist in full, as they exist in part, in England, and as obligatory regulations, instead of being left to the discretion of chemists, we should not hear of so many dreadful accidents and mistakes as occur every year in this country'.[11]

When it came to medical labelling, accidents and mistakes there were aplenty. The *Atlas* reported on 9 July 1826 that an inquest into the death of Mrs Sarah Coates had been held the Thursday before. She was the wife of 'a respectable livery-stable keeper', George Coates, one of whose horses had been ill. He

> applied to Mr. Fenton, a veterinary surgeon, giving him a bottle, to contain the medicine, with the label, 'the draught to be taken directly. Mrs. Coate's.' This Mr. Fenton did not see, and having filled it, he sent to the house of Mr. Coates.

The bottle in question belonged to the Coateses, already labelled from a previous prescription, and was being recycled. Because Coates himself was not home when the medicine arrived, his child intercepted it and, reading the old label which remained fixed to the bottle, 'supposed her mother was to take the draught, conceiving it to be medicine for her'. As the *Atlas* points out, poor Sarah Coates knew it was poison as soon as she drank it, exclaiming 'I am poisoned', 'and in fact the medicine was composed of the most deleterious poison'. The jury returned a verdict of accidental poisoning.[12] Had the apothecary applied his own label, perhaps the accident might have been averted.

Even when labels were applied, however, there remained an issue with their legibility. When apothecary's assistant John Merrell was indicted for the murder of Mary Rocher Latter on 11 April 1833, the jury heard how he had mistaken hydrosiamus for hydrocyanic acid, both of which had been abbreviated in prescriptions in a manuscript day-book of the surgeon and apothecary Henry Thomas Clapham. Clapham was then interrogated for requesting too much of an assistant who might not fully understand Latin terminology and therefore the minute but deadly difference between prussic acid (hydrocianic acid) and tincture of myrrh (hydrosiamus).[13] Merrell was found not guilty.

Latin labels were sometimes as ineffective as no labels at all, given the likelihood that the people administering medicines in this period were unfamiliar with Latin terminology which remained standard in pharmaceutical descriptions. In 1839 an enquiry was launched into the tragic death of five-week-old Henry Love at Axminster Workhouse. He had been administered emetic tartar instead of magnesia by the nurse, who had been unable to understand the Latin labels on the bottles in the medicine cabinet. As a result, the Assistant Poor Law Commissioner determined that the Master and Matron be replaced and that 'all bottles left out should be labelled with the common and familiar name of the medicine' to 'prevent any similar error'.[14] Labels could save lives, but were most likely to be effective when composed in the vernacular.

There was growing concern about the unrestricted availability of potentially poisonous substances and their irregular labelling. In 1819, at a meeting of chemists and druggists, their committee identified medical labels as a key tool to ameliorating dispensing practice and defending the standards of their professions:

> First – That no arsenic, oxalic acid, or corrosive sublimate, be issued by any vendor, without a printed label of the name of the article, and the word 'POISON' being affixed to every wrapper, box, bottle, or other vessel containing the same.
>
> Secondly – That on every wrapper or vessel containing any drug or preparation likely to produce serious mischief, if improperly used, the name of the article be affixed in a legible form; and as many persons can read print who cannot read writing, they would recommend that printed labels be used where possible, in preference to written ones.[15]

This was ultimately a bid to put a stop to impending government regulation through the adoption of voluntary labelling, and it was effective: a poison labelling law would not be passed until 1868.[16] The year before, Elizabeth Cox advertised catalogues of preprinted and bespoke medical labels in both Latin and English which she had printed using letterpress and copperplate technology. She was the printer-publisher of *Cox's Companion to the Medicine Chest* (c.1829), up to sixty editions of which were published during the first half of the nineteenth century.[17] The pamphlet included a short but informative summary of each item included in a standard cabinet as well as a pull-out sheet of printed labels for the clear identification of chemicals using their vernacular names. It constituted a major printing innovation, with the labels helping to defend against accidental poisoning and to promote accurate medical labelling at home, in the workplace and in the colonies. Her *Cabinet* labels enabled lay people – even those on long sea voyages – to administer and self-administer medicines as safely as possible.

Elizabeth Cox, medical bookseller

Elizabeth Cox took on, in name, the medical publishing business of her husband, Thomas Cox, bookseller and engraver, when he died in 1806. As with many other women in family businesses, it is likely that she also took a leading role in its management before her husband's demise. The Coxes sold and loaned out medical volumes from their premises, which was a library as well as a bookshop.[18] In the early days, when Thomas had been alive, the business had seemed to suffer something of a crisis of identity, selling at one stage taxidermy, though it seems that this may have been a favour for a friend.[19] As was usual for the period, as a bookseller Cox also stocked medicine, being the wholesaler and retailer of Cullen's Edinburgh Cerate for the Ring-Worm and Scald-Head between 1810 and 1812.[20] Booksellers were often stockists of branded medicines, countersigned by either the bookseller or the medicine maker. The most notable example of a female bookseller and medicine vendor is perhaps Elizabeth Newbery (fl. 1780–1821), but a preliminary search of the *British Book Trade Index* throws up several lesser known examples including Miss Bowden in Ilfracombe, Devon, in 1797, Miss Dixon in Deal, Kent (trading 1772–78), Mrs Dodge of Exeter in 1790, Mrs Pike of Ashford in Kent (trading 1772–74) and Mrs Sarah Booth of Wednesbury, Staffordshire, working in 1845.[21] Few booksellers, male or female, marketed themselves as 'medical booksellers', indicating a distinctive specialism in publishing and/or selling material of a specifically medical nature. Cox's rivals included John Callow of Princes Street, Soho (trading 1799–1828), and Samuel Highley (trading 1796–1856), who had a shop on Fleet Street, and who also sold entry tickets to the Theatre of Anatomy and Medicine from an office adjoining the theatre.[22]

Elizabeth Cox inherited, honed and grew a specialist enterprise that was of national significance in the early nineteenth century. Thomas's will suggests that he intended the business to help his wife provide for their children during their minority:

> to permit and suffer my said dear Wife Elizabeth Cox to have and enjoy all my said Stock and Utensils in Trade household furniture and all other my Estate and Effects and to carry on the said Trade for the maintenance and Education of my Children until they shall respectively attain the Age of twenty one years.[23]

This was a family business with Elizabeth at its head, whereby, upon coming of age, the children were encouraged to 'use their best Endeavors and Assistance in the said Trade', but ultimately the business would remain in her hands. This was indeed the case: she helped her three sons to establish themselves as independent entities in the medical bookselling business, but she ultimately retained her hold over her own premises on St Thomas's Street, Southwark. Her shop brought together as a network the major players of the medical world, including Thomas Wakley of the *Lancet* and leading medical practitioners of the day, Sir Astley Cooper and Bransby Cooper.[24] As her apprentice would later remember it, the premises 'was immediately adjoining Guy's and St. Thomas's Hospitals, and became the daily resort of the lecturers and numerous students of the schools'.[25] Her location and her trade contributed to the shop's appeal, which stocked the largest collection of medical books in the country. The second edition (1832) of *Cox's Druggist's Price Book*, for instance, advertised a range of 'valuable medical' works published by Cox, followed by the astonishing announcement that 'E. Cox has on Sale upwards of Thirty Thousand Second-hand and Scarce Medical Books'.[26] She also published and sold fine art prints of medical practitioners who wrote the works she sold in her bookshop, and she later expanded to publish non-medical portrait prints.[27] After her husband's death, the Cox establishment went from strength to strength, extending to specialist stationary, and printing bespoke labels for medicine bottles.

Elizabeth Cox remains unrecognised by scholars of the book and of the history of medicine, other than entries in the usual book trade directories.[28] But she does make an appearance in Maurice Quinlan's study of the poet William Cowper, as the 'obscure' publisher of one of two editions of the poet's memoir, both published in 1816. Quinlan goes on to suggest that she was a nonconformist, and probably a Baptist, making a connection between the James Churchill of Ditton, Surrey, to whom Cox dedicates Cowper's *Memoir* ('as a small tribute to Unvarying Friendship and Exemplary Piety by his affectionate friends the Publishers'), and the Reverend James Churchill, who edited at least three of the religious works she published alongside her largely medical corpus.[29] It is unlikely to be a coincidence that many prominent women in the book trade preceding Cox were also dissenters, such as Tace Sowle, Elinor James, Mary Fenner, Mary Lewis and Mary Cooper.[30] As Timothy Whelan has argued, though nonconforming women of the eighteenth and nineteenth centuries could be seen as doubly repressed, as both women and as dissenters deprived of civil liberties, 'Nonconformity may well have been more conducive to women engaging in political discourse in the home, in private coteries, and even in print than any other segment of British society'.[31]

Cox's dispensing labels

Cox was certainly a prominent player in the London book trade. As a medical bookseller who employed her son as an engraver, she would have been aware of the recent emergence of mass-produced engraved labels. Since the seventeenth century, wine, ale and medicine sellers had used glass bottles for their wares, rather than casks or flagons, and by the nineteenth century the scale of bottle production meant that there was a hitherto unsurpassed need for labelling.[32] This led to the establishment of some of the earliest label printers, of which the Cox establishment was one. Cox was also sufficiently familiar with the medical profession and conscious of their concerns to identify medical labelling as a major concern, announcing her medical labels in 1818:

TO SURGEONS, APOTHECARIES, and CHEMISTS. – COX'S NEWLY INVENTED LABELS, for tying round Phials; comprising upwards of One Hundred different Directions, which are generally used by Medical Practitioners, neatly written and engraved in a small intelligible running hand. Price 5s. per thousand. Sold by Cox and Son. St. Thomas's-street, Southwark.[33]

Cox was joining an emerging market. Since 1815, a reasonably priced set of a thousand labels had been available from various stockists across London and directly from a factory in Westminster, for three shillings and sixpence. This was 'a cheaper rate than paper can be purchased of the same quality, they being formed from the torn sheets of an extensive paper manufactory', at the 'New' premises on Charles Street.[34] And yet even with Cox's product, the market was not saturated. Callow would also join the game in 1818, advertising medical labels 'cheaper than anyone can make them' at 4,000 for £1, available at Apothecaries' Hall.[35] Nevertheless, Cox and Callow seemed to remain on good terms, or at least determined to continue to collaborate for their mutual benefit, as demonstrated by Callow stocking in 1818 a medical portrait print published and also sold by Cox.[36]

Cox advertised her labels in the press and in a series of catalogues which included samples on both plain and coloured paper.[37] She took care to map her labels onto the latest version of the *Pharmacopeoia Londinensis*, published in 1815 and recently reprinted, and much updated since the original by Nicolas Culpeper. In a large advertisement in *The Times*, Cox set out her portfolio:

TO SURGEONS, APOTHECARIES, and CHEMISTS. This Day are Published, by E. COX and SON, St. Thomas's-street. Borough,
ORNAMENTED LATIN LABELS, for Drawers and Bottles, in two Sizes, according to the last Edition of The London Pharmacopoeia. With neat emblematical borders, neatly engraved, and printed on various coloured papers.
Set on White, of one size - - - - £1 1 0
-- -- -- -- -- £1 8 0
Set on Green, Yellow, or Pink Paper, of one size 1 10 0
Ditto, Ditto, two sizes 2 0 0
Two Supplementary Sheets, containing Labels which were omitted in the Set, will be ready in a few days, and may be had gratuitously by the Purchasers of the Sets specified above.
The following are of another pattern, in a semi-circle form, containing the names of The New London Pharmacopoeia:–
Complete Set, in three sizes, on White Paper – £1 16 0
Complete Set, in three Sizes, on Green or Yellow Paper 2 10 0
Set of Large Size, White Paper — 0 18 0

– Large Size, on Green or Yellow Paper — 1 4 0
– Second Size, White Paper — 0 14 0.[38]

The catalogue from 1828, while it represents the labels ten years later, gives us a sense of what this portfolio would have looked like (Figure 8.1). It includes a sheet of bright green paper, upon which potentially poisonous substances are printed in Latin in three sizes and decorated with gold-painted borders: 'PAPAV. CAPS.' (poppy capsules, representing label size 1 – the largest), 'ACID. NITRIC.' (nitric acid, representing size 2), and 'EXT. STRAMON.' (stramonium extract, representing the third and smallest size label). It also includes dispensing instructions, 'The Pill to be taken at bed time' and 'A Draught to be taken night & morning'. The second sample page is printed on white paper and includes a range of labels aimed at dispensing practitioners (such as the Latin label in three sizes for 'ACET. COLCH.', or colchicum acid, a poison, or the plain rectangular label for 'RHUBARB POWDER') as well as at vendors or wholesalers of medicines and cosmetics (like the labels for 'PAREGORIC ELIXIR', used

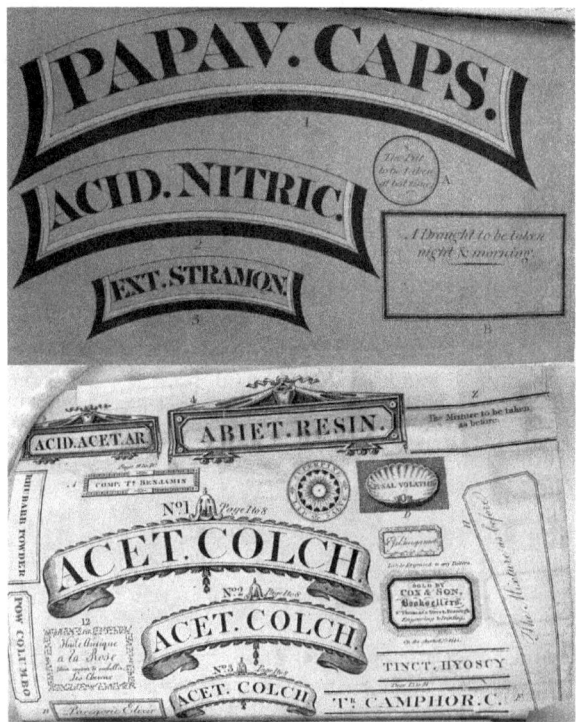

Figure 8.1 Cox's Medical Labels, from the 1828 catalogue. Wellcome Library. Public Domain.

to treat diarrhoea, and the decorative French label for 'Huile Antique a la Rose', to nourish and embellish the hair). All labels were engraved, rather than printed with moveable type, probably by Cox's son Benjamin, the in-house engraver. The Cox & Son establishment was itself advertised on the sample page: '*Labels Engraved to any Pattern*, SOLD BY COX & SON, Booksellers, St. Thomas's Street, Borough. *Engraving & Printing. On the shortest Notice*'.[39]

Erica M. Storm has explored how the senses helped users to navigate potentially dangerous medicines: 'colour, shape and flavour offered patients the assurance of a standard, safe and effective product'.[40] Colour could be remarkably fixed, denoting authenticity, because printing using multiple colours did not become possible at large scale until 1835.[41] Colour also assisted with the safe dispensing of drugs. Storm warns against accepting the monochrome world of the periodical advertisement and reveals the technicolour sensory experience that (patent) medicines offered their eighteenth-century consumers. For instance, she reveals that the most common colour for the labels of patent medicines was red with white lettering.[42] However, while much work has been done on patent medicines and their counterfeits, an analysis of the labelling of unbranded medicines has yet to be undertaken.[43] Within this context, it is clear that Cox's provision of labels on differently coloured backgrounds enabled pharmacists and druggists to adopt systems of their own. They could choose yellow, green, pink or white labels according to what might be most visible on their particular bottles, or perhaps choosing one colour for their stores of ingredients, and another for medicines made up.

Cox was keen to point out that Latin labels should not be fixed to bottles intended to be used by untrained staff, distinguishing between her first and second patterns, the first taken from the latest version of the Latin *Pharmacopoeia Londinensis* (1618; 1815), and the second from its translation: 'N.B. The Labels of the first Pattern are designed principally for the Uses of Surgeons and Apothecaries'.[44] Her catalogue included dispensing labels as well as labels for carboy bottles (huge vessels holding up to 60 litres) in gold, green and yellow for the use of apothecaries, surgeons and chemists, engraved by her son in copperplate, with his distinctive calligraphy contributing to the visual culture and mythology of the dispensary. Cox also sold 'chemical characters', presumably small blocks for printing chemical characters or labels printed from them, and gold paper labels (for ready money only, rather than on credit, due to their cost).[45] She was catering for a professional market which she knew well and to which she had to constantly adapt her printing and bookselling practice.

The work of the medical label publisher was unending, requiring up-to-date knowledge of the latest developments in medicine and technology.

On or before 1828, Cox adapted her portfolio from labels for tying on to vials to labels 'gummed at the Back, and ready for immediate Use'.[46] Because paper was damp at the point of printing, to enable the weave to accept the pressure of the printing press without breaking, gum was applied when the paper was dry.[47] Rollers, or large stippling brushes like those used to colour sheets of paper, were used to apply the coating, a process which would not be mechanised until around 1886. Professionally produced gummed labels tended to be most commonly used in this period for book labels, attendance stickers, posters and office labels.[48]

Perhaps the most recognised use for gummed paper in its earliest days was for stamps. On 2 October 1839, the *London Evening Standard* printed that 'It is the current report at the Post Office, that stamped labels saturated with gum, and to be affixed on the direction side of the letter, will be the means used for carrying the New Penny Postage Act into operation'.[49] Gummed stamps were first produced by James Chalmers in Dundee in 1834.[50] Cox was using the latest technology at a time when Rowland Hill was first considering gumming the backs of English postage stamps, a project he had proposed in 1837, though gummed stamps would not appear in England until 1840.[51] There were, however, complaints about the effectiveness of the Penny Post and its innovations:

> Stamps! – And loud resounds the yell of the stationer 'who is to find me capital? How am I to keep the various sizes of paper? Will you give me credit?' 'I should think not!' ... growls the chancellor.
> Labels! – 'How am I to stick them on, asks the delicate lady; am I to keep a paste-pot in my writing desk?'
> Gummed Labels! – 'They won't stick'; cries every body, and Rowland Hill scratcheth his head, and government forthwith offers two hundred pounds to any one who will get him out of his scrape. We are afraid Government will keep the two hundred pounds, and Rowland Hill remain in full possession of his dilemma.[52]

Nevertheless, gumming was perceived to be sufficiently reliable to be used in the context of the dispensary. As Michael Fairley and Tony White point out, 'Few realise ... that a further traditional use for gummed paper labels was for prescription labelling of medicine bottles, etc, in chemists shops and in identification of "Poison" bottles'.[53] Perhaps in no other sector could paper technology and its ability to defend against mislabelling be quite so important. While Cox was not the first to offer gummed medical labels – Wheeler's System of Labelling had been advertised at least as early as 1818 – this was nevertheless cutting-edge technology; gummed labels of any kind would not be introduced to America until 1864.[54]

The perils of mislabelling

While Cox's labels were intended to aid transparency in the production of medicines, they were produced by a hand that had been found guilty of fraudulent practice. Benjamin, Cox's son, was a 'copper-plate printer, residing in the Borough, very generally employed by oilmen, perfumers, and others in London, to print their labels'. He was also the defendant of Lazenby v. Cox at the Court of King's Bench, in an action of damages against Elizabeth Lazenby, proprietor of her father's 'Harvey's Fish Sauce' from her shop near Portman-square.[55] Lazenby accused Cox of having made and sold a large quantity of her labels to a rival sauce seller. He claimed unknowingly to have struck off a fraudulent plate for 'Harvey's Fish Sauce' in 1811 or 1812. He was found out when the young boy of eleven who was sent to deliver the new labels accidentally delivered them to Lazenby, who at that point became aware of and reported the crime. Harvey's Fish Sauce was a household name, and the case was covered in journalism across the nation in the metropolitan and provincial press. In 1820, the Chief Justice summing up for the jury, observed that 'the law would not warrant him in selling such article under the name of another, without his authority, nor would it warrant any man to aid him in such an imposition; it was in proof, that the defendant had aided others to vend a spurious composition of their own, in the name and as the production of the plaintiff, and therefore he must be responsible in such damages as the Jury should deem reasonable': the charges were damages 40 shillings; costs 40 shillings.[56]

We cannot know whether Elizabeth as business manager at this time was privy to, or part of, the fraud. Lazenby certainly thought so. She would continue to have problems with counterfeit sauce sellers, and so, ten years later, inserted a notice in the *Globe* of 17 September 1829 raking over old ground:

> TO COPPER-PLATE ENGRAVERS AND PRINTERS. E. LAZENBY and SON feel it their duty to caution the Trade in general against engraving or selling Labels to imitate those used for their genuine HARVEY'S FISH SAUCE. E. L. and Son having on 15th of February, 1820, obtained a verdict, with full costs, against Cox and Son, engravers and printers in the Borough. And as from a recent trial (Lazenby v. Wingrave, before Lord Tenterden, at Guildhall, 28th July, 1829) it is evident that Labels are selling without their authority.[57]

Pleading for witnesses to come forward to support her lawsuits, Lazenby meanwhile reminded the printing community of the less than salubrious history of Cox's son, directing the blame not just at Benjamin but at his mother, too, through the invocation of their trading name at this time,

'Cox and Son'. This was not a good look for a brand predicated on ideal values of transparency, authenticity and trust.

But the fish sauce scandal did not sour business. In fact, Cox's capacity to produce ephemera which consolidated her name as a brand leader continued to grow. She was an early producer of a near essential item: the medicine chest booklet. The earliest known advertisement for the *Companion* is 16 November 1829, in the *Morning Chronicle*, in a note appended to Cox's publication notice for her 'Elegant Gold Labels':

> "Cox's Companion to the Family Medicine Chest," with plain rules for taking the Medicines in the Cure of Diseases, in a style adapted to every capacity, by a Member of the Royal College of Surgeons, with the Labels annexed for each article, price 1s. Also, "A Sea Medicine Chest," of the same description, with labels added, price 1s.[58]

Medicine chest booklets, as J. K. Crellin and J. R. Scott argue, 'were exceedingly common' in the 1800s, and *Cox's Companion to the Family Medicine Chest* (c.1829) the most successful pamphlet of the century.[59] Medicine chest booklets were small pamphlets which accompanied the nineteenth-century equivalent of the first aid kit. As *Cox's Companion* pointed out:

> A judicious and discerning public have long experienced, and repeatedly acknowledged, the inestimable advantage derived from a portable dispensary; but it must be obvious to all, that without full and perspicuous directions how to proceed, for the relief of the multiplied forms of human misery, to which the humane part of mankind may administer assistances, the advantages would be much curtailed.

Companions to medical chests, therefore, filled an important gap in supplying the information on compounding and applying medicines in appropriate doses, 'as cannot fail to render a Medicine Chest more extensively useful'.[60] Medical chests had recently become must-have items.[61] Heather Hayley has traced their status as essential equipment of the naval surgeon to an object of luxury, promoted, in part, through the distribution of trade cards, of which Cox and Co. were also producers.[62] The Cox enterprise, therefore, sold medicines, produced trade cards for medical cabinets, and published the accompanying pamphlets which made the medicines and the cabinets all the more saleable. One such cabinet was recently sold by antiques dealer Graham Smith (Figure 8.2).

Cox was not the originator of the medical cabinet booklet genre. One of the earliest had been apothecary Hugh Smith's *The Family Physician* (London, 1760), which was printed for the author 'at his Chymical Warehouse', and on sale alongside his remedies.[63] Another was Doctor Thomas John Graham's *Modern Domestic Medicine* (1826), which

Mislabelling and the medical printer-publisher 165

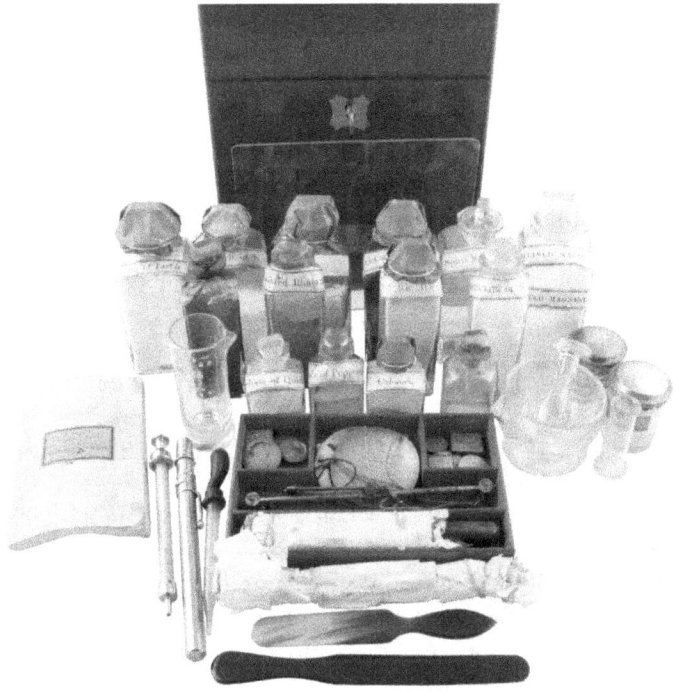

Figure 8.2 A medicine cabinet (h 22 cm × w 18 cm × d 16 cm), *c*.1850, sold by Graham Smith Antiques, complete with the booklet, 'Cox's Medical Cabinet', and the accompanying labels cut and stuck to the bottles.

included 'approved prescriptions adapted to domestic use' and a table of doses.[64] Early pamphlets to explicitly brand themselves as medicine chest 'companions' include Richard Reece's *Domestic Medical Guide* (London: Longman, 1802), which from its 1803 editions was subtitled the *Complete Companion to the Family Medicine Chest*, and publisher James Tindal's *Companion to the Medicine Chest* (1804). Cox's success perhaps derived from three things: detail, branding and labels. The extensive detail Cox provided was unusual, outlining doses for ages under 1, 2, 3, 4, 7, 14 and 20 years and over 21, over 65 and over 80.[65] Cox also undertook to describe the properties of individual medicine ingredients as well as their compounds, meaning it was particularly suited to the layperson attempting to administer medicines. Hers was also the only booklet to be associated with a female producer.

In terms of branding, Cox's *Companion* took many slightly altered forms. The pamphlet aimed at families covered only 'Such medicines as are safe, useful, or convenient for a medicine chest'. On medicines that were included in chests solely for the convenience of medical practitioners, 'it was thought proper to remain silent, both as to their virtues and application in the cure of diseases, lest such comments should lead to a misapplication in practice, and consequent mischief to the patient'. Cox chose to print 'The names to which the public have been most familiarized ..., as being better calculated to prevent mistakes'.[66] As a label printer she well understood the need to cater both for the learned practitioners and for those unaccustomed to the Latin terms. Cox pivoted towards markets other than the family, too. *Cox's Companion to the Sea Medicine Chest* had an extended title which made clear that it was *Particularly Adapted for Captains of Merchant Vessels, Missionaries, and Colonists* (c.1836). This companion included a section 'On the Venereal Disease' which did not feature in the family edition.[67] Her ability to adapt her pamphlet to different markets meant that Cox was pioneering in establishing what would become the medical cabinet companion's most popular iteration.

In the seventeenth edition of her booklet (1833) Cox writes, 'This small Work', 'intended principally for Domestic Use, is respectfully dedicated to the Heads of Families in England, Scotland and Ireland, By their Obedient Servant, The Publisher'.[68] In this personal note, Cox spoke directly to her readers, which, in the absence of an author's name on the title page, served to indicate her editorial agency over the project. Her work quickly became a recognisable brand, known by the Cox name, as was customary for ephemera produced by medical booksellers, identified as much by their publisher as by their titles and authors.[69] One thing that her competitors could not do, or at least offer efficiently, was to combine their companions with gummed labels. For Cox, it was important that labels were not only for professional use but also provided (with accompanying instructions) for laypeople intending to handle or administer drugs. Like her instructions, her cabinet bottle labels were printed in the vernacular. Perhaps Cox's most pioneering intervention into the cabinet companion genre was her incorporation of her characteristic pull-out attachment of labels, merging the practices – of bookselling, printing and engraving – in which her establishment excelled.[70]

A misremembered legacy

Cox developed key works other than the *Companion*: handbooks more squarely aimed at the medical practitioner. She was the publisher of chemist and druggist Robert Oliver Wilkinson's *Druggists' Price Book* (1832?), known as *Cox's Druggist's Price Book* on its label.[71] And she innovated in other respects pertaining to medical publishing which combined her own skills as entrepreneur with those of her son as engraver in order to reach wider audiences. She established two botanical periodicals, *Medical Botany* (1819) and *Flora Domestica; or, History of Medicinal Plants Indigenous to Great Britain* (1836), making botanical information and engravings more readily available to a range of readers. She also republished William Smellie's *Set of Anatomical Tables* as a small, more affordable, pamphlet after recommissioning the engravings accordingly. As Ruth Richardson notes, the scandal of his teaching female anatomy to large mixed classes of men and women at his midwifery school, accompanied by these affordable tables, produced using the relatively quick and inexpensive method of etching, contributed to Smellie's renown.[72]

But despite the mark left upon nineteenth-century medical bookselling by Elizabeth Cox, she suffered from misinformation in her lifetime and beyond. She was misgendered as 'Messrs. Cox and Son' in an advertisement in the *New Times* of 5 May 1818 and in Henry Curwen's *History of Booksellers, the Old and the Young* (1874).[73] Her *Companions* are widely catalogued as having been written by Edward Cox, 'Writer on Medicine'.[74] No particular person tends to be indicated by that appellation, but it might be associated with Edward Cox Mann (1850–1908), who wrote *A Manual of Prescription Writing* (1880) and *A Manual of Psychological Medicine and Allied Nervous Diseases* (1883), though he was not yet born when Elizabeth Cox was trading. Given that Cox herself died in 1841, it remains clear that any work published by her before her death would be unlikely to be by an 'Edward Cox', with Elizabeth falling prey to the mislabelling she worked to counter in her business. While we cannot know how much Cox herself contributed to the *Companions*, the false attribution of the booklets to an 'Edward Cox' demonstrates a widespread misunderstanding of the nineteenth-century meanings of these pamphlets, with the intervention of publishers in their creation being considered tantamount to (co-)creators in the public imagination.

After her death, posthumous editions of Cox's *Cabinet* continued to flourish, and from 1845 (the twentieth edition) onwards were 'revised, and considerably enlarged', by R. Davis, 'Member of the Royal College of Surgeons' and published by 'E. Cox, St. Thomas's street'. Elizabeth outlived all of her children. Benjamin Rane Cox (1787–1828) had been a medical bookseller but predeceased her and left her his estate.[75] John Cox, another son, had a medical bookselling business in Berners-Street, Oxford Street (trading 1822–26), serving the new Middlesex Hospital, but he died aged 30 at his mother's home.[76] A daughter, Mary Johanna Cox, had also died young.[77] It would be her sons Daniel and Thomas junior who would have a family and to whose descendants Cox would ultimately bequeath her business. In her will, she instructed trustees to enable her daughter-in-law, Ellen Frances Cox, and her granddaughter, the daughter of Thomas, Emily

Eliza Cox, to live in her premises and inherit her household estate.[78] The 'E. Cox' of 1845 could be either Ellen or Emily, or perhaps both, or trustees working for their benefit.

Cox also left a professional legacy. For the customary seven years, she had apprenticed the son of the Reverend James Churchill, John Spriggs Morss Churchill (1801–75), who, after a brief stint at Longmans, would go on to purchase Callow's business and became a leading medical bookseller in his own right, issuing an annual catalogue. Thanks to expertise learned from Cox, he would publish his own works, including Liston's *Practical Surgery* (1837), and he would take over the publication of the *Lancet* between 1842 and 1847.[79]

As Stanley C. Hollander wrote in his 1956 *History of Labels*: 'While labels have been used for many odd and interesting purposes over the centuries, the student will find that the ways in which people until recently, failed to use labels were far more curious and significant'.[80] Elizabeth Cox, medical bookseller and publisher, made a career out of what had been a lack of formal medicine labelling at the beginning of the nineteenth century. Despite her success, until now Cox's contribution to both professional and home-based medical practice has been either misidentified, misgendered or entirely overlooked. Though her son, as copperplate engraver, was involved in a case of fraud by mislabelling, the Cox & Son establishment was nevertheless one that became a prominent brand, and seller of the most successful pamphlet of the nineteenth century, in the form of *Cox's Companion to the Medicine Chest* and its various iterations, all of which were accompanied by the family's distinctive copperplate labels.

Notes

1 Helen Smith, *'Grossly Material Things': Women and Book Production in Early Modern England* (Oxford: Oxford University Press, 2012), p. 109; Paula McDowell, *The Women of Grub Street: Press, Politics, and Gender in the London Literary Marketplace 1678–1730* (Oxford: Clarendon, 1998), p. 35.

2 James Raven's *The Publishing Business in Eighteenth-Century England* (Woodbridge: Boydell, 2014) has been important in arguing for the value of jobbing printing to individual businesses and to the wider economy. Recent work to recover women entrepreneurs in the book trade includes Hannah Barker's *The Business of Women: Female Enterprise and Urban Development in Northern England, 1760–1830* (Oxford: Oxford University Press, 2006) and the essays collected in Cathleen A. Baker and Rebecca M. Chung (eds), *Making Impressions: Women in Printing and Publishing* (Ann Arbor, MI: Legacy, 2020). On female entrepreneurship more broadly, see Jennifer Aston, *Female Entrepreneurship in Nineteenth-Century England: Engagement in*

the Urban Economy, Palgrave Studies in Economic History (Basingstoke: Palgrave, 2016).
3 Michael Harris, 'Printed Ephemera', in Michael F. Suarez, S.J. and M. R. Woudhuysen (eds), *The Oxford Companion to the Book*, 2 vols (Oxford: Oxford University Press, 2010), vol. 1, pp. 120–128: p. 120. Gillian Russell's work on *The Ephemeral Eighteenth Century: Print, Sociability, and the Cultures of Collecting* (Cambridge: Cambridge University Press, 2020) provides a thorough history of ephemera studies. See esp. p. 4.
4 McDowell, *Women of Grub Street*, pp. 45–46.
5 Raven, *Publishing Business*; Russell, *Ephemeral Eighteenth Century*.
6 Leslie Howsam, 'In My View: Women and Book History', *SHARP News* (1998); Michelle Levy, 'Do Women Have a Book History?', *Studies in Romanticism* 53:3 (2014): 297–317; Sarah Werner, 'Working Towards a Feminist Printing History', *Printing History New Series*, 27/28 (2020): 11–25; Kate Ozment, 'Rationale for Feminist Bibliography', *Textual Cultures* 13:1 (2020): 149–178.
7 J. K. Crellin and J. R. Scott, 'Pharmaceutical History and its Sources in the Wellcome Collections: II. Drug Weighing in Britain, *c*.1700–1900', *Medical History* 13:1 (1969): 51–67, at p. 58 n. 38.
8 'State of the Medical Profession in St Petersburgh', *London Medical Gazette, or Journal of Practical Medicine* 2:52 (1828): 815–816, at 816.
9 Stuart Anderson, 'From "Bespoke" to "Off-the-Peg": Community Pharmacists and the Retailing of Medicines in Great Britain 1900–1970', in Louise Hill Curth (ed.), *From Physick to Pharmacology: Five Hundred Years of British Drug Retailing* (Aldershot: Ashgate, 2006), pp. 105–142, at p. 108.
10 Ibid.
11 'State of the Medical Profession in St Petersburgh', p. 816.
12 *The Atlas* (9 July 1826).
13 *Old Bailey Online*, 11 April 1833, reference number t18330411-209, available at https://www.oldbaileyonline.org/browse.jsp?name=18330411, last accessed 30 October 2023.
14 Letter from William Gilbert, Assistant Poor Law Commissioner to the Poor Law Commission, regarding the Death of a Child [Henry Love] in the Workhouse in consequence of an improper medicine having been administered by mistake. Plymouth, 7 March 1839. Devon Poor Law Unions: Axminster 76. The National Archives, [MS] MH12-1-2096.
15 Report from the meeting of 24 June 1819, quoted in Jacob Bell and Theophilus Redwood, *Historical Sketch of the Progress of Pharmacy in Great Britain* (London: Pharmaceutical Society, 1880), pp. 70–71.
16 Stanley C. Hollander, *History of Labels: A Record of the Past Developed in the Search for the Origins of an Industry* (New York: Hollander, 1956), pp. 7–8.
17 The earliest surviving edition is a thirteenth edition held by Indiana Historical Society Library: [by a 'Member of the Royal College of Surgeons' and E. Cox], *Companion to the Medicine Chest: with Plain Rules for Taking the Medicines in the Cure of Diseases*, 13th edn (London: Cox, 1830). The next is at the Wellcome Library: [Elizabeth Cox & Son and a 'Member of the Royal College

of Surgeons'], *Companion to the Medicine Chest, with Plain Rules for Taking the Medicines in the Cure of Diseases*, 15th edn (London: Cox, 1832). Both feature six leaves of engraved bottle labels.

18 Joseph Fox's *Natural History of the Human Teeth* was advertised as published by 'Thomas Cox (at his Medical Library), St. Thomas's-street, Borough' in the *London Courier and Evening Gazette*, 9 March 1804.
19 *London Courier and Evening Gazette* (1 April 1816).
20 *Morning Advertiser* (29 September 1810); *Oxford Journal* (6 October 1810); *Northampton Mercury* (26 December 1812).
21 *The British Book Trade Index*, from here on abbreviated to '*BBTI*', available at http://bbti.bodleian.ox.ac.uk/#, last accessed 28 July 2022.
22 *BBTI*.
23 Will of Thomas Cox, Bookseller and Engraver of Southwark, Surrey (1806), National Archives, PROB-11-1444-260.
24 P. W. J. Bartrip, 'Churchill, John Spriggs Morss (1801–1875)', *Oxford Dictionary of National Biography*, ed. H. C. G. Matthew and Brian Harrison (Oxford: Oxford University Press, 2004), vol. 11, pp. 634–635.
25 James Morss Churchill, in Henry Curwen, *A History of Booksellers, the Old and the New* (London: Chatto & Windus, 1874), pp. 339–340.
26 Robert Oliver Wilkinson, *The Druggist's Price-Book, or a Catalogue of the Drugs, Chemicals, and Perfumery Generally Sold by Chemists & Druggists, with the Doses and Old Names Annexed*, 2nd edn (London: Cox, 1832), p. 54.
27 Sir Antonio More after Robert Thew (engraver), *Sir Thomas Gresham, Founder of the Royal Exchange* [engraving, uncoloured] (London: Elizabeth Cox, 1823).
28 See the *BBTI* for a comprehensive list.
29 Maurice J. Quinlan (ed.), 'Memoir of William Cowper', *Proceedings of the American Philosophical Society*, 97:4 (1953): 359–382.
30 McDowell, *Women of Grub Street*; Paula McDowell (ed.), *Elinor James: Printed Writings 1641–1700* (London: Routledge, 2005); Alison McNaught, 'Two Nonconformist Women Printers and Booksellers in the Mid-Eighteenth Century', *Bunyan Studies* 24 (2020): 65–84; Timothy Whelan, 'Mary Lewis and her Family of Printers and Booksellers, 1 Paternoster Row, 1749–1812', *Publishing History* 85 (2021): 31–67.
31 Timothy Whelan, Introduction, *A Tradition of Nonconformist & Dissenting Women Writers, 1650–1850*, available at https://www.nonconformistwomen writers1650-1850.com/introduction, last accessed 30 June 2022.
32 Michael Fairley and Tony White, *The History of Labels: The Evolution of the Label Industry in Europe* (London: Tarsus, 2014), pp. 1–2.
33 *New Times* (23 November 1818). Stockists included H. Burtershaw on St Martin's Lane and Thomas Woodham in High Holborn.
34 'Labels', *Kentish Gazette* (1 September 1815).
35 *BBTI*. 'Medical Blank Labels', in the *London Morning Herald* (23 February 1819). As the advert notes, these were labels aimed at 'houses of extensive practice'.
36 *New Times* (5 May 1818).

37 A sample of the green paper labels can be found in the 1828 catalogue preserved in the Wellcome collection.
38 *New Times* (28 May 1818).
39 *Cox's Catalogue of Dispensing Labels, as per Specimens, at 2s. 6d. per Thousand, Gummed at the Back, and Ready for Immediate Use* (London: Cox, 1828). Wellcome Trust b31909401.
40 Erica M. Storm, 'Gilding the Pill: The Sensuous Consumption of Patent Medicines, 1815–1841', *Social History of Medicine* 31:1 (2018): 41–60, at p. 46.
41 Ibid.; Helen Williams, *Laurence Sterne and the Eighteenth-Century Book* (Cambridge: Cambridge University Press, 2021), p. 125.
42 Storm, 'Gilding the Pill', p. 52.
43 George Griffenhagen and Mary Bogard, *History of Drug Containers and Their Labels* (Madison, WI: American Institute of the History of Pharmacy, 1999); Louise Hill Curth (ed.), *From Physick to Pharmacology: Five Hundred Years of British Drug Retailing* (Aldershot: Ashgate, 2006); Roy Porter, *Health for Sale: Quackery in England, 1660–1850* (Manchester: Manchester University Press, 1989).
44 *New Times* (28 May 1818). The Royal College of Physicians' *Pharmacopoeia Londinensis* (1618), which by the Royal Proclamation of King James I made it illegal to sell a drug that did not appear in this book. It was an essential guide for every apothecary and druggist in England, though it had only emerged from an anxiety around the establishment in 1617 of the Worshipful Society of Apothecaries, which took away the power of the physicians to regulate their activities. The volume was first translated into English by apothecary Nicolas Culpeper in 1649.
45 Catalogues from 1828 and 1836, Wellcome Library.
46 Catalogue 1828. See also *Cox's Catalogue of Dispensing Labels, at 2s. 6d. per thousand, Gummed for Immediate Use* (London: Cox, 1836), Wellcome Library b30387826.
47 The adhesive tended to be made from gum arabic, rather than dextrin, because it was considered purer. Later, when gum arabic became expensive, starch-based adhesives were used, made from potatoes or corn and converted into dextrin, and animal-based glues when a higher tack was required.
48 Fairley and White, *History of Labels*, pp. 34–36.
49 *London Evening Standard* (2 October 1839).
50 Patrick Chalmers, *The Adhesive Postage Stamp* (London: Wilson, 1886).
51 Ibid., p. 29.
52 'The Penny Post System', *Roscommon & Leitrim Gazette* (5 October 1839).
53 Fairley and White, *History of Labels*, pp. 35–36.
54 *Morning Post* (25 March 1818). Griffenhagen and Bogard, *History of Drug Containers*, p. 34. Gummed labels had been used by Nottingham Dispensary since at least December 1838, though it is not clear who had made or sold them. 'Important Case', *Nottingham and Newark Mercury* (29 December 1838).
55 *Globe* (14 January 1819); *Saunders's News-Letter* (23 February 1820).

56 *Saunders's News-Letter* (23 February 1820).
57 *Globe* (17 September 1829).
58 *Morning Chronicle* (16 November 1829).
59 Crellin and Scott, 'Pharmaceutical History', p. 58 n. 38. The earliest advertisement for the *Companion* is from 16 November 1829, in the *Morning Chronicle*, in a note appended to Cox's publication notice for her 'Elegant Gold Labels': '"Cox's Companion to the Family Medicine Chest," with plain rules for taking the Medicines in the Cure of Diseases, in a style adapted to every capacity, by a Member of the Royal College of Surgeons, with the Labels annexed for each article, price 1s. Also, "A Sea Medicine Chest," of the same description, with labels added, price 1s.' *Morning Chronicle* (16 November 1829).
60 'Preface', in *Companion to the Medicine Chest* (London: Cox, 1843), p. v.
61 A diagram of one can be seen in the frontispiece to Richard Reece's *Domestic Medical Guide* (London: Stower, 1803). Wellcome Trust.
62 See the trade card for Christopher Woodhouse, apothecary, druggist and medicine chest fitter, which survives in the British Museum, 'DRAFT Trade card of Christopher Woodhouse, Chemist', Museum Number Heal, 35.84. Heather Hayley, '"Convenient in Any Exigency": The Transcendence of the Medicine Chest from the Professional to the Domestic in the Early Nineteenth Century', *Global Maritime History*, 3 July 2017, available at https://globalmaritimehistory.com/convenient-exigency-transcendence-medicine-chest-professional-domestic/, last accessed 22 July 2022.
63 Hugh Smith, *The Family Physician: Being a Collection of Useful Family Remedies*, 8th edn (London: Printed for the author, 1770–1775?).
64 Thomas John Graham (1826), *Modern Domestic Medicine*, 3rd edn, much enlarged (London: Published for the author, 1827).
65 Crellin and Scott, 'Pharmaceutical History', p. vi.
66 'Preface', in *Companion to the Medicine Chest*, pp. vi–vii.
67 *Cox's Companion to the Sea Medicine Chest* (London: Simpkin, Marshall & Co., 1845), available at https://www.abebooks.co.uk/servlet/BookDetailsPL?bi=30870412362&searchurl=kn%3Dcox%2Bmedical%2Bbookseller%26sortby%3D17&cm_sp=snippet-_-srp1-_-title14, last accessed 22 July 2012.
68 *Companion to the Medicine Chest with Plain Rules for Taking the Medicines in the Cure of Diseases*, 17th edn (London: Cox, 1833) [pharmecutical remedy booklet], Accession Number, 1954.3.2, Kingston Museum of Healthcare University Health Network – Academy of Medicine Collection (available at https://mhc.andornot.com/en/permalink/artifact15264, last accessed 20 October 2023).
69 Druggists' price books, such as Anderson's (1825), Armstrong's (1826) and Jameson's (1830).
70 All of Cox's *Companions* seemed to have included labels, from the 1829 advertisement onwards, where they are explicitly advertised, as in the 1836 druggists' price book, which noted that her 'new edition' of *Cox's Companion to the Sea Medicine Chest* and the fifteenth edition of the *Companion to the Medicine Chest* both had 'Labels Annexed'. Rival editions featuring labels included Henry

Gregory's *A Companion to the Medicine* Chest (London: Butler, 1837), though I have found none earlier.

71 Robert Oliver Wilkinson, *Druggists' Price Book*, 3rd edn (London: Cox, 1736), British Library RB23.a.12230.

72 Ruth Richardson, *The Making of Mr. Gray's Anatomy: Bodies, Books, Fortune, Fame* (Oxford: Oxford University Press, 2008), p. 101.

73 *New Times* (5 May 1818); Curwen, *A History of Booksellers*, p. 339.

74 See, for example, the British Library copies of the *Companion to the Medicine Chest*, 32nd edition, 1845, the *Companion to the Family Medicine Chest*, 33rd edition, 1845, and the *Companion to the Sea Medicine Chest*, 20th edition, 1844. At the Wellcome Library the following editions are linked to his name: *Cox's Companion to the Sea Medicine Chest*, 1st American from the 33rd London edition (1851) and *Cox's Companion to the Family Medicine Chest*, 48th edition (1887), available at https://wellcomecollection.org/works/dz6e4qvv, last accessed 22 July 2022.

75 Neither Benjamin nor John appear in the *BBTI*. For the former, see Will of Benjamin Rane Cox, 11 October 1828, Medical Bookseller and Publisher of Saint Thomas Street, National Archives, PROB 11/1746/276.

76 Ian Maxted, 'Thomas Cox', *The London Book Trades 1775–1800: A Preliminary Checklist of Members*, Exeter Working Papers in British Book Trade History (Folkstone: Dawson, 1977); For the latter, see the newspaper article which reported John's death: 'Thursday, at the house of his mother, St. Thomas-street, Southwark, aged 30, Mr. J. Cox, medical bookseller of Berners-street, London', *Hereford Journal* (25 January 1830). See also the fire insurance records for John: 4 April 1822: 'Insured: John Cox 11 Berners Street Oxford Street bookseller', Records of the Sun Fire Office, Policy Register, London Metropolitan Archives MS 11936/493/989752.

77 Will of Elizabeth Cox, 6 February 1841, Medical Bookseller of Brewers Court Saint Thomas Street Southwark, PROB-11-1940-300.

78 Ibid.

79 Bartrip, 'Churchill, John Spriggs Morss'.

80 Hollander, *History of Labels*, p. 5.

9

The uneasy relationship between traditional and orthodox medicine in the works of Elizabeth Gaskell

Barbara Witucki

Though 'the work of Elizabeth Gaskell (1810–65) is not often seen as a source for the student of medical history',[1] her first novel, *Mary Barton: A Tale of Manchester Life*, incorporates a general exposition of the status quo of the healing arts, both traditional and orthodox, in Manchester in the late eighteenth and early nineteenth centuries. Her succeeding works include a surprising number of details that illustrate both the development of orthodox medicine from hereditary knowledge and the fabric of irrational beliefs and myths found in traditional medicine, and the friction that ensues as the orthodox slowly supersedes the hereditary and traditional. Thus, just as it has been said that Gaskell 'has preserved for future generations the manners, customs, and characters which were in vogue in provincial towns during the early part of the Victorian era',[2] it can also be said that she has preserved the daily practice of the healing arts.

Through the corpus of her longer fiction, Gaskell traces the transition from traditional plant lore through domestic medicine to nascent pharmacology and medicine founded on scientific principles, and the transition from practitioners dependent on irregular training to druggists, doctors and surgeons who have completed systematic training and certification. Throughout, her intent appears to be descriptive rather than evaluative. Nonetheless, the arc from the death of Alice Wilson in Gaskell's first novel, the only folk herbalist in her longer works, to the life of Mr Gibson, the general practitioner portrayed in her last novel, *Wives and Daughters*, suggests that she recognises the changes in the healing arts not as an unmasking and correction of deficiencies by later generations, but as an evolution from ignorance to understanding through advances in scientific knowledge. Mr Gibson is a socially acceptable gentleman. He is also the product of the newer, systematic medical training, and he remains abreast of developments not only in medicine but in all fields of scientific inquiry through publication and professional interactions.[3] Gaskell thus conjectures that one era's knowledge becomes mythic ignorance of the next as human knowledge and consequent understanding increase.

The persistent presence of healing practitioners in Gaskell's fiction reflects their presence in her own life.[4] While growing up in provincial Knutsford, she spent much time at the home of her uncle, Peter Holland, the surgeon for Knutsford and the surrounding area.[5] She is remembered as having 'accompanied him on his rounds in his gig whenever possible'.[6] Her uncle also links Gaskell to the lore of the Manchester medical establishments and surgeons. Peter Holland was considered 'the most celebrated' of the many apprentice surgeons and man-midwives taught by Charles White, who was himself 'the originator of lectures to medical students in Manchester, the founder of the science of anthropometry, and for half a century the most original, able, and prominent surgeon in the town [Manchester]', and served as Honorary Surgeon to the Manchester Infirmary, 1752–90.[7] Though Charles White provides a prototype for the training and practice of medical professionals, it is Gaskell's uncle who is frequently mentioned as the original for 'Dr. Hoggins in *Cranford*, Dr. Morgan in *Mr. Harrison's Confessions*, and the kind Dr. Gibson in *Wives and Daughters*'.[8] Similarly, 'Dr. Peter Colthurst, the novelist's great-uncle, who was the doctor at Knutsford in an earlier age (he died in the year 1769)' is also suggested as a model 'for some of the medical characters'.[9] Likewise, Peter Holland's son and Mrs Gaskell's cousin, Henry, who served as Physician-in-Ordinary to Queen Victoria and became Sir Henry Holland, is considered a source for 'information which enabled [Gaskell] to give the conventional representation of a past type of medical student'.[10] This blending of the real and the fictional is perhaps clearest when the good ladies of Cranford, though they wish that 'Queen Adelaide or the Duke of Wellington being ill ... would send for Mr. Hoggins', wonder what they would do 'if Mr. Hoggins had been appointed physician in ordinary to the Royal Family' (2.11.124).[11]

In addition to her relatives, Gaskell encountered Dr Anthony Thomson, the brother of her father's second wife, Catherine Thomson, while visiting her father. Dr Thomson played an 'influential' role in 'the transformation of the traditionally tripartite medical community' into its modern form with the evolution of the general practitioner trained equally in medicine, surgery and apothecary.[12] Following her marriage to William Gaskell in 1832, Gaskell moved to Manchester, where she continued her acquaintance with Dr Thomson and his wife. Further, her brother-in-law Samuel Gaskell trained at the Royal Manchester Infirmary and in Edinburgh, and practised medicine at the 'cholera hospital' in 'Swan Street, Ancoats' during the 1832 cholera outbreak in Manchester. Later, he worked at the Manchester Royal Infirmary and Lunatic Asylum.[13] Gaskell also became friends with James Phillips Kay. Though usually cited as the author of *The Moral and Physical Condition of the Working Class Employed in the Cotton Manufacture in*

Manchester, prior to turning to social and education reform, Kay worked as a doctor at the Ardwick and Ancoats Dispensary.[14] The son of James Phillip Kay, later Sir James Phillips Kay-Shuttleworth, remembers the visits of his father's 'remarkable friends', including those of Mrs Gaskell.[15]

In Manchester, the medical men played a significant role in establishing natural knowledge as a major factor in the cultural life of the city.[16] They were the driving force behind the founding of the Literary and Philosophical Society in 1781, and its development as a force for sharing scientific and medical advances with professionals and the general public as well as a centre for traditional cultural events. Participation in the society and its administration became a means for medical men to build status in the community as well as to serve as 'guardian[s] of the politer virtues in an industrializing world'.[17] Through social and cultural events, therefore, Gaskell would have kept abreast of current events and topics of interest in medicine and natural science. Even this brief overview of Gaskell's relatives, friends and acquaintances who were medical professionals and of her social environment suggests an extensive first-hand knowledge of the current trends in the healing arts, which, in turn, find a little noted but persistent place in her fiction.[18]

Herbalist, druggist, physiognomist and doctor

Gaskell's first novel, *Mary Barton: A Tale of Manchester Life* (1848),[19] tells the story of John Barton,[20] a mill worker, his daughter Mary, and a small circle of the Barton's friends. This circle incorporates different aspects of Manchester life: exploration through the travels of a sailor, Will Wilson, the amateur study of natural science in Job Legh, a mill worker, 'folk' music through Job's granddaughter Margaret, the police and the legal system in the trial of Jem Wilson, a foundry worker, the mill owners, through Mr Carson, and the mill workers themselves through John Barton and his friends. Notwithstanding the importance of medical men as healers as well as leaders in Manchester's cultural and social life, Barton's circle lacks a representative of the medical professions. Gaskell fills this void with Alice Wilson, a traditional herbalist and aunt to Will Wilson and his cousin Jem Wilson. Though medical men appear in the novel, Gaskell obscures them by leaving them anonymous and undeveloped consequently minimising orthodox medicine and its practitioners. Conversely, she privileges the traditional healing arts by naming Alice Wilson and making her part of the Barton circle.

Gaskell begins *Mary Barton* with the traditional healing practices based on a 'regionally differentiated tradition of folk and domestic medicine'.[21]

She pictures domestic herbalism, which evolved when a 'knowledge of plant medicines' served a vital role in daily life,[22] through a domestic garden surrounding a farmhouse located in 'some fields near Manchester ... [that] speaks of other times and occupations'. This garden is 'crowded with a medley of old-fashioned herbs and flowers, planted long ago, when the garden was the only druggist's shop in reach ... roses, lavender, sage, balm (for teas), rosemary, pinks and wallflowers, onions and jessamine (1.1.1–2). Gaskell stresses the past – 'other times', 'old-fashioned' and 'long ago' – and acknowledges the waning use of traditional herbal remedies coincident with the expansion of urban centres in the eighteenth and nineteenth centuries.[23] She acknowledges the historic shift from domestic herbalism to the druggist with the clause, 'when the garden was the only druggist's shop within reach' (1.1.2). The druggists, who had initially served as a supply source for apothecaries, began to sell directly to the public, but in doing so, posed a threat to the apothecary and the surgeon-apothecary.[24] They, in turn, considered the dispensing druggist 'ignorant, uneducated, and a public menace' and denounced him as 'a quack or irregular all the more dangerous because the public could be deluded into believing he was just another, but cheaper, form of medical practitioner'.[25]

Gaskell represents this conflict through John Barton's trip to the druggist seeking medicine to help the critically ill and starving Ben Davenport, a mill worker. Unable to take Davenport to the infirmary immediately, Barton turned to the druggist for advice. The druggist concluded the illness was typhus, and made 'up a bottle of medicine, sweet spirits of nitre, or some such innocent poison, very good for slight colds, but utterly powerless to stop ... the raging fever'. Contrary to the narrator's statement of the potion's impotence, Barton had a 'comfortable faith in the physic' and, like others 'of his class', belief that every physic 'is equally efficacious' (1.6.70). Both characters fit an historic type: Barton seeks the advice of the druggist as a substitute for a doctor and accepts the physic with blind faith in it; the druggist, with no mandated training or licensing, diagnoses the illness and concocts a physic.[26] The narrator remarks on Barton's ignorant belief in the efficacy of the physic and on the druggist's knowledge in correctly diagnosing typhus, but does not clarify if the druggist also knew his physic was 'powerless'. The druggist could be ignorant and acting in good faith, or he could knowingly be perpetuating a form of misinformation.

In addition to the domestic garden, Gaskell also introduces traditional, or folk, herbalism in the earliest chapters of *Mary Barton*. Alice Wilson, a domestic servant, '[gathered] wild herbs for drinks and medicine' from whatever fields and meadows she could reach on foot and was known for her 'considerable knowledge of field simples' (1.2.15).[27] Her one-room cellar home 'was oddly festooned with all manner of hedge-row, ditch, and field plants' which were 'strewed and hung to dry' (1.2.15). The narrator notes that 'we are accustomed to call [these plants] valueless', but that they were 'much used among the poor' because of their 'powerful effect for good or for evil' (1.2.15). She was summoned 'by the neighbours [... when] this one was ill, and that body's child was restless' (1.17.225) thus modelling the poorer practitioners of herbalism who treated their families 'with simple herbal medicines extending similar help to neighbours, and acquiring some local reputation as an herbalist'.[28] Alice Wilson embodies the care and personal attention implicit in traditional folk herbalism as opposed to the 'naked arrogance and elitist aspirations' of the regular practitioners.[29] Late in the novel, she suffers a lingering death as she slowly loses her senses of hearing and sight, suffers a stroke, and finally slips into dementia and death. The enfeeblement and death of Alice Wilson parallels the slow displacement of traditional folk herbalism by domestic herbalism, medical botany and homoeopathy.

Gaskell also touches on the then popular practice of physiognomy, which derived from Greek thought and flourished in England 'from the sixteenth to the early nineteenth century'.[30] As *Mary Barton* opens, the narrator analyses the faces of the factory girls noting their 'irregular features' but 'acuteness and intelligence of countenance' (1.1.3). She then reads John Barton's 'wan, colourless face' as revealing 'scanty living' in his childhood, and his regular but 'strongly marked features' as 'resolute either for good or evil' (1.1.4). Finally, Jem Wilson's trial becomes a demonstration of the 'science' of physiognomy, when the narrative shifts from the opening statements to 'a physiognomic debate' among audience members over what character the physical aspects of Jem's face signalled: murderer or not. The debate itself 'replicates ... the most common characterological controversies of early- and mid-nineteenth century England'.[31] In *Mary Barton*, then, Gaskell introduces three contemporary forms of irregular medicine: the druggist, the herbalist and the physiognomist. She also alludes to a continuum between the traditional and the modern through the transition from the herbalist to the druggist,[32] and from Greek thought to physiognomy.

When Gaskell turns to the orthodox practitioners of medicine, she mentions them anonymously as the 'doctor' and the 'surgeon', but never pictures them treating patients. Early in the novel, John Barton fetches the doctor in the middle of the night to help his wife through a difficult birth. By the time they reach Barton's home, however, his wife and unborn child are dead and the doctor, 'very sleepy', returned home (1.3.20). Gaskell does not clarify whether Mrs Barton was preparing for the birth with help from female acquaintances, a midwife, or the doctor as man-midwife, the three common forms of birth at the time. The lack of specificity leaves all possibilities open, thus suggesting an overview of the range of practices and practitioners. Similarly, when Barton recounts the death of his son, Tom, following a bout with scarlet fever, he recalls that the doctor merely says that 'good nourishment' was necessary 'to keep up the little fellow's strength' (1.3.25). The summons for the doctor to 'treat' Harry Carson already dead from a bullet wound (1.18.237) reinforces the image of doctors as necessary, though not necessarily serving a productive outcome. Throughout *Mary Barton*, Gaskell never shows doctors actively practising medicine and never notes their training or qualifications (or lack thereof). Though she includes doctors, her avoidance of detail echoes the conditions in the early nineteenth century when 'there was no uniformity, no control, no clear public distinction between the educated regular practitioner and the other practitioners, and no guarantee to the public that their local doctor had any sort of proper preparation'.[33]

Gaskell also references orthodox practitioners in medical facilities through references to the infirmary (Manchester Infirmary – Manchester Royal Infirmary after 1830). John Barton recounts his in-patient experience at the infirmary for fever, but he does not discuss the facilities, treatment or practitioners. Instead, he explains how he was invited to stay an extra week to assist the 'surgeon' since he could write. Through this work, Barton learned that most mill accidents occurred in the last two hours of work, and the surgeon told Barton that he was 'going to bring that fact to light' (1.8.93). Here, Gaskell references the significance of medical men in the drive for social improvement, particularly for the mill workers, through the use of facts,[34] and the growing dissemination of information through publications. Thus, Gaskell outlines the organisation of the orthodox British medical profession into physic, surgery, pharmacy and midwifery in the early nineteenth century[35] in *Mary Barton*. Simultaneously, she sketches three forms of irregular medicine, the druggist, herbalist and physiognomist, and charts the waning dependence on traditional folk and domestic herbalism.

Mr Harrison and Mr Gibson

Although Gaskell treats the medical practitioners as almost interchangeable in *Mary Barton*, she developed two later works each based on the life of a provincial doctor: Mr Harrison of *Mr. Harrison's Confessions* (1851)[36] and Mr Gibson of *Wives and Daughters: An Everyday Story* (1866).[37] Both works focus on the doctor's role in society more than the doctor *qua* doctor,[38] but they also incorporate much factual information about the changing medical profession. Both describe an aging practitioner in a provincial town taking a young doctor as a partner. The eponymous Mr Harrison follows the traditional path to becoming a medical professional: an apprenticeship through which he earned a certificate to practice,[39] then partner, and finally successor in an established practice. He followed his apprenticeship with further instruction, attending lectures and 'walking the hospitals' (5.1.405) for which there was no standard syllabus or examinations, though the students generally earned a certificate of attendance.[40] At the conclusion of his training, Mr Harrison was taken on as partner by Mr Morgan, an aging doctor with a 'capital country practice', on the basis of a 'good account ... from an old friend of his, who was a surgeon at Guy's' (5.1.406). Although the training of Mr Gibson in *Wives and Daughters*, published fifteen years later, is not detailed, his hiring by Mr Hall is described in much the same way as Mr Harrison's, yet on a more professional basis. Mr Hall sought a successor through 'advertising in medical journals, reading testimonials, sifting character and qualifications' (8.3.30). Thus, he was able to assure his patients that Mr Gibson had 'professional qualifications ... as high as his moral character, and that both were far above average' (8.3.31). Mr Hall hired Mr Gibson after a broad search through professional channels, rather than depending on friends like Mr Morgan.

Gaskell marks the growing tension between the generations of medical professionals through Mr Harrison and Mr Gibson, who are both more modern than the beloved and trusted country doctors who preceded them, Mr Morgan and Mr Hall. When faced with a patient who suffered a badly broken wrist, Mr Morgan says they must amputate, an approach Mr Harrison characterises as 'the rough and ready surgical practice' of Mr Morgan's day (5.14.453). He suggests 'an improved treatment' that would allow them to save the arm (5.14.453). The two have a second disagreement over the treatment of a patient with a potentially fatal fever. Mr Harrison is convinced that the 'measures [Mr Morgan] was adopting were powerless to check so sudden and violent an illness' (5.26.482). Therefore, he consults a London specialist who 'recommended a new preparation, not yet in full use' (5.26.482) as the only chance to save the patient. Initially, Mr Morgan refused to use the medicine since he had 'never tried it' and 'it must be very powerful' (5.26.483–484). When he has no other recourse, he administers it as the only chance for recovery (5.27.485). In both instances, Mr Harrison proves correct in his course of treatment, saving both the arm of the one and the life of the other. Mr Morgan bases his decisions on empirical knowledge while Mr Harrison suggests more modern methods based on scientific advances. Through this fictional dispute, Gaskell replicates the early nineteenth-century shift in which 'medical treatments had replaced operation for many surgical conditions'[41]. In the end, Mr Morgan characterises himself as 'an old fool' (5.28.486).

In contrast to Mr Harrison, Mr Gibson in *Wives and Daughters* faces no such conflicts, doubtless because his senior partner, Mr Hall, retired within a year leaving him the sole doctor, whereas Mr Morgan has a multiyear agreement of gradually turning over his practice to Mr Harrison. Unlike Mr Harrison, who temporarily became a social pariah, Mr Gibson was accepted socially. He not only socialises with the local gentry, he also forms a friendship with Lord Hollingford, the local heir, who had earned 'much reputation in the European republic of learned men' (8.4.38). Through this friendship, he begins to mingle with 'the leaders of the scientific world' which motivates him to contribute his own research 'to the more scientific of the medical journals' (8.4.41). Though Mr Harrison, too, publishes his treatment of the broken wrist 'in the *Lancet*' (5.14.452), he lacks a collegial professional environment.

One of Mr Gibson's qualifications was that 'his moral character ... [was] far above the average' (8.4.31), something Mr Hall had established before introducing Mr Gibson to his patients. Within a year, Mr Gibson 'earned respect for his professional skill' (8.4.31) and a reputation as 'a clever surgeon' (8.4.34), but he was also accepted for his 'genteel appearance' and 'elegant figure' (8.4.31). In contrast, Mr Morgan gently chastises Mr Harrison on his first day at work for his choice of attire, and asks him to change into something 'professional' with a reminder that 'black is the garb of our profession' (5.2.411). Mr Harrison's friend, Jack, also contributes to his social missteps by regaling the locals gathered at a party with some of Mr Harrison's youthful misdeeds, including betting losses, temporary imprisonment and practical jokes. Although Mr Morgan accepts Mr Harrison's explanation of what really happened, he warns Mr Harrison that because of the damage done to his reputation, 'it may require some short time to overcome a little prejudice' (5.9.444). Once the people begin to distrust Mr Harrison's good character, they also lose faith in his medicine. Though he assures a patient that he is following standard procedure and that the medicine 'was sure to be successful', the patient wonders whether Mr Morgan would 'know more about it' (5.13.450). The disagreement between the two doctors over the best treatment for the broken wrist perhaps did the greatest harm to Mr Harrison's medical credibility. Though Mr Harrison's non-surgical treatment was successful, local rumour led to false beliefs of the patient's illness and death before the fully cured patient re-emerged publicly. In fact, Mr Harrison's professional reputation sinks so low that he is no longer summoned to treat patients until public opinion is reversed at the end of the novel. Thus, through different means, both Mr Harrison and Mr Gibson illustrate the truth of Mr Morgan's claim, 'It is, in fact, sir, manners that make the man in our profession' (5.2.416). In addition to illustrating the position of medical men in local society through

Mr Harrison and Mr Gibson, Gaskell uses them to illustrate conventional eighteenth- and early nineteenth-century medical training, and to suggest the initial development of pharmacology, the burgeoning of local, national and international cooperation between medical professionals, and, through Dr Gibson, the growing interconnections between medical men and natural scientists.

From *Mary Barton* to *Wives and Daughters*

Throughout her longer fiction, Gaskell references the following trends in orthodox medicine to a greater and lesser degree: standardisation of medical training and greater differentiation in the respective fields of surgeon, physician and apothecary together with the rise of the general practitioner and specialist. In *Ruth* (1853),[42] Gaskell returns to medical training and the prevailing practice of apprenticeship, previously described through Mr Harrison, in the character of Mr Davis, 'the first surgeon in Eccleston' who is well-respected by all classes of Eccleston society (3.34.434). He asks the eponymous Ruth to allow him to foster her illegitimate and ostracised son, Leonard. Once Leonard completes grammar school, Mr Davis intends to take him as an apprentice without requiring the usual premium. Following completion of the apprenticeship, Mr Davis will take him on as his partner, and then as successor to his practice (3.34.433–434). He does this not only to honour Ruth for her work nursing typhus patients, but also to give Leonard a chance in life. Mr Davis admits that he, too, had been an illegitimate child and knows the difficulty of overcoming such a heritage. He acknowledges that the practice of medicine had allowed him to become a respected member of society, which he foresees will also be the outcome for Leonard.

Despite this positive reflection on the value of a medical apprenticeship, Gaskell subtly acknowledges the current conflict over the use of apprenticeships as a training tool in the medical professions. In *Wives and Daughters*, Mr Gibson follows the tradition set by Mr Hall and takes two apprentices at a time who are 'bound by indentures' and paid 'a handsome premium to learn their business' (8.3.34). Mr Gibson, however, is troubled by the apparatus of teaching and providing accommodations for the apprentices. Therefore, despite 'his reputation as a clever surgeon' which attracted pupils and conferred 'prestige' on them at the completion of their training (8.3.34), he decides that his current apprentices will be 'the last of the race of pupils' (8.15.205). Mr Gibson's discontent with the system draws attention to the controversy over the 'education and licensing of medical professionals'[43] confronting the nineteenth-century medical profession. Though the practice of apprenticeships was longstanding and deemed effective in its intention of providing 'practical clinical experience in treatment of disease' and 'experience making up bottles of medicine', in reality it was not thought to accomplish its goals and was ultimately 'abolished by the Medical Act of 1858'[44] only a few years before the publication of *Wives and Daughters* in 1866.

In addition to her consideration of the controversy over the value of apprenticeships, Gaskell also examines the ongoing evolution of the surgeon. In *Ruth*, she initially places the surgeon in virtually the same category as the shopkeepers. Both find themselves working in what had become a 'dark' and 'dingy' street where the shopkeepers could not 'show off their goods to advantage' and the surgeon could not see 'to draw his patients' teeth' (3.1.3).[45] By this placement, she allocates the surgeon to a rank perhaps not far from his origins as barber-surgeon. In *Wives and Daughters* she hints at another antecedent of the surgeon when, in the absence of an available doctor, old Robin, 'a knowledgeable man among dumb beasts' is summoned 'till th' regular doctor came' as second only to the surgeon in knowledge of the body (8.51.642).

Even though Gaskell seems to be suggesting an increasing standardisation in the medical professions, she hints that it is more myth than reality through her continuing use of ambiguous terminology. In *Cranford* (1853),[46] the ladies consider their doctor, Mr Hoggins, 'a very worthy man' and 'a very clever surgeon', and they 'were rather proud' of him 'as a doctor' and 'as a surgeon' (2.11.124). Here, Gaskell employs 'doctor' and 'surgeon' seemingly interchangeably. Likewise in *Ruth*, Mr Davis 'the doctor' is further described as 'the clever, prosperous surgeon of Eccleston' (3.25.434), and 'Mr. Wynne (the parish doctor)' as 'Mr. Wynne, the parish surgeon' (3.29.384,6). In *North and South* (1855),[47] when Margaret Hale is wounded in the incipient riot, and there is a rush to get 'the doctor' (4.22.215), but Mrs Thornton returns with 'the nearest surgeon' (4.22.218). Even Mr. Gibson in *Wives and Daughters* is initially described as 'the younger doctor' (8.3.31) and 'the handsome young surgeon' (8.3.32). By blurring the titles, Gaskell suggests the controversy developing between surgeons and physicians over spheres of treatment, training and credentials. More significantly, she suggests the emerging development of the general practitioner with training and experience in all three branches of medicine, physic, surgery and apothecary,[48] and the coincident development of specialist physicians and surgeons in major metropolitan areas available for consultation. Mr Harrison rushes to London to consult with a specialist about the patient with a deadly fever. Likewise, in *Ruth*, when a wealthy tourist falls ill in rural Wales, a London specialist is summoned to treat the patient in place of Mr Jones, the local doctor. Nonetheless, the locals knowingly remark that the patient will face the crisis before the 'fine London doctor' arrives, but that he 'will get all the credit, and honest Mr. Jones will be thrown aside' (3.7.81). Though Margaret Hale in *North and South* finds the local Dr Donaldson caring and competent in the treatment of her 'seriously indisposed' mother (4.15.128), her brother questions whether '[their mother] should have some other advice – some London doctor … [a] great London surgeon' (4.30.295). Mr Brown, who treats the eponymous Cousin Phillis for a kind of brain seizure, sends for another doctor from the city to consult when he considers 'fresh symptoms' unfavorable (7.4.102). Even Mr Gibson in *Wives and Daughters* seeks specialty consultation about Osborne Hamley's ominous symptoms (8.29.375–377). Like their historic counterparts, Gaskell begins to differentiate her fictitious medical men into generalists and specialists, the former associated with the more provincial areas and the latter with larger urban areas.

While noting the incipient changes in orthodox medical training and practice, Gaskell simultaneously preserves the interplay between them and the traditional healing arts, often referencing the forms of traditional healing introduced in *Mary Barton* as touchstones. Through John Barton's belief that 'any' physic was helpful, Gaskell adapted the time-honoured belief in the efficacy of charms and magic as a means of healing; that is, a trust in the mysterious and irrational. She alludes to these older practices in *The Moorland Cottage* (1850)[49] when Nancy, an elderly servant, realises that her comments on the dead and dying have distressed young Maggie Browne. She tries to comfort Maggie through her reminiscences about a girl cured 'by a charm', and remarks that perhaps they 'could hear of a doctor who could charm away illness' such as there had been in her 'glory days' (2.3.292). Nancy, despite her desire to console Maggie Brown, concludes, 'I don't think people are so knowledgeable now' (2.292), showing a more traditional understanding of knowledge than the contemporary orthodox medical men. As with Alice Wilson and folk herbalism, using an elderly servant as the advocate for healing by charm implies a vestige of past rather than contemporary practice.[50]

Nonetheless, even the modern practitioners as depicted by Gaskell depend on the ignorant and superstitious nature of the patients, though for a different reason. In *Ruth*, for example, the doctor prescribes 'care and quiet, and mysterious medicines' (3.10.105). Part of the mystery of medicine lay in the prescriptions being written in Latin, a language unknown to the larger population. Ruth, who from a slightly educated orphan apprentice seamstress matures into a self-educated woman, asserts, 'I can read prescriptions which doctors would prefer you not do' (3.29.385), suggesting the elitism of the doctors seeking to keep their knowledge arcane.[51] However, it also implies a continuum between the old and the new.

Gaskell continuously interweaves the thread of the older, traditional medicine throughout her longer fiction. While cleaning out the attic, Miss Matty Jenkins of *Cranford* reads letters sent from her mother to her father when she was a young child. In these, her mother writes 'about the poor in the parish; [describing] what homely domestic medicines she had administered; what kitchen physic she had sent' (2.5.55). Though brief, Gaskell acknowledges the significance of the tradition of domestic medicine for the poor, but she also acknowledges its hereditary significance. *Sylvia's Lovers* (1863),[52] like *Mary Barton*, begins with a description of the countryside surrounding a town (Monkshaven), and the narrator reverts to what it was a century ago (6.1.1). She lists the herbs a farmer's wife or daughters would have cultivated in a domestic garden in 'the last century': 'A few "berry" bushes, a black current tree or two (the leaves to be used for heightening the flavour of tea, the fruit as medicinal for colds and sore throats), ... a bush of sage, and balm, and thyme, and marjoram, with the possibly a rose tree, and "old man"' (6.1.5).[53] Later in the novel, Sylvia, who has married and moved from the country into Monkshaven, seeks to calm her dying mother with a traditional herbal remedy. She returns to Haytersbank Farm, her now abandoned childhood home, to find 'a plant of balm ... in a sheltered corner' in the remains of the kitchen garden she had planted as a child (6.33.395). From experience, she knew that balm tea would calm her mother and reflected that 'it might be that the herb really possessed some sedative power; it might be only early faith, and often repeated experience, but it had always had a tranquillizing effect' (6.33.395). Gaskell describes Sylvia's mix of empirical knowledge of the medicinal effects as well as her irrational faith in the remedy and suggests that the plant contains an innate power. The 'sedative *power*' (italics added) that Sylvia recognises hints at the discovery of an 'active principle' that chemists could separate from the rest of the plant matter'.[54] Once separated, they could use the 'pure matter' to develop 'accurate dosage' and to eliminate 'toxic effects due to impurities in crude drugs'.[55] Thus, chemists could produce 'a pure substitute for the variable original' of the plant.[56] In a few words, Gaskell describes how advances in natural science were transforming traditional herbalism into the emerging study and practice of pharmacology.[57]

In *Mary Barton*, Alice Wilson implies that she gained her knowledge of herbs from her mother. She, in turn, shared her skill through nursing and preparing remedies for others. Gaskell continues to reference the use and transmission of hereditary family remedies throughout her fiction. Mrs Purkiss of rural Helstone in *North and South* says, 'My mother and my grandmother before me ... took salt and senna when anything ailed them; and I must e'en go on in their ways' (4.46.463). Despite Mrs. Purkiss's trust in senna, historically, its mythic powers were reviled in the *Lancet* as being 'wildly, excessive claims for efficacy.[58] Her belief in the traditional is echoed in her complaint that her mistress 'does not want to give me comfts instead of medicine, which, as she says, is a deal pleasanter, only I have no faith in it' (4.46.463). Likewise, *My Lady Ludlow* (1858)[59] illustrates a common mode of hereditary transmission for herbal remedies through reference to a compendium of the traditional medicinal herbs and remedies, Buchan's *Domestic Medicine*, that Lady Ludlow's female dependents referenced to prepare 'physics' for her tenants and neighbours since there was no doctor close by.[60] Maggie Dawson, one of the female dependents, considered their physic 'as good as what comes out of the druggist's shop' (5.2.27). Nonetheless, she notes that 'if any of our physics tasted stronger than usual, [they were bid to] let it down with cochineal and water' until they 'had very little real physic in them'. Further, she admits to having 'sent off many a bottle of salt and water coloured red' (5.2.27). Like John Barton's urban druggist, the rural Lady Ludlow provides a harmless physic as medicine, but she does so knowingly.

In addition to physic, Lady Ludlow's dependents make 'bread-pills' which were reputed to be 'very efficacious' (5.2.27).[61] Maggie Dawson describes an old man 'who took six pills a-night ... to make him sleep' and if 'he was out of his medicine, he was so restless and miserable ... he was like to die' (5.2.27–28). According to her, belief in the medicine and the healing powers of nature itself had more to do with healing than anything else. Similar to Ruth's reflection on the mysteriousness of Latin prescriptions, Maggie Dawson notes how carefully they put labels on the physic, 'which looked very mysterious to those who could not read, and helped the medicine to do its work' (5.2.27). She concludes her memories of making medicine with the reflection, 'I think ours was what would be called homoeopathic practice now-a-days' (5.28). This marks first, the unscientific and irregular nature of physic and healing practices characteristic of Maggie's youth with Lady Ludlow, and second, the slow shift from traditional herbalism to homoeopathy, one of the newer forms of herbalism to emerge in the nineteenth century. Unlike the traditional forms of herbalism, homoeopathy was marked by the same professionalisation and standardisation then transforming regular medicine.[62]

Gaskell further acknowledges the ongoing eclipse of past practices by modern in her portrayal of the conflict between regular and irregular practitioners in *My Lady Ludlow*. The village surgeon, Mr Prince, who has 'a grand pharmacopoeia' and thus appears to be a traditional surgeon-apothecary, and Miss Galindo, a herbalist who has 'her queer, odd recipes', meet in a sickroom. Miss Galindo is the preferred 'medical attendant', either because of her approach to the ill or her free services. She marks her contempt for Mr Prince's abilities by remarking that Lady

Ludlow had also sent Doctor Trevor to the sickroom who 'looked well after that old donkey of a Prince, and saw that he made no blunders' (5.10.158). Although Miss Galindo values her own herbal contribution to healing more than that of the surgeon-apothecary, she acknowledges the skill of the more modern Doctor Trevor.

Gaskell shows true inclusivity of the great variety of medical practices trending in the first half of the nineteenth century by including forms of alternative healing other than traditional domestic and folk herbalism. As mentioned previously, she incorporates physiognomy in *Mary Barton*, a topic she returns to in *Wives and Daughters* through the narrator's suggestion that 'a physiognomist ... would have read ... defiance and anger, and perhaps also a little perplexity' in the expression on Cynthia's face (8.26.341). Gaskell also references mesmerism, which 'was popularized in Britain in the 1830s', twice in *Wives and Daughters*:[63] first when Lady Cumnor replies to her husband's claim at having a hand in Mr Gibson's second marriage, 'You must be strongly mesmeric, and your will acted upon theirs ...' (8.12.157), and later when Cynthia asks Molly Gibson, 'Have you ever heard of strong wills mesmerizing weaker ones into submission?' (8.37.474). Like physiognomy's root in ancient Greek thought, mesmerism contained 'threads from western society's inheritance of religion and magic'.[64] All of these movements 'combined fresh elements with older ones ... but the older practices lacked formal organization'.[65] As the nineteenth century progressed, homoeopathy, phrenology,[66] mesmerism and other movements in alternative medicine embraced and mimicked the emerging formal apparatus of orthodox medicine and natural science in establishing societies, presenting lectures, publishing journals, newsletters, and pamphlets and formalising training and treatment.[67]

Thus, though the fiction of Elizabeth Gaskell is not often cited as a source for medical history, she provides a rich source for it. While it is easy to see how the 'medical' part of 'medical men' is eclipsed by the social in her fiction, she does much more than portray the character and place of provincial doctors in society. An investigation of her longer fiction reveals a narrative picture of the melange of practitioners and practices at work in the healing arts in turn of the century Britain. Gaskell recognises historic antecedents to the more modern practices and records shifting trends, but she does not overtly prioritise the past or the present. Instead, she depicts the slow eclipse of the traditional and irregular by orthodox medicine. The traditional folk and domestic herbal medicine particularly as personified in Alice Wilson, anonymous doctors, and the amateur natural scientist Job Legh, all from *Mary Barton*, are replaced by a succession of doctors and scientists. These culminate in Mr Gibson, who is systematically trained and certified, examines and treats patients, participates in his local scientific network as well as professional exchanges and publications, and the publicly funded scholar and explorer, Roger Hamley, who inhabits professional scientific circles in *Wives and Daughters*, which, due to Gaskell's sudden death, became her final novel.

Through an accumulation of detail, Gaskell creates a living portrayal of the interaction between the traditional and the orthodox, and the regular and the irregular in medicine in her works. Rather than stopping at a single point on this constantly shifting continuum, she seems content to explore the continuum and examine how what is considered knowledge in time is revealed to be misinformation and becomes the stuff of myth. Though Mr Gibson and the medical and scientific world he participates in appears more scientific and rational than the world of John and Mary Barton, his world, too, stands to become recognised as founded on misinformation and considered mythic further down the continuum. Gaskell celebrates the nature of progress, rather than evaluating the individual steps.

Notes

1. Christopher Hilton, 'Elizabeth Gaskell and Mesmerism: An Unpublished Letter', *Medical History* 39:2 (1995): 219–235, at 219.
2. Mrs Ellis H. Chadwick, *Mrs. Gaskell, Haunts: Homes & Stories* (New York: Frederick A. Stokes, 1911), p. 52.
3. Linda K. Hughes, '"Cousin Phillis", *Wives and Daughters*, and Modernity', in Jill L. Matus (ed.), *The Cambridge Companion to Elizabeth Gaskell* (Cambridge: Cambridge University Press, 2007), pp. 98–101.
4. See J. H. Ross, 'Elizabeth Gaskell (1810–1865) and the Medical World', *Journal of Medical Biography* 24:2 (2016): 215–219.
5. John Chapple, *Elizabeth Gaskell: The Early Years* (Manchester: Manchester University Press, 1997), p. 58.
6. Thomas Beswick, 'Local Associations with Mrs. Gaskell', *Knutsford and Mrs. Gaskell*. Issued by The Gaskell Committee, 1960 (Derby: New Centurion), p. 15.
7. Edward Mansfield Brockbank, *Sketches of the Lives and Works of the Honorary Medical Staff of the Manchester Infirmary from its Foundation in 1752 to 1830 When it Became the Royal Infirmary* (Manchester: Manchester University Press, 1904), p. 27.
8. Beswick, 'Local Associations', p. 15 and Brockbank, *Sketches*, p. 61.
9. Chadwick, *Mrs. Gaskell*, pp. 58–59.
10. Ibid., pp. 7, 270.
11. *The Works of Elizabeth Gaskell in Eight Volumes*. Knutsford Edition (1906; Reprint, New York: AMS Press, 1972), Vol. 2: *Cranford and Other Tales*.

All references to Gaskell's works will be taken from this edition and cited by volume, chapter and page number.

12 David Innes Williams, 'Anthony Todd Thomson and the Rise of the General Practitioner', *Journal of Medical Biography* 10:4 (2002): 206–214, at 206. See also Carol A. Bock, 'Elizabeth Gaskell's "Useful" Relatives: Katharine and Anthony Todd Thomson and the Society for the Diffusion of Useful Knowledge', *Gaskell Journal* 22 (2008): 72–85.
13 Chapple, *Elizabeth Gaskell*, pp. 420, 95.
14 Ibid., p. 421.
15 Frank Smith, *The Life and Work of Sir James Kay-Shuttleworth* (London: John Murray, 1923), p. 333.
16 Arnold Thackray, 'Natural Knowledge in Cultural Context: The Manchester Mode', *American Historical Review* 79:3 (1974): 672–709.
17 Ibid., pp. 684–685.
18 Marie Fitzwilliam, 'Mr. Harrison's Confessions: A Study of the General Practitioner's Social and Professional Dis-ease', *Gaskell Society Journal* 12 (1998): 28–36, examines the social role of the general practitioner in Gaskell's *Mr. Harrison's Confessions*.
19 *Mary Barton: A Tale of Manchester Life*, in *The Works of Elizabeth Gaskell*, Vol. 1.
20 Gaskell originally titled the novel *John Barton*, and planned to write 'a tragic poem', based on the 'life of an ignorant thoughtful man of strong power of sympathy, dwelling in a town so full of striking contrasts'. J. A. V. Chapple and Arthur Pollard (eds), *The Letters of Mrs. Gaskell* (Manchester: Manchester University Press, 1967), letter 39.
21 Charles E. Rosenberg, 'Medical Text and Social Context: Explaining William Buchan's *Domestic Medicine*', *Bulletin of the History of Medicine* 57:1 (1983): 22–42, at 27.
22 Gabrielle Hatfield, *Memory, Wisdom, and Healing: The History of Domestic Plant Medicine* (Stroud: Sutton, 1999), p. 4.
23 Hatfield, *Memory*, p. 161, and S. W. F. Holloway, 'The Orthodox Fringe; The Origins of the Pharmaceutical Society of Great Britain', in W. F. Bynum and Roy Porter (eds), *Medical Fringe and Medical Orthodoxy, 1750–1850* (Kent: Croom Helm, 1987), pp. 129–157, at p. 154.
24 Irvine Loudon, 'The Vile Race of Quacks with which this Country is Infested', in W. F. Bynum and Roy Porter (eds), *Medical Fringe and Medical Orthodoxy, 1750–1850* (Kent: Croom Helm, 1987), pp. 106–128, at p. 108.
25 Irvine Loudon, *Medical Care and the General Practitioner 1750–1850* (Oxford: Clarendon, 1986), p. 137.
26 Elizabeth Gaskell, *Mary Barton: A Tale of Manchester Life* (New York: Penguin, 1996), p. 402 n. 11, references 'the working class's resort to quack remedies and medical charlatans' in Friedrich Engels (1845), *The Condition of the Working Class in England* (London, Panther 1969), pp. 134–135.

27 Holloway, 'The Orthodox Fringe' mentions Alice Wilson as a representative of 'folk medicine' (p. 154), as does Edgar Wright, *Mrs. Gaskell: A Basis for Reassessment* (London: Oxford University Press, 1965), pp. 78, 95.
28 P. S. Brown, 'Herbalists and Medical Botanists in Mid-Nineteenth-Century Britain with Special Reference to Bristol', *Medical History* 26:4 (1982): 405–420, at 414.
29 Roger Cooter, 'Alternative Medicine, Alternative Cosmology', in Roger Cooter (ed.), *Studies in the History of Alternative Medicine* (Hampshire and London: Macmillan, 1988), pp. 62–77, at p. 65.
30 T. M. Parssinen, 'Popular Science and Society: The Phrenology Movement in Early Victorian Britain', Journal of Social History 8:1 (1974): 1–20, at 7.
31 Christie Harner, 'Physiognomic Discourse and the Trials of Cross-Class Sympathy in *Mary Barton*', *Victorian Literature and Culture* 43:4 (2015): 705–724, at 705–706.
32 Hatfield, *Memory*, p. 161, and Holloway, 'The Orthodox Fringe', p. 154.
33 Loudon, *Medical Care*, p. 131. Peter Gaskell, in *Artisans and Machinery: The Moral and Physical Condition of the Manufacturing Population Considered with Reference to Mechanical Substitutes for Human Labour* (1836; Reprints of Economic Classics, New York: Kelly, 1968), p. 207, notes the dependence on quacks, domestic medicine, and inexperienced physicians and surgeons who treated without charge.
34 See Christopher O'Brien, 'The Origins and Originators of Early Statistical Societies: A Comparison of Liverpool and Manchester', *Journal of the Royal Statistical Society* 174:1 (2011): 51–62.
35 Loudon, *Medical Care*, p. 18.
36 *Mr. Harrison's Confessions*, in *The Works of Mrs. Gaskell*, Vol. 5, *My Lady Ludlow and Other Tales*, pp. 405–491.
37 *Wives and Daughters: An Everyday Story*, in *The Works of Mrs. Gaskell*, Vol. 8.
38 Loudon, *Medical Care*, p. 271, references various nineteenth-century authors and their fictional doctors to support the claim that although fiction is not useful in terms of describing 'illnesses and diagnoses', it was an effective mode of transmitting 'the character of medical practitioners and especially what their patients thought of them'. He does not include Gaskell.
39 Brockbank, *Sketches*, p. 27.
40 Loudon, *Medical Care*, p. 35.
41 Ibid., p. 191.
42 *Ruth*, in *The Works of Mrs. Gaskell*, Vol. 3, *Ruth and Other Tales*, pp.1–454.
43 Loudon, *Medical Care*, p. 148.
44 Ibid., pp. 179–180.
45 Suzie Grogan, *Death, Disease & Dissection: The Life of a Surgeon-Apothecary, 1750–1850* (South Yorkshire: Pen & Sword, 2017), pp. 4–7, gives a brief overview of the origin of barber-surgeons.
46 *Cranford*, in *The Works of Mrs. Gaskell*, Vol. 2, *Cranford and Other Tales*, pp. 1–195.

47 *North and South*, in *The Works of Mrs. Gaskell*, Vol. 4.
48 Loudon, *Medical Care*, p. 148.
49 *The Moorland Cottage*, in *The Works of Mrs. Gaskell*, Vol. 2, *Cranford and Other Tales*, pp. 267–383.
50 Brown, 'Herbalists', pp. 406–407, summarises the persistence of magical traditions in Britain and particularly Bristol through the mid-nineteenth century.
51 Cooter, 'Alternative Medicine, Alternative Cosmology', p. 65, generalises the Victorian turn to alternative medicine as a response to 'the naked arrogance and elitist aspirations of the orthodox practitioners'.
52 *Sylvia's Lovers*, in *The Works of Mrs. Gaskell*, Vol. 6, *Sylvia's Lovers Etc.*, pp. 1–530.
53 'Old man' (southernwood) is mentioned again in the same garden (20.231). Footnote 1 for p. 231 describes southernwood as 'formerly much cultivated for medicinal purposes' (p. 525).
54 Barbara Griggs, *Green Pharmacy: A History of Herbal Medicine* (New York: Viking, 1981), p. 220.
55 Holloway, 'The Orthodox Fringe', p. 144.
56 Griggs, *Green Pharmacy*, p. 222.
57 Holloway, 'The Orthodox Fringe', p. 154, concludes, 'The rise of the chemist and druggist is an aspect of the adaptation of folk medicine to industrial, urban society'.
58 Roy Porter, *Health for Sale: Quackery in England 1660–1850* (Manchester: Manchester University Press, 1989), p. 223.
59 *My Lady Ludlow*, in *The Works of Mrs. Gaskell*, Vol. 5, *My Lady Ludlow and Other Tales*, pp. 9–217.
60 Buchan's *Domestic Medicine* (1769) was one of two widely used compendiums from the eighteenth to the nineteenth centuries. See C. J. Lawrence, 'William Buchan: Medicine Laid Open', *Medical History* 19:1 (1975): 20–35. For the second compendium, see Deborah Madden, *'A Cheap, Safe and Natural Medicine': Religion, Medicine and Culture in John Wesley's Primitive Physic* (Amsterdam and New York: Rodopi, 2007).
61 See Porter, *Health for Sale*, p. 225, for bread pills.
62 Glynis Rankin, 'Two Interpretations of Homoeopathy', in Roger Cooter (ed.), *Studies in the History of Alternative Medicine* (Hampshire and London: Macmillan, 1988), pp. 46–62, discusses the constitution of the British Homoeopathic Society, founded 1844, and the English Homoeopathic Association, founded 1845.
63 Noted by Hilton, 'Elizabeth Gaskell', p. 230.
64 Fred Kaplan, '"The Mesmeric Mania": The early Victorians and Animal Magnetism', *Journal of the History of Ideas* 35:4 (1974): 691–702, explains the relationship between phrenology and mesmerism.
65 Logie Barrow, 'Why were Most Medical Heretics at their Most Confident Around the 1840s? (The Other Side of Mid-Victorian Medicine)', in Roger French and Andrew Wear (eds), *British Medicine in an Age of Reform* (London and New York: Routledge, 1991), pp. 165–185, at p. 164.

66 J. G. Spurzheim, in the Introduction to *Phrenology, in Connexion with the Study of Physiognomy*, 1st American edn (Boston, MA: Capen & Lyon, 1833), pp. 1–8, explains why the study of phrenology was a prerequisite to physiognomy.
67 Thackray, 'Natural Knowledge', pp. 698–709, gives an overview of the societal affiliations of successive generations of Mancunians.

10

Medical men recommend them: branded medicines and the myth of the medical moral economy c. 1876–80

Laura Robson-Mainwaring

With the passing of the Trade Marks Registration Act, 1875, a register for proprietary marks was created for the first time, established at the Patent Office. Previously, there had not been any legislation specifically covering trademarks, with registration taking place under copyright law. In May 1876, only five months after the central register came into force, Dr Henry Hanks applied to register 'Neuralgia and Nerve mixture' as a trademark (no. 5491).[1] Hanks was no quack: he was a qualified medical practitioner, passing examinations to become a Member of the Royal College of Surgeons (MRCS) in 1851, and obtaining the Licentiate of the Society of Apothecaries (LSA) in 1858.[2]

The nineteenth century was a period of change for the medical profession. With the passing of the Medical Act in 1858, there was a move to regulate medical practice and improve education standards. A statutory body, in the form of the General Medical Council, was formed to manage the provisions of the Act, including the creation of an annually published register for those who qualified as an apothecary, physician or surgeon. Common narratives of the nineteenth-century marketplace have centred on quacks and how, as medical practice professionalised, the profession sought to self-regulate the sale and supply of medicines in response to rising competition and concerns over quackery.[3] Print media, namely in the form of professional advice literature and medical journals, was utilised to establish a shared set of values, mythologizing an image of professional respectability that was opposed to commercial undertakings. Yet, while the medical profession and advertising of branded medicines have been traditionally seen as diametrically opposed, some of the most popular patent medicines were linked to members; Dr James's Fever Powders, for instance, originated at the hands of an eminent physician in the eighteenth century. Lori Loeb has pointed out that the *British Medical Journal* (*BMJ*) carried advertisements for patent medicines despite publishing editorials opposed to them.[4] Medical men like Henry Hanks, who engaged in the commercial sale of remedies, further complicate this narrative.

Using contemporary newspaper advertisements, medical journals, trademark registers, census records, medical registers and directories, this chapter examines a selection of medical practitioners who registered trademarks shortly after the passing of the Trade Marks Registration Act, 1875. This chapter illustrates that, not only were qualified practitioners prescribing branded medicines and talking about branded medicines in medical literature, they also registered their own trademarks for remedies and devices and promoted them for sale. Significantly, these findings displace the myth that only quacks or fringe practitioners were engaging in the selling and promotion of medical products. It also serves to demonstrate the significance of the commercial world for medical practice, which in turn added to the myth-making of the eminent medical practitioner.

This chapter considers the representations of trademarks registered in the first four years after the Trade Marks Registration Act, 1875, in registers that were originally maintained at the Patent Office and are now held at the National Archives.[5] These volumes of representations do not, as a general rule, contain details of the proprietor registering the mark. Only four registers relating to the volumes survive, thus the *Trade Marks Journal* held at the British Library needs to be consulted to ascertain proprietorship. Roger Price and Frazer Swift have, however, compiled a catalogue of medical trademarks that were registered in the early years of the Act, listing the name, address, firm or occupation of the proprietor, and details of when the mark was applied for. The marks identified by Price and Swift relate to products with a medical use, including soap, disinfectants and invalid foods, as well as surgical, dental and vision aid devices.[6] Fifty material classes were established by the Trade Marks Registration Act, 1875. Of primary interest here is Class Three, comprising 'Chemical substances used in medicine and pharmacy'.

This chapter takes these sources and cross-references them with contemporary medical registers to determine whether the proprietor was a qualified medical practitioner. An emblematic selection of trademarks registered by practitioners will be discussed; however, interpreting the representations is problematic, as it is difficult to determine whether the marks were used commercially. It is possible that these remedies were promoted via the likes of bill stickers and posters, which were ubiquitous at the time, but unlikely to be extant due to their ephemeral nature. Nonetheless, in the majority of cases it has been possible to trace print advertisements within the lay and medical press, indicating that the marks were indeed used to market and sell remedies.

Building on observations by Frampton and Wallis that medical journals helped to shape the medical marketplace, this chapter will refer to a number of publications, like the *Medical Press and Circular*, the *Medical Times and*

Gazette, the *British Medical Journal*, and the much-studied *Lancet*.[7] These journals featured commentary on professional and commercial activities as a form of self-regulation, helping to protect against misinformation that could circulate within promotional copy. Proprietaries were often critiqued in comment sections. For example, the *BMJ* wrote that there was 'nothing remarkable' about the sample of 'Maori Cigarettes', indicated for the cure of chest complications, 'except that "none are genuine without the registered trade-mark"' and that they are prepared only by T. Kennedy Douglas, who describes himself as "M.B., C.M., etc., Edinburgh University"'.[8] Further to commentary about new products, Frampton found that medical periodicals were 'self-declared upholders of professional ethics'.[9] The medical journal the *Lancet*, for example, was used as a mouthpiece by medical reformers to impose regulation on the market in an attempt to improve medical practice.[10]

This chapter begins with an overview of the medical marketplace in the nineteenth century, looking at the development of commercial legislation as well as regulation of the medical profession that served to mythologise the ideal practitioner. It then explores the use of trademarks as a new socio-economic opportunity for practitioners in a marketplace defined by competition, showing that professional medicine was not remote from the commercial world despite codes of medical ethics perpetuating this myth. It concludes that scholars should not ignore the significance of trademark legislation for uncovering the realities of nineteenth-century medical practice.

Historiographical context: professional ideals and the sale of medicines

The significance of the world of print to the medical market has been clearly established by scholars. Patent medicines were among the most heavily advertised products in the early modern marketplace and drew in extensive revenue for newspaper proprietors. Their popularity also meant that it was common for newspaper proprietors to advertise their own nostrums in their own papers.[11] The nineteenth century has been characterised by the principle of individual liberty, with an emphasis on free trade over protection. As a result of this freedom, it was common for advertisements to employ hyperbole – to construct myths of efficacy – which have amused and somewhat dominated the studies of subsequent commentators.[12] Contemporaries were aware of the problems associated with excessive claims attached to medicines; ineffective remedies were commonly mocked in satirical illustrations and poison scandals were relayed in the press.[13] This association between patent medicines and myth and misinformation meant that the profession wanted to distance itself from advertising and thus from any notion of quackery.

The demise of the 'golden age' of quackery in the eighteenth century has traditionally been associated with the onset of professionalization.[14] The supply of drugs also began to be regulated in the nineteenth century: the Arsenic Act (1851) required vendors to record every sale of arsenic, and the Pharmacy Act (1868) controlled the selling of poisons, like strychnine and opium, requiring that registered chemists, or qualified practitioners who had obtained the LSA, label them as poison and record sales. However, professionalisation and the expansion of regulation did not curb quackery nor the increasing dominance of pre-packaged medicines.[15]

Patent medicines had their formula disclosed and registered at the Patent Office. Proprietary medicines, on the other hand, referred to all non-patented medicines using a secret formula. Under the Medicine Stamp Act, 1804, proprietaries with undisclosed formula became liable for duty and had to be registered at the Stationery Office. The two terms, however, have been used interchangeably as the term 'patent medicine' was applied to all medicines that required a medicine stamp. An editorial from the *BMJ* (1867) opined that, ethically, a medical patent only differed to a secret remedy to a degree: 'It proclaims the remedy, but says, you shall get it only through the inventor, who may effectually check any improvement by a threat of action for infringement of patent right, and thus defeat the sacred claims both of medicine and humanity'. Confronting concerns about commercial motivations, the editor continued, 'we thank God that … boastful self-assertion has not yet become the rule of our order; and that we have not yet adopted a system of trade-marks for every medicine discovered or newly applied, or for every instrument invented by ingenious members of our profession'.[16]

Patenting medical apparatus and procedures conflicted with medical ethics. In 1878, medical man Jukes de Styrap wrote that it was derogatory to professional character for a practitioner to hold a patent for a medicine or surgical instrument, noting that it was

> extremely reprehensible for a practitioner to attest the efficacy of patent or secret medicines, or, in any way, to promote their use; … It is likewise degrading for a medical man to enter into compact with a druggist to prescribe gratuitously or otherwise, and, at the same time, share in the profits arising from the sale of medicine.[17]

However, reputation and claims of ownership could be established in other ways. Sally Frampton and Claire Jones have identified the importance of eponymising procedures or tools as well as publishing or writing opinion articles in the medical press as common ways of establishing credit.[18]

Authorship, as a means to establish reputation, was not seen to contravene the ideal of the respectable practitioner, and ultimately served to mythologise the eminence of individual practitioners. In an editorial, the *BMJ* asserted that 'authorship is the most effectual way, not of securing to himself, but of putting the whole world in possession of the fruits of the labour and experience and matured thought of many years'.[19]

Advertisements for medical texts, prevalent in the press, also seemed acceptable within the moral economy of the profession. However, ethical codes were in flux and some organisations pressed for a more hard-line stance. For example, the *Medical Times and Gazette* reported that a resolution was passed in 1876 by the Metropolitan Counties Branch of the British Medical Association to discourage doctors from advertising their publications in non-medical papers.[20] As Jones has observed, codes of conduct were an ideal and not the reality, highlighting that the patenting of medical devices and surgical instruments by medical practitioners was not unheard of.[21] Indeed, Robert Burrell and Catherine Kelly have shown that around one-fifth of patents taken out for medical apparatus between 1800 and 1852 were by medical practitioners.[22] Trademarks, however, may have been used instead of, or in conjunction with, registered patents by the medical profession, and their significance within the medical marketplace has been the subject of limited scholarship.[23] In her study of medical advertising in the Georgian period, Hannah Barker has identified branding as the dominant promotional tactic – citing names, signatures and embossed bottles as examples.[24] However, these studies analyse branding in earlier periods, before the codification of trademark law.

The nature of branding changed significantly in the nineteenth century. Before the Merchandise Marks Act, 1862, made it illegal to counterfeit any trademark or use a trademark with intent to defraud, judicial proceedings involving trademarks were carried out under common law.[25] Many firms had to take matters into their own hands and threaten would-be imitators with legal action, citing examples from common law precedents. This was the case for Perry Davis and Son, whose 'Painkiller' trademark was infringed on a number of occasions, inducing the company to compile a treatise that served a pedagogic purpose and cautioned potential infringers.[26] The Trade Marks Registration Act, and subsequent revisions to patent and trademark legislation in 1883, 1888 and 1905, would help to define what could be protected. Business historians have shown how trademark legislation influenced developments in the market, with many including drug vendors within studies. However, there has been limited discussion of the medical market itself.[27] Elsewhere, the common use of trademarks has been commented on by Jones, who highlighted their presence within price lists and catalogues circulated to the profession.[28]

Large-scale manufacturing, advertising and distribution, expansion of urban centres and developments in retail practices aided the expansion of the proprietary medicine industry.[29] However, with the depersonalisation of the marketplace, characterised by the separation of producer and consumer in the distribution chain, proprietors needed to find ways to communicate reputation and authority.[30] Successful product lines were at risk of imitation and proprietors sought to distinguish them. In the absence of a straight-forward, affordable patent system in the period, alternative forms of branding were sought. Alan Mackintosh has demonstrated, for example, that the medicine stamp was used to denote authority and brand products.[31] Trademarks also offered an alternative to patenting, allowing proprietors to establish priority without having to disclose ingredients or processes. This would have particular value for the medical market, which was plagued with imitation and misinformation. Using Roland Cox's *Manual of Trade Mark Cases* (1881), which detailed 464 products involving multiple trademark cases between 1862 and 1880, Paul Duguid has highlighted that the largest category comprised medical products, with a total of forty-six.[32] The attractiveness of trademarks to combat imitation and promote health products is also evidenced by examining copy designated for retailers found in the trade periodical the *Chemist and Druggist*, where entire advertisements were centred on the announcement of a registered trademark.[33] In a full-page advertisement, the proprietor of Clarke's Blood Mixture quoted the trademark certificate, threatening to take immediate proceedings against all persons pirating his Trade Mark, that was 'fully protected under the Trade Marks' Registration Act of 1875'.[34] Advertising discourse was an important tool for the mythologising of remedies. For example, many featured a common tagline 'Medical Men Recommend Them', giving the impression there would be not only demand for the product, but that they were efficacious.

Competition has been cited as a reason for the profession's stance against patent medicines. Historians have suggested that the medical marketplace in the nineteenth century was overcrowded, with orthodox and unorthodox practitioners competing to supply medical care alongside increasing competition from chemists and druggists, an occupation that emerged in the late eighteenth century.[35] The competitive medical marketplace was not just centred on commercial products, but extended into the profession, with health practitioners vying for patients.[36] Sydney Holloway has demonstrated how self-interest led to intra-professional rivalry in an attempt to retain a monopoly over healthcare provision in the market.[37] This self-interest suggests that there was a significant demarcation between apothecaries (general practitioners), physicians and surgeons. However, the reality was that many practitioners qualified in more than one area or identified more broadly. For example, George Pearse Sargent was listed as a 'General Practitioner' in the 1871 census, a 'surgeon' in 1881, a 'surgeon and apothecary' in 1891, a 'medical practitioner' in 1901 and, lastly, as a 'medical man registered' in the 1911 census.[38] Distinction between medicine provided by a member of the profession and an unlicensed vendor was also minimal, as the therapeutic arsenal used by unqualified proprietors was essentially the same as that of the profession.[39] Indeed, scholars have found that the medical profession commonly prescribed branded medicines as they had a similar efficacy to their own remedies.[40] However, despite widespread scholarly recognition of the profession's complicated relationship with branded medicines there has been no discussion of members of the profession registering their own trademarks to brand medicines and sell them on the market.

The medical profession and trademarks

To register a trademark a proprietor had to send an application to the Patent Office. The *Trade Marks Journal* was an important tool in the process to prevent mis-selling, with a mark only considered registered if there were no objections to its announcement in the weekly journal (Figure 10.1).[41]

Price and Swift's catalogue includes details of 1,285 trademarks for health-related products registered in the first four years of the Trade Marks Registration Act. It shows that a varied range of market participants were registering marks in the category relating to health products: namely large wholesalers and manufacturers, unlicensed practitioners and ad hoc proprietors. Cross-referencing the names of the proprietors with the *Register of Pharmaceutical Chemists and Chemists and Druggists*, *The Dentist Register* and *The Medical Register* reveals that just under a third of medical trademarks in the first four years of the Act were registered by proprietors that could be found in a practitioner register (see Figure 10.2). This finding has significant implications for our perception of the medical marketplace, of which it has traditionally been said that branded medicines were solely connected to quackery and fringe groups. The reality is that a diverse array of medical practitioners, registered and unregistered, were using trademarks to protect and promote their products. Of the 31 per cent of proprietors found in a practitioner register, unsurprisingly the largest group were chemists and druggists or pharmaceutical chemists (29 per cent);[42] 1 per cent could be found in the *Dentist Register*, and the remaining 1 per cent were made up of qualified medical men.

The 1 per cent equates to fifteen qualified medical practitioners, who registered seventeen trademarks between them. In order to further dismantle

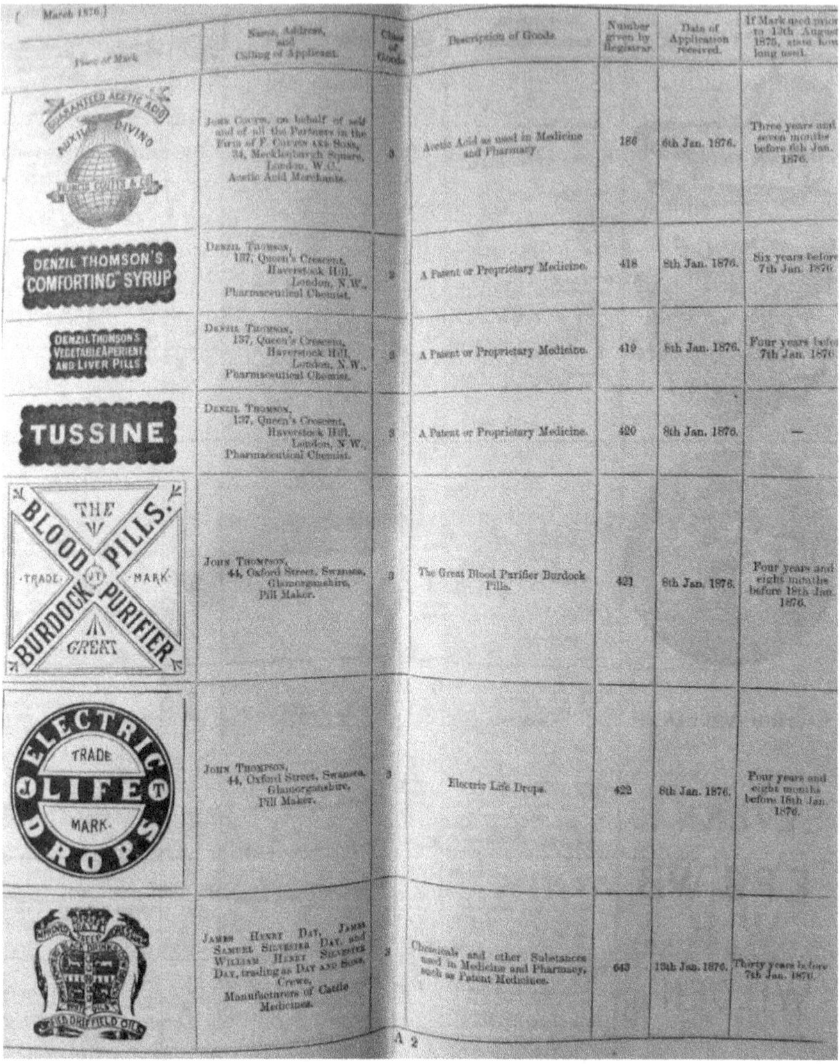

Mark	Name, Address, and Calling of Applicant.	Class of Goods	Description of Goods	Number given by Registrar	Date of Application received.	If Mark used prior to 13th August 1875, state how long used.
GUARANTEED ACETIC ACID / FRENCH COUTTS & CO.	John Coutts, on behalf of self and of all the Partners in the Firm of F. Coutts and Sons, 34, Mecklenburgh Square, London, W.C., Acetic Acid Merchants.	3	Acetic Acid as used in Medicine and Pharmacy.	186	6th Jan. 1876.	Three years and seven months before 6th Jan. 1876.
DENZIL THOMSON'S "COMFORTING" SYRUP	Denzil Thomson, 137, Queen's Crescent, Haverstock Hill, London, N.W., Pharmaceutical Chemist.	3	A Patent or Proprietary Medicine.	418	8th Jan. 1876.	Six years before 7th Jan. 1876.
DENZIL THOMSON'S VEGETABLE APERIENT AND LIVER PILLS	Denzil Thomson, 137, Queen's Crescent, Haverstock Hill, London, N.W., Pharmaceutical Chemist.	3	A Patent or Proprietary Medicine.	419	8th Jan. 1876.	Four years before 7th Jan. 1876.
TUSSINE	Denzil Thomson, 137, Queen's Crescent, Haverstock Hill, London, N.W., Pharmaceutical Chemist.	3	A Patent or Proprietary Medicine.	420	8th Jan. 1876.	—
THE GREAT BLOOD PILLS BURDOCK PURIFIER TRADE MARK	John Thompson, 44, Oxford Street, Swansea, Glamorganshire, Pill Maker.	3	The Great Blood Purifier Burdock Pills.	421	8th Jan. 1876.	Four years and eight months before 18th Jan. 1876.
ELECTRIC LIFE DROPS TRADE MARK	John Thompson, 44, Oxford Street, Swansea, Glamorganshire, Pill Maker.	3	Electric Life Drops.	422	8th Jan. 1876.	Four years and eight months before 18th Jan. 1876.
DRIFFIELD OILS	James Henry Day, James Samuel Silvester Day, and William Henry Silvester Day, trading as Day and Sons, Crewe, Manufacturers of Cattle Medicines.	3	Chemicals and other Substances used in Medicine and Pharmacy, such as Patent Medicines.	643	13th Jan. 1876.	Thirty years before 7th Jan. 1876.

A 2

Figure 10.1 A selection of trademarks registered in class three in the first issue of the *Trade Marks Journal* (3 March 1876). The National Archives, STAT 12/1/19.

the myth that the medical profession were hostile towards intellectual property, the remaining sections of this chapter will look at how a selection of practitioners interacted with the medical market, looking at their career paths, the make-up of their households and whether they promoted their products.

The myth of the medical moral economy 201

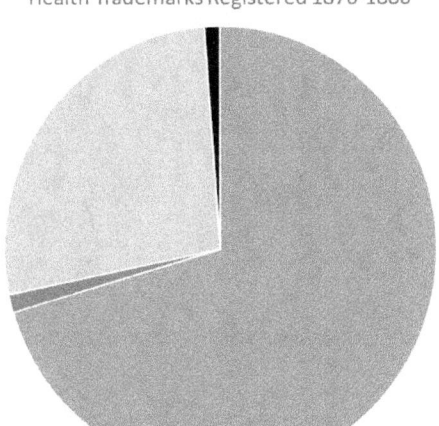

Health Trademarks Registered 1876-1880

■ No of trademarks registered by vendors without a medical qualification
■ No of trademarks registered by a member of the medical profession
▨ No of trademarks registered by Chemist and Druggists/Pharmaceutical Chemists
■ No of trademarks registered by practitioners on the Dentists Register

Figure 10.2 Graph showing proportion of trademarks registered by professional medical practitioners.

What kind of medical practitioner was registering trademarks?

Dr Herbert Tibbits registered 'Dr. Herbert Tibbits' Medical Battery' as a trademark in December 1877 (Figure 10.3). This battery theoretically emitted a low electrical current, which could be used on a variety of medical devices, such as medical belts. Tibbets was a licentiate of the Royal College of Physicians (RCP), obtaining both the LSA and MRCS in 1865.[43] Takahiro Ueyama explored the conflict between commerce and professional ideals with a case study of Tibbit's involvement with the Medical Battery Company and the inclusion of his name in laudatory advertisements. The Censor's Board of the RCP was active in attempting to quash interaction with commerce, particularly with regards to any connection with a company providing treatment for profit. In correspondence with Tibbits the RCP cited bylaws passed in the 1880s to this effect. Tibbits responded that, as he had become a member before the passing of the bylaws, he was not bound to them. This led to a drawn-out battle with the Censor's Board, eventually resulting in his removal from the medical register in 1895, sending out the message that the profession took a strong stance against practitioners using their positions for commercial gain.[44]

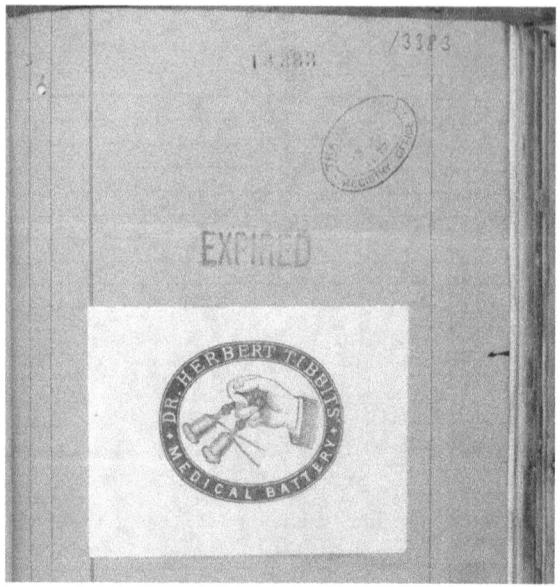

Figure 10.3 Representation of the trademark 'Dr. Herbert Tibbits' Medical Battery', The National Archives, BT 82/54, no. 13383.

Tibbits was clearly a man who challenged orthodox medical ethics. Yet, as Ueyama predicted, 'many doctors were quietly engaged in profitable activities; whatever the College said to the contrary'.[45] Other medical professionals in this sample highlight the more nuanced ways in which doctors promoted and sold branded medical products.

The motive for professional medical men to engage in commerce is unclear, particularly as their financial situation can be difficult to ascertain. However, as Jenkinson noted, the employment of servants was an indicator of middle-class status in Victorian society.[46] Census records show that the number and type of servant varied over time of the sample, indicating a fluctuating income or family arrangement and perhaps a motive for undertaking commercial activities.

Looking at practitioners who identified themselves within journal correspondence, Jones found that those who carried out patenting tended to be young, not as experienced with the ethics of orthodox practice, and practised outside London – with many holding appointments abroad.[47] These observations, however, are not entirely reflected in the sample gathered for this chapter (Table 10.1). None of the sample were below the age of 30 when they applied for a trademark and, taken together, the average age of application was 42.2. Moreover, many of the sample were fully engaged in the medical community, held reputable positions within the

Table 10.1 Table of medical practitioners who registered trademarks 1876–80, showing qualifications and highest number of servants in household*

Name of medical practitioner	Qualifications	Registered trademark (Number; date)	Age when registered TM	Number of servants (highest known number in household)
Adolphus Hahnemann Allshorn (1844–89)	LRCS Edinburgh (1865) LRCP Edinburgh (1865) MD University of Edinburgh 1866	Synthesis (1674; 17 May 1876)	32	4
Mark French Anderson (1835–85)	MRCS 1860 LRCP Edinburgh 1860	Tissue Phosphate of Mineral Food (20327–20328; 28 May 1879)	44	2
William Batchelour (1813–78)	LSA 1834 MRCS 1835	Faith. Hope. Charity (6487; 15 Nov 1876)	63	2
Arthur James Mcdonald Bentley (c.1850–1911)	MB Master Surgeon 1871 MD University of Edinburgh 1889 MRCS 1871	Mentholeum (22139; 21 July 1880)	30	Not known
Benjamin Browning (1835–)	MRCS 1860 LRCP 1866	Dr Browning's Mistura Bismuthi Composita (21118; 1 October 1879)	44	4
John Andrew Ferris (1835–97)	MRCS 1861	Barton's Tyrodont or United Service Tooth Cream (22974; 10 November 1880) Parnell's Chalybeate Saline (14948; 4 December 1878)	43	2

Table 10.1 (continued)

Name of medical practitioner	Qualifications	Registered trademark (Number; date)	Age when registered TM	Number of servants (highest known number in household)
Peter Gowan (1847–1902)	MB Master Surgeon 1871 MD University of Edinburgh 1873	Peptoleine (15985; 30 April 1879)	32	1
Henry Greenway (1829–99)	MRCS 1851 LSA 1851	Spirolene (14352; 5 February 1879)	50	3
Henry Hanks (1828–82)	MRCS 1851 LSA 1858 LRCP Edinburgh 1860	Neuralgia and Nerve Mixture (5491; 4 October 1876)	48	2
Alfred Harvey (1827–1914)	LSA 1852 MRCS 1859 MD University King's College Aberdeen 1860	Steel (9266; 14 February 1877)	50	4
John Robert Samuel Hayward (1835–1913)	MRCS 1857 LSA 1859	Maltese Cross (15106; 16 October 1878)	43	1
Henry Stone Hutcheon (1838–90)	MRCS 1859 LRCP Edinburgh 1860	Dr York's Pills (12635; 26 September 1876)	38	1
Charles Calthrop Mitchinson (1838–1914)	MRCS 1859 LSA 1860	Zoolac (11361; 9 May 1877)	39	2

| George Pearse Sargent (1839–) | Licentiate of the Faculty of Physicians and Surgeons, Glasgow 1862
MD University of St Andrews 1862
LSA 1863 | Dr Sargents (20397; 16 Apr 1879) | 40 | 1 |
| Herbert Tibbits (1840–97) | LRCP 1865
LSA 1865
Member of the RCP Edinburgh 1874, and Fellow 1876
MD University of St Andrews 1881 | Dr Herbert Tibbits' Medical Battery (13383; 5 December 1877) | 37 | 5 |

* Price and Swift, *Catalogue*; Medical Directories 1845–1942 Collection, Wellcome Library, Ancestry.co.uk, last accessed 29 March 2022); UK Census Collection, Ancestry.co.uk, last accessed 29 March 2022.

206   *Myth and (mis)information*

locality, attended meetings of medical organisations and wrote articles for the medical press.

Arthur James McDonald Bentley MD, for example, was a man of national and international reputation. He was a president of the Royal Medical Society Edinburgh and a member of the Medical Society of Java. He also held a number of house appointments at the Edinburgh Royal Infirmary. In addition, he had experience abroad as a surgeon to the Lock and Chinese Hospital, visiting surgeon to the Leper Hospital at Singapore, medical advocate to the Government of Johore, physician to the Sultan, and as the colonial surgeon to the Straits Settlements. He also lectured on tropical diseases in Britain and published a number of articles in the medical press.[48] His remedy, Mentholeum, 'the wonderful cure for Headache, Neuralgia, Colic, and Tic-Douloureux', was advertised in the *London and China Express* and the *London Evening Standard*, with a prompt for the audience to 'Observe the Trade Mark'.[49] There was, however, nothing in the advertisement explicitly linking him to the remedy. Distribution was aided by agents, including the wholesalers Francis Newbery and Sons in London, which gave Bentley the option to market the remedy without having to attach his details. A trademark offered him statutory protection for a brand, while enabling him to stay incognito within promotional material.

Conversely, Dr Henry Hanks advertised his 'Neuralgia and Nerve mixture' alongside his name and address in the trade and lay press shortly after it was officially registered in October 1876 (Figure 10.4). A year prior, Hanks had also received a Royal Patent.[50] The formula of the remedy would have been disclosed to the Patent Office and Hanks showcased its 'royal' status within advertisements as a means of idealising the product.

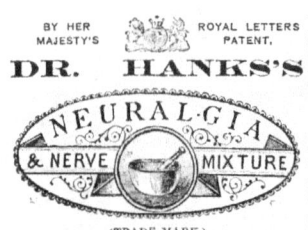

Figure 10.4 Advertisement for Dr. Hank's Neuralgia & Nerve Mixture, Chemist & Druggist, 15 February 1881. Wellcome Library.

Keen to distance the product from quackery, in an advert in the *Chemist and Druggist* the nerve mixture was described as 'no Quack Imposture, but a genuine, truly useful, *boná-fide* medicine'.[51] The long list of illnesses that the product claimed to cure, including toothache, sciatica and nervous disorders, would suggest otherwise to the modern eye. On the surface this looks like a man who had no concern for medical ethics. However, in his early career Hanks had written to the *Lancet* to say quackery 'is the most intolerable bugbear which besets us'.[52] He went on to take specific umbrage against practitioners who advertised their services:

> Let anyone start from Whitechapel Church, walk to Cheapside, wind round St. Paul's, and thence in a line to Trafalgar-square, with his hand as a receptacle for folded bills, and he will possess a precious assortment of surgeons of eminence, on paper, which surgeons and their eminence may be nullified by the London Medical Registration Association.[53]

Moreover, he was an active correspondent in the pages of medical journals, covering a range of medical topics, including 'On Teething of Infants', which featured an expose on the dangers of teething powders.[54] Hanks was a man of contradiction, attempting to use his status to perpetuate the myths of his seemingly elite product while at the same time fighting against misinformation within the medical marketplace. Hanks's advertisements and correspondence implies that professional opposition to branded medicines was indeed as complex as some historians have suggested.

Financial opportunities and competition in the medical marketplace

Studies of the medical marketplace have explored how competition pushed practitioners into commercial ventures in order to make a living. There were numerous forms of remuneration available to practitioners, through the likes of contract practice, provident dispensaries, medical aid companies, doctors' clubs, Friendly Society schemes, or by acting as a Poor Law medical officer or sanitary inspector.[55] Anne Digby has established that the oversupply of practitioners in relation to demand led to the development of specialisms.[56]

Henry Greenway was one such specialist. His obituary in the *Lancet* stated that he studied medicine at King's College Hospital, obtaining both the MRCS and LSA in 1851. He subsequently became assistant surgeon to the Plymouth Provident Dispensary and, later, was appointed the medical officer of health of Plymouth. After he retired, he retained consulting positions.[57] In 1868, Greenway wrote to the *BMJ* relaying his experience of treating constitutional syphilis by carbolic acid. He advised prescribing five doses of glycerinum acidii carbolici in one ounce and a half of water, three times a day. In order to protect against mis-selling he asserted that the drug should be made with the 'colourless acid of the *Pharmacopeia*', referring to an official text that set national pharmaceutical standards. Greenway continued, 'I mention this as some of my prescriptions have been dispensed with an inferior drug (made with the brown crystals of commerce), which is too offensive for internal exhibition'.[58] Greenway's correspondence suggests that he was opposed to proprietary medicines, yet, he registered 'Spirolene' as a trademark for a cough mixture in February 1879. It does not appear to have been advertised in the lay or medical press, but that is not to say it was not promoted via other media. It is likely that Greenway did use the trademark commercially as he later registered an alternative graphic device for 'Spirolene' as a trademark in November 1888. The logo included space for doctors to insert dosage instructions (Figure 10.5).

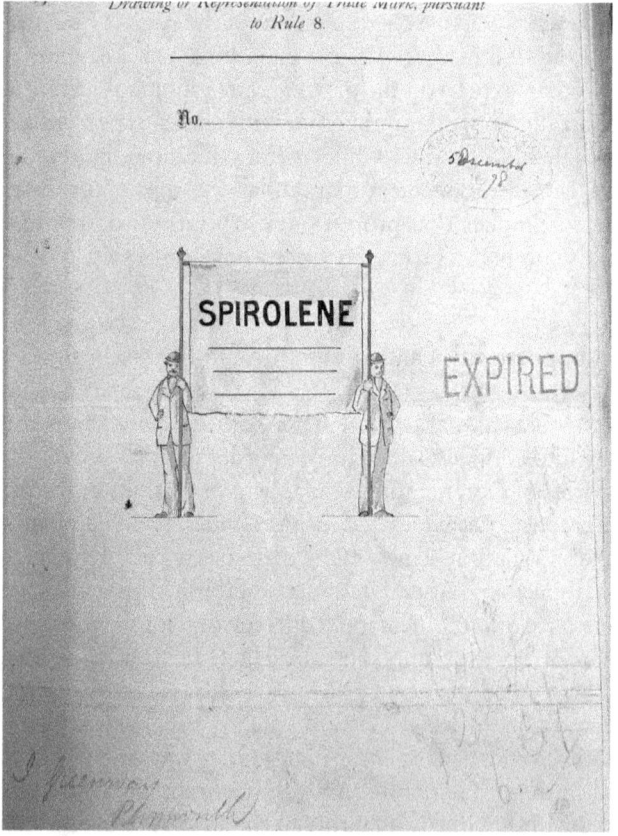

Figure 10.5 Representation of 'Spirolene' trademark, The National Archives, BT 82/54 no. 79,648.

In 1874, Greenway wrote to the *BMJ* on the treatment of pneumonia and bronchitis by carbolic acid, again sharing his preferred formula.[59] This suggests that Greenway did not conceal the ingredients of Spirolene, perhaps indicating that his motive for trademarking was to prevent mis-selling and substitution.

Sharing the formula of a remedy was conceivably one way in which practitioners could justify selling a medicine commercially, as it legitimised the product in the eyes of the profession. This was the case for Dr Benjamin Browning's Mistura Bismuth Composita, a tonic digestive which contained 'Bismuth in its most concentrated form', and featured the formula on the label.[60] 'Peptoleine', registered as a trademark by Scottish-born practitioner Dr Peter Gowan on 30 April 1879, was similarly marketed (Figure 10.6).[61] In the weeks leading up to registration, Burgoyne, Burbidges, and Co, manufacturers and wholesalers, began advertising the product in the vovelties section of the *Medical Press and Circular*, where it was disclosed that Peptoleine was 'An emulsion made with gum acacia, balsam of Peru and phosphate of soda, with 50% oil'.[62] Gowan's medical credentials and publications were noted, including that he was the 'Late Physician and Surgeon to the King of Siam'.[63] The advertisement also referenced Peptoleine's registered status, with the declaration that 'None is genuine unless bearing our Trade Mark and Signature', suggesting that the mark was an important mechanism for communicating authenticity.

It is difficult to ascertain the motives of practitioners for engaging in the sale and advertisement of branded medicines. Gowan and Bentley had prestigious appointments overseas, suggesting that they already enjoyed a good income, and Browning had served in the Royal Navy as an assistant surgeon and surgeon since 1856, likely retiring on a pension in 1869.[64] Jones makes the point that retirees or those with overseas appointments may have had less to fear in terms of retribution from professional bodies for engaging in trade.[65] Indeed, a number of the practitioners in the sample began their careers in the military. Charles Calthrop Mitchinson was an assistant surgeon in the Royal Navy, serving from 1861 and retiring in February 1870

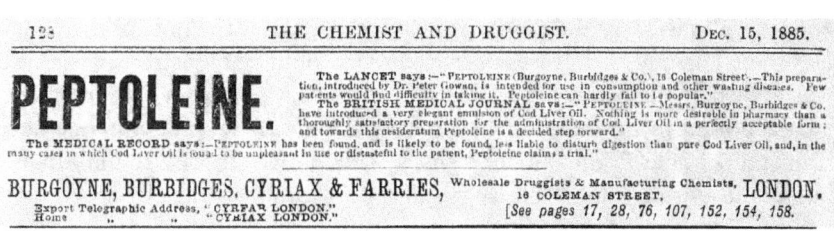

Figure 10.6 Advertisement for Peptoleine, *Chemist and Druggist*, 15 December 1886, p. 128.

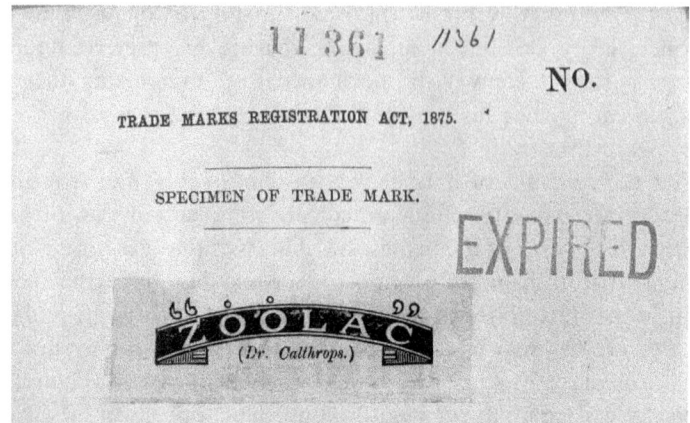

Figure 10.7 Representation of 'Zoolac' trademark, The National Archives, BT 82/46 no. 11,361.

on a pension of four shillings a day.[66] Mitchinson registered 'Zoolac' as a trademark on 9 May 1877, advertising his product widely in the lay press (Figure 10.7).[67] However, while the earliest advertisements for Zoolac made reference to 'Dr Calthrops', any identifier was shortly after dropped.

Nonetheless, Mitchinson was not cautious enough. Like Tibbits, he also caused a controversy by becoming overtly embroiled in commercial activities. In 1884 he attended the City Police Court in Manchester alongside the Reverend Silverton, charged with conspiracy to defraud. Silverton had made announcements in the local press that he would attend the Free Trade Hall 'with his physician', who could be consulted for free daily. Hyperbolic language was used in Silverton's advertisements, referring to 'wonderful cures of deafness' as well as cures for the likes of indigestion, blood diseases, consumption and general weakness. Aggrieved patients accused Silverton and Mitchinson of selling inefficacious medicine to the public. The defence argued that 'There, in one newspaper, side by side with Mr. Silverton's, was an advertisement of "Clarke's World-famed Blood Mixture," which was good for all diseases, and cure was guaranteed, and if the time of the Court was to be taken up with cases of that kind it would be monstrous'. The case was eventually thrown out.[68] The liquidation of Mitchinson's business was later reported in the London Gazette.[69] Mitchinson was the only member from the sample found on the census who did not have servants in his household during adulthood, suggesting he was not financially secure and had been pushed into commercial ventures to make a living.[70]

Digby has highlighted the difficulty of practitioners making a living and the precariousness of extracting financial reward from medical positions pushing them into commercial ventures.[71] Mark French Anderson, a practitioner from the sample, had come from a financially stable household, having been born in Trinidad to a barrister. He had been able to obtain medical positions early in his career, acting as the honorary medical officer to the Coventry and Warwickshire Hospital from 1863 and joining the 2nd Warwickshire Rifle Volunteer Corps as assistant surgeon in 1864.[72] Throughout the 1860s and 1870s Anderson worked with local boards of health to treat sewage.[73] He also applied for patents for the improvement of sewage, reflecting previous findings by scholars that the medical profession used patenting as a means of establishing credit and reputation.[74] In this case, however, patenting was, in part, done for financial gain. In 1871 he sold a patent for utilising sewage to the General Sewage and Manure Company for a hefty £50,000, half being in the form of shares.[75] His business ventures paid off. At the time of the 1871 census Anderson was living in Coventry with his wife, four children and three servants.[76] However, in 1877, like Mitchinson, Anderson entered a form of liquidation under the Bankruptcy Act.[77] Financial precarity may have led Anderson to take advantage of the new opportunity to register a trademark, as two years later he registered two trademarks for 'Tissue Phosphate or Mineral Food' in May 1879. Just one month prior, Anderson put up a notice in the *London Evening Standard* outlining his aspirations:

> A Medical Man and Analyst desires a PARTNER, with Capital, to develope [sic] the sale of a new proprietary medicine, from which a large fortune will be made. – Principals of solicitors only address Dr. M.A., 58, Upper Gloucester-place, N.W.[78]

Notably his name was not given in full, perhaps to distance himself from the advertisement if the need arose. Indeed, Jones found that practitioners tended to ask for patent application advice anonymously through the correspondence columns of journals like the *BMJ*, usually marked with their initials or pseudonyms.[79] There were a number of phosphate foods on the market in the period and it has not been possible to establish a link between Anderson and those found in advertisements, likely due to conscious anonymising. It is difficult to ascertain whether Anderson was successful in selling a commercial remedy; however, he was able to leave £402 19s 11d in his will.[80]

In 1877, Anderson published a medical text on the chemical composition of phosphates, referring to the branded proprietary Parrish's Food. He observed that 'The phosphates in such a combination as that of Parrish's serve as a useful medicine in many cases'.[81] Anderson's writings highlight that some medicines were widely recognised by the profession by their trade names rather than their therapeutic or chemical name. Anderson, a medical man, recognised the efficacy of a branded proprietary product.

Through the use of advertisements the proprietor could influence the medical practitioner and retail chemist to refer to medicine by its trademarked name, rather than by its chemical substance. There is evidence that the use of trademarks led to changes in medical terminology. In 1880 the *BMJ* urged caution around prescribing certain remedies under their trademarked name, as it meant that only the named proprietary, sold by a specific firm, could be dispensed. Doctors were reminded that remedies like antipyrine and lanolin were registered trademarks, but they could be 'manufactured by other than the patented methods'. To solve dispensing limitations the substances were added to the pharmacopeia under new names, rechristening the substances in question.

> Thus antipyrin is designated as phenazone and lanolin as adeps lanae hydrosus. The new names will be a little strange at first, but there are undoubted advantages in using them in preference to names which, although more familiar, are yet the special property of particular firms of manufacturers.[82]

Registered trademarks thus had an impact on the market beyond their existence in advertisements and as a means of establishing trust and controlling imitation.

Conclusion

This chapter contributes to socio-economic studies of the relationship between the medical profession and commerce in the late nineteenth century. While professional codes of conduct and legislation explicitly laid out the unethical nature of commerce, this study has shown that this did not dissuade some practitioners from engaging in commercial activities. It demonstrates that the professional ethics of medical practice were a myth and that medical practitioners of the period were far from homogenous.

The sample used only references members of the profession who registered a trademark in the first four years after the passing of the Trade Marks Registration Act. The sample did not include any medical professionals who qualified overseas, and it was not clear whether Charles Harwood Greene, a registered surgeon and apothecary, was perhaps the same Harwood Greene who registered Zooloo as a trademark in 1877, although it is likely. The years following this time-frame have not been assessed and it is very likely more names could be uncovered, such as that of Thomas Kennedy Douglas, who advertised his registered 'Maori Cigarettes' in the *BMJ* in 1888.[83] Moreover, further marks may be found for the practitioners already identified, as was the case for Greenway, who registered a second 'Spirolene' mark in the 1880s. There was no requirement to register a trademark for a remedy in order to sell it in the marketplace, indicating that those who did were seriously engaged in commerce and valued it as means to communicate reputation and authority in the market. This also suggests that many more medical practitioners unofficially branded and sold their own remedies, particularly as a large cohort of them were still actively dispensing medicines in this period. Indeed, in 1887 the *Chemist and Druggist* reported that dispensing by doctors was on the increase, with the majority doing their own dispensing.[84]

The reappraisal of trademarks as an economic asset in the late nineteenth century played a significant role in the development of commodity branding. The use of legally protected brands gave proprietors novel ways to evoke credibility in the market, imbuing a sense of ownership and traceable origins, which appealed to consumers throughout the buying and selling chain to tackle misinformation and mis-selling. This perhaps held greater appeal for medical practitioners, who could obtain ownership over a product without having to explicitly link themselves to it. The increased presence of manufacturers and wholesalers in the market aided developments in distribution and meant that doctors could effectively sell their products via these middlemen, obscuring themselves entirely from promotional material in order to satisfy the moral economy of the medical profession. Subsequently this anonymity served to perpetuate the myth that the profession did not engage in commercial trade.

Building on scholarship that has shown that practitioners could not ignore the trends of the marketplace and would not be averse to prescribing branded medicines, this chapter highlights that some were even manufacturing and promoting branded medicines, albeit in most cases invisibly. This study has implications for our current understandings of the competitive medical market in the nineteenth century, suggesting that the profession's relationship with patent and branded medicines needs to be explored in more detail as the sale of them was not confined to those struggling to make a living or young inexperienced medical men practising on the margins of the profession.

Notes

1 Entry for 'Neuralgia and Nerve Mixture' in Roger Price and Frazer Swift (eds), *Catalogue of Nineteenth-Century Medical Trade Marks 1800–1880* (London: Science Museum, 1988).
2 *Medical Directory* (London: J. & A. Churchill, 1878), p. 115.
3 Roy Porter, *Quacks: Fakers & Charlatans in English Medicine* (London: Tempus Publishing, 2003); M. Jeanne Peterson, *The Medical Profession in Mid-Victorian London* (Berkeley, CA: University of California, 1978); Ivan

Waddington, *The Medical Profession in the Age of the Industrial Revolution* (Dublin: Gill and Macmillan, 1984).

4 Lori Loeb, 'Doctors and Patent Medicines in Modern Britain: Professionalism and Consumerism', *Albion: A Quarterly Journal Concerned with British Studies* 33:3 (2001): 404–425, at 408.

5 The Patent Office, *A Century of Trade Marks 1876–1976* (London: HMSO, 1976).

6 Roger Price and Frazer Swift, *Catalogue of Nineteenth-Century Medical Trade Marks 1800–1880* (London: Science Museum, 1988).

7 Sally Frampton and Jennifer Wallis, 'Reading Medicine and Health in Periodicals', *Media History* 25:1 (2019): 1–5.

8 *BMJ* (5 December 1885), p. 1070.

9 Sally Frampton, 'Honour and Subsistence: Invention, Credit and Surgery in the Nineteenth Century', *Owning Health: Medicine and Anglo-American Patent Cultures*, Special Issue of *British Journal for the History of Science* 49:4 (2016): 561–576, at 571.

10 Roger Jones, 'Thomas Wakley, Plagiarism, Libel, and the Founding of *The Lancet*', *Lancet* 371:9622 (2008): 1410–1411.

11 Terence R. Nevett, *Advertising in Britain* (London: Heinemann, 1982), p. 71; Thomas Richards, *The Commodity Culture of Victorian Britain: Advertising and Spectacle 1851–1914* (California: Stanford University Press, 1990).

12 Leonard de Vries, *Victorian Advertisements* (London: John Murray, 1968); Keith Souter, *Medical Meddlers, Mediums and Magicians: The Victorian Age of Credulity* (Stroud: History Press, 2012).

13 Kate Arnold-Forster and Nigel Tallis, *The Bruising Apothecary: Images of Pharmacy and Medicine in Caricature* (London: Royal Pharmaceutical Society, 1989).

14 Porter, *Quacks*.

15 Sydney W. F. Holloway, *Royal Pharmaceutical Society of Great Britain, 1841–1991* (London: Pharmaceutical Press, 1991), p. 247.

16 *BMJ* (2 November 1867), p. 385.

17 Jukes de Styrap, *A Code of Medical Ethics* (London: J. & A. Churchill, 1878), p. 28.

18 Sally Frampton, 'Patents, Priority Disputes and the Value of Credit: Towards a History (and Pre-History) of Intellectual Property in Medicine', *Medical History* 55:3 (2011): 319–324; Claire L. Jones, 'A Barrier to Medical Treatment? British Medical Practitioners, Medical Appliances and the Patent Controversy, 1870–1920', *British Journal for the History of Science* 49:4 (2016): 601–625.

19 *BMJ* (2 November 1872), p. 385.

20 *Medical Times and Gazette* (1 April 1876), p. 361.

21 Jones, 'A Barrier to Medical Treatment?', p. 2.

22 Robert Burrell and Catherine Kelly, 'Myths of the Medical Methods Exclusion: Medicine and Patents in Nineteenth-Century Britain', *Legal Studies* 38:4 (2018): 607–626.

23 For discussion of trademarks in the American medical market, see Joseph M. Gabriel, *Medical Monopoly: Intellectual Property Rights and the Origins of the Modern Pharmaceutical Industry* (Chicago, IL: University of Chicago Press, 2014).

24 Hannah Barker, 'Medical Advertising and Trust in Late Georgian England', *Urban History* 36:3 (2009): 379–398, at 396.
25 Lionel Bently, 'The First Trade Mark Case at Common Law? The Story of Singleton V. Bolton (1783)', *U. C. Davis Law Review* 47:3 (2014): 969–1013.
26 For more on Perry Davis, see Ross D. Petty, 'Pain-Killer: A 19th Century Global Patent Medicine and the Beginnings of Modern Brand Marketing', *Journal of Macromarketing* 39:3 (2019): 287–303.
27 Mira Wilkins, 'The Neglected Intangible Asset: The Influence of the Trade Mark on the Rise of the Modern Corporation', *Business History* 34:1 (1992): 66–95; John Mercer, 'A Mark of Distinction: Branding and Trade Mark Law in the UK from the 1860s', *Business History* 52:1 (2010): 17–42.
28 Claire L. Jones, *The Medical Trade Catalogue in Britain, 1870–1914* (London: University of Pittsburgh Press, 2013), p. 45.
29 Nevett, *Advertising in Britain*, p. 15.
30 Stuart Anderson, 'From "Bespoke" to "Off-the-Peg": Community Pharmacists and the Retailing of Medicines in Great Britain 1900 to 1970', *Pharmacy in History* 50:2 (2008): 42–69.
31 Alan Mackintosh, *The Patent Medicines Industry in Georgian England: Constructing the Market by the Potency of Print* (Basingstoke: Palgrave, 2016), pp. 48–54.
32 Paul Duguid, 'Developing the Brand: The Case of Alcohol, 1800–1880', *Enterprise & Society* 4:3 (2003): 405–441.
33 Laura Mainwaring, 'Profit and Paratexts; The Economics of Pharmaceutical Packaging in the Long Nineteenth Century', in Hannah C. Tweed and Diane G. Scott (eds), *Medical Paratexts from Medieval to Modern: Dissecting the Page* (Basingstoke: Palgrave, 2018), pp. 75–90.
34 *Chemist and Druggist* (15 April 1879), p. 14.
35 Irvine Loudon, *Medical Care and the General Practitioner* (Oxford: Clarendon Press, 1986), pp. 208–227; Hilary Marland, 'The "Doctor's Shop": The Rise of the Chemist and Druggist in Nineteenth-Century Manufacturing Districts', in Louise Hill Curth (ed.), *From Physick to Pharmacology: Five Hundred Years of British Drug Retailing* (New York: Routledge, 2002), pp. 79–104.
36 Marguerite W. Dupree, 'Other Than Healing: Medical Practitioners and the Business of Life Assurance during the Nineteenth and Early Twentieth Centuries', *Society for the Social History of Medicine* 10:1 (1997): 79–103; Anne Digby, *Making a Medical Living: Doctors and Patients in the English Market for Medicine, 1720–1911* (Cambridge: Cambridge University Press, 1994).
37 Holloway, *Pharmaceutical Society*, p. 67.
38 The National Archives, London (hereafter TNA), Census for England and Wales, RG10/1659/69/21; RG11/582/11/20; RG12/1646/48/45; RG13/1993/69/3; RG14/269/18.
39 J. W. Estes, 'The Pharmacology of Nineteenth-Century Patent Medicines', *Pharmacy in History* 30:1 (1988): 3–18.
40 Loeb, 'Doctors and Patent Medicines', pp. 404–425.
41 TNA, 'Preparations for publication of the Trade-Marks Journal', *STAT 12/1/19*, 25 February 1876.

42 On the significance of trademarks for retail chemists, see Laura Robson-Mainwaring, 'Branding, Packaging and Trade Marks in the Medical Marketplace *c*.1870–*c*.1920', unpublished PhD thesis, University of Leicester (2019).
43 *Medical Register* (1883), p. 858.
44 Takahiro Ueyama, 'Capital, Profession and Medical Technology: The Electro-Therapeutic Institutes and the Royal College of Physicians, 1888–1922', *Medical History* 41:2 (1997): 150–181.
45 Ibid., p. 180.
46 Jacqueline Jenkinson, 'More "Marginal Men": A Prosopography of Scottish Shop-Keeping Doctors in the Late Nineteenth and Early Twentieth Centuries', *Social History of Medicine* 29:1 (2015): 89–111, at 105.
47 Jones, 'A Barrier to Medical Treatment?', p. 24.
48 *The Scotsman* (22 April 1911), p. 10.
49 *London and China Express* (16 July 1880), p. 25.
50 *London Gazette* (19 November 1875), p. 5531.
51 *Chemist and Druggist* (15 February 1881), p. 64.
52 *Lancet* (10 September 1859), p. 277.
53 Ibid.
54 *BMJ* (15 March 1862), p. 265.
55 Dupree, 'Other Than Healing', p. 81; David G. Green, *Working-Class Patients and the Medical Establishment* (Aldershot: Gower, 1985), pp. 8–14.
56 Digby, *Making a Medical Living*, pp. 33–35.
57 *Lancet* (2 December 1899), p. 1523.
58 *BMJ* (19 December 1868), p. 635.
59 Henry Greenway, 'Treatment of Pneumonia and Bronchitis by Carbolic Acid', *BMJ* (18 July 1874), p. 75.
60 *Friend of India and Statesman* (29 December 1880), p. vi.
61 *Medical Register* (1879), p. 276.
62 *The Medical Press and Circular* (21 May 1879), p. 416.
63 *The Medical Press and Circular* (23 April 1879), p. vii.
64 TNA, Officer's Service Records, Browning, ADM 196/9/258.
65 Jones, 'A Barrier to Medical Treatment?', p. 19.
66 TNA, Mitchinson, ADM 196/9/532.
67 Example, Advertisement for Zoolac, *Southend Standard and Essex Weekly Advertiser* (15 February 1878).
68 *Chemist and Druggist* (14 June 1884), p. 259.
69 *London Gazette* (19 August 1884), p. 3769.
70 It has not been possible to trace Bentley in the census as he resided in Cairo for half the year.
71 Digby, *Making a Medical Living*.
72 *Bell's Weekly Messenger* (17 October 1863), p. 5; *London Gazette* (10 May 1864), p. 2518.
73 *Inverness Courier* (28 February 1861), p. 7; *Nuneaton Advertiser* (8 August 1874), p. 4.
74 *London Gazette* (28 May 1875), p. 2820.

75 *Morning Journal* (Kingston) (25 July 1872), p. 2.
76 TNA, 1871 Census, RG 10/3180/11/16/88.
77 *London Gazette* (19 June 1877), p. 3758.
78 'Partnership', *London Evening Standard* (18 April 1879), p. 8.
79 Jones, 'A Barrier to Medical Treatment?', pp. 610–611.
80 'Mark French Anderson, 1885', in England & Wales, National Probate Calendar (Index of Wills and Administrations), 1858–1995, available at https://probatesearch.service.gov.uk/, last accessed 30 March 2022.
81 M. F. Anderson, *Phosphates: Their Chemical Composition and Uses in the Different Tissues of the Body* (Coventry: Robertson and Gray, 1877), p. 24.
82 'Additions to the British Pharmacopeia', *BMJ* (13 December 1880), pp. 1389–1390.
83 *BMJ* (5 December 1885), p. 1070; *Medical Register* (1891), p. 371.
84 *Chemist and Druggist* (26 November 1887), pp. 672–673.

11

Dissecting Venus: popular consumption of flap anatomies, 1890–1910

Jessica M. Dandona

At the end of the nineteenth century, widespread access to reproductive technologies such as colour lithography and halftone printing were quickly transforming medicine into a profoundly visual profession. These advances made anatomical and medical literature available to a wider audience than ever before, facilitating the rapid circulation of knowledge, text and image between professional and private spheres. One of the most striking examples of this new emphasis on scientific popularization and visuality is that of nineteenth-century 'flap anatomies' – layered, printed illustrations of human anatomy. Produced in brilliant colour and composed of dozens of separate superimposed images, flap anatomies decorated the walls of physicians' offices, the desks of medical students and the bookshelves of middle-class families in both Britain and the United States.

Widely circulated works such as *Dr. Minder's Anatomical Manikin of the Female Human Body* (c.1905) (Figure 11.1), examined here, offered readers the opportunity to engage in a virtual dissection as they folded back layered illustrations of the body. The centrepiece of *Dr. Minder's* is a paper 'manikin', or 'a model of the human body, made of papier-maché or other material, commonly in detachable pieces, for exhibiting the different parts and organs, their relative positions, etc'.[1] The work also includes a legend identifying labelled structures and a short explanatory text describing the structures depicted in greater detail.

Nineteenth-century flap anatomies such as *Dr. Minder's* offered lay audiences access to detailed and comprehensive knowledge on topics rarely discussed in the drawing room, from digestion to human reproduction. In the process, they reinscribed older forms of knowledge, including the 'secrets of women',[2] within the framework of modern medical practice. Even as such works democratised access to information about the human form, they also affirmed the privileged status of anatomy as a visual and textual language for describing the body. Popular flap anatomies thus articulated a new, medicalised body: an impossible ideal of health, youthfulness and fertility against which the bodies of living patients would be measured.

Popular consumption of flap anatomies 219

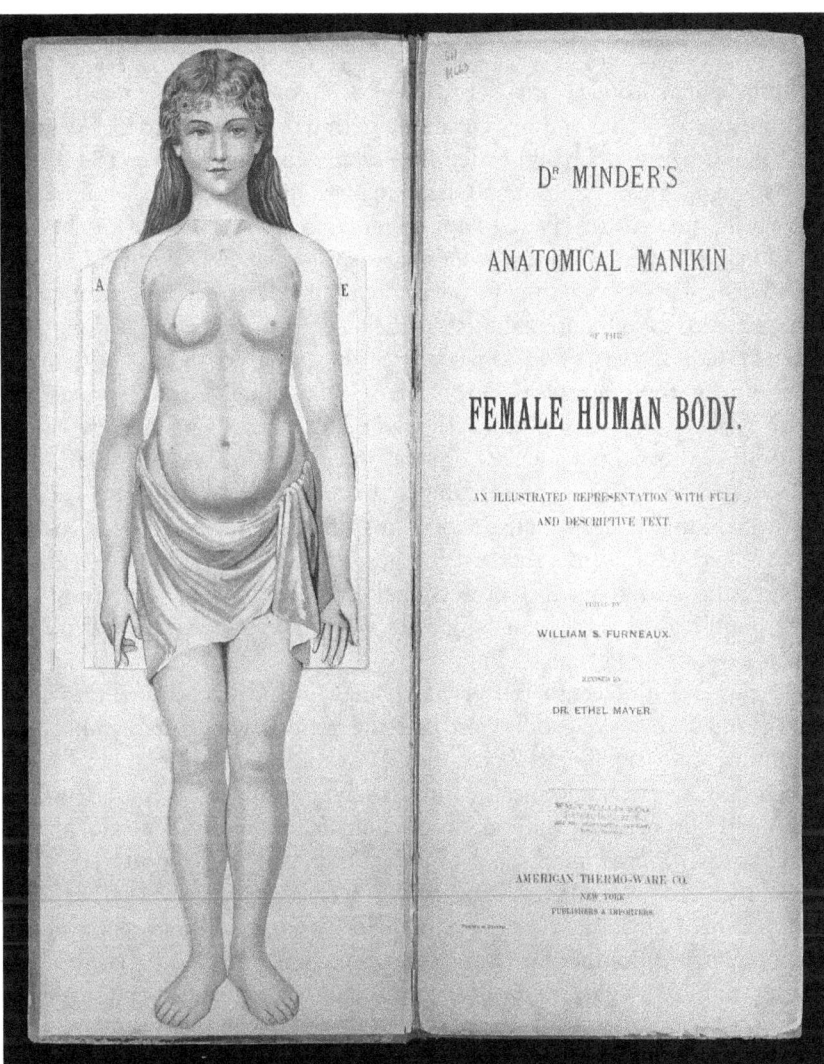

Figure 11.1 William S. Furneaux (ed.) and Ethel Mayer (rev.), *Dr. Minder's Anatomical Manikin of the Female Human Body: An Illustrated Representation with Full and Descriptive Text* (New York: American Thermo-Ware Co., c.1905). Drexel University Legacy Center.

A short history of flap anatomies

Publishers of anatomical atlases had long been pioneers in the realm of printmaking and book illustration, beginning with the work of Andreas Vesalius (1514–64), whose richly illustrated *De humani corporis fabrica* (1543) set a new standard for naturalism and detail in anatomical imagery. Vesalius was among the first to use layered flaps to represent the interior of the human body in his more economical, summary edition of *Fabrica*, the *Epitome* (1543). Similar works dating to the sixteenth and seventeenth centuries are often referred to as 'fugitive sheets', as they were issued as a single print or in pairs. Perhaps the earliest known of these is Heinrich Vogtherr's *Anothomia, oder abconterfettung eines Weybs leyb* (1538), copied and reprinted by Jacob Frölich in 1544 (Figure 11.2), which illustrates a female figure whose torso lifts to reveal her internal organs. Vogtherr's innovation was to pair his work's anatomical content, familiar to readers from woodcuts used to illustrate bloodletting, with the paper flaps employed for *volvelles* in cosmological diagrams.[3] Works such as Vogtherr's likely appealed to a broad, lay public rather than to medical professionals or students:[4] many fugitive sheets were published in vernacular languages and the knowledge they deployed was often outdated or misleading.[5]

By the late nineteenth century, advances in mechanisation, transportation and industrial production laid the groundwork for a publishing revolution and made producing full-colour versions of flap anatomies easier and more economical. Chromolithography, a technique widely employed for printing greeting cards, illustrated children's books, and trade cards, offered publishers of scientific volumes new strategies for attracting a broad audience. Companies such as American Thermo-ware in the United States and Baillière, Tindall & Cox in Britain soon began employing chromolithography to produce complex pictorial atlases of the human body with dozens or even hundreds of flaps, each painstakingly assembled by hand.

Flap anatomies such as *Dr. Minder's* employed double-sided colour printing, which allowed publishers to create multiple folded flaps from a single sheet. The logic of flap anatomies was additive and multiple, and their creation required careful collaboration between authors, illustrators and printers.[6] In order to create the layered effect, publishers began with a substrate, often representing the skeleton, and individual flaps were then added one at a time, with attention paid to their complex interleaving. Rather than a simple progression from the top layer to the bottom (or vice versa), flap anatomies often involved folding overlapping flaps up, down, left and right. Any error in the book's assembly, meanwhile, could mislead readers or invalidate its claim to scientific accuracy.

Popular consumption of flap anatomies 221

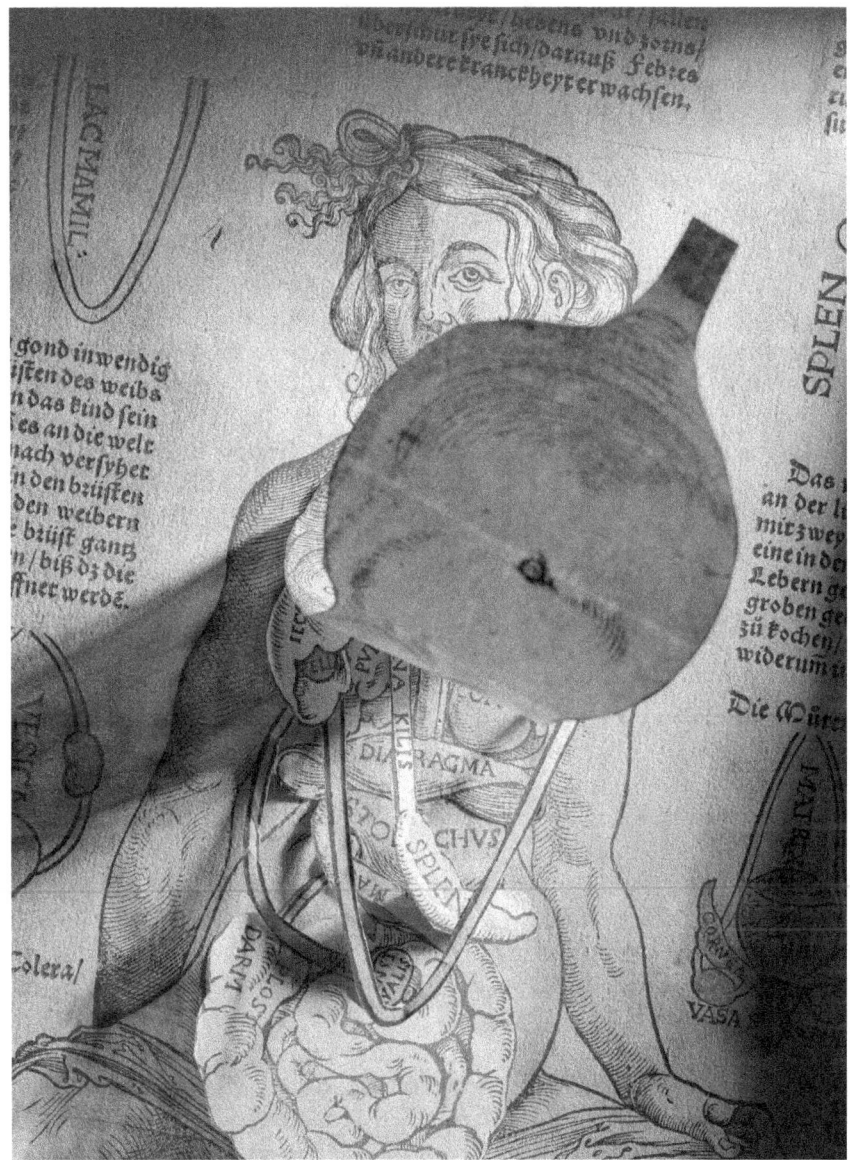

Figure 11.2 *Anathomia oder abconterfettung eines Weibs leib, wie er inwendig gestaltet ist* (Strasbourg: Jacob Frölich, [1544]). Wellcome Collection.

Dr Minder's anatomical manikins

Vaguely reminiscent of old-fashioned greeting cards and 'Victorian' storybooks, *Dr. Minder's Anatomical Manikin of the Female Human Body* appears in collections throughout the English-speaking world. In Britain, a well-known family of map publishers, George Philip & Son,[7] published a slightly less expensive version of the work as *Philips' Anatomical Model of the Female Human Body* (c.1903–58).[8] The use of different titles for what were virtually identical publications reflects not only changing publishers, but also an attempt to extend the work's commercial viability without substantially recreating its time-consuming, elaborate illustrations. Neither American editions of *Dr. Minder's* nor British editions of *Philips'* are dated, a strategy no doubt intended to ensure the works' longevity and to protect against accusations of copyright infringement. *Philips'* offered readers a glimpse of the enclosed female figure on its cover, while *Dr. Minder's* limited all images to the interior of the volume, but the illustrations and text of the two editions are otherwise nearly indistinguishable – with one exception.

While both American and British editions contained the same illustrations, only *Philips'* and the 'Students Edition' of *Dr. Minder's* offered readers a written description of the female reproductive organs. This curious omission extended to similar editions representing the male body, which appeared in Britain as *Philips' Anatomical Model* (c.1893) and in the United States as *Dr. Minder's Anatomical Manikin of the Human Body* (c.1900). Publishers advertised the latter work as 'sexless', suggesting both that it served as a universal human figure and, more specifically, that the publication omitted any depiction of the male reproductive organs. Such works cast human sexuality as a matter of medical concern, allowing the flap anatomy to function in both educational and domestic contexts where frank discussion of sexuality and reproduction was constrained on moral and religious grounds.

The exact identity of 'Dr Minder' remains elusive, although a German author of that name published an atlas on the anatomy of the child in 1901.[9] American editions of *Dr. Minder's* were edited by William S. Furneaux (1855–1940), a British author of popular texts on natural history, biology and anatomy, many of which were marketed to students. Furneaux is also associated with a number of other flap anatomies, including *Whittaker's Anatomical Model* (c.1893), *Hammond's Anatomical Model of the Female Human Body* (c.1899), *Whittaker's Anatomical Model of the Female Human Body* (c.1902)[10] and *Hammond's Popular Manikin* (c.1919).

Both *Dr. Minder's Anatomical Manikin of the Female Human Body* and the 'Students Edition' of *Dr. Minder's Anatomical Manikin of the*

Human Body credit Dr Ethel Mayer (b. 1877; fl. 1895–1905) with revising Furneaux's work. Mayer is likely a woman physician who graduated from Cornell Medical College in 1901.[11] Displaying the name of a woman physician on the book's cover served two purposes: it signalled the work's modernity, as women were only just entering American medical schools in large numbers,[12] and in the case of the female manikin, may also have persuaded readers of the work's anatomical accuracy as well as its inherent modesty. The inclusion of Mayer's name also entailed risks, however, for women seeking to enter the medical profession were often viewed as unnatural beings who risked being 'de-sexed'[13] through their study of subjects such as anatomy.

No artist is credited with creating the images for *Dr. Minder's*, although one might infer that the potentially fictitious 'Dr Minder' provided the original drawings. Some editions of *Dr. Minder's* bear the words 'Printed in Germany', while others read 'Printed in Bavaria'. This likely refers to the work's colour illustrations, as Germany was a well-established centre for chromolithographic printing in this era.[14] The manikin may have been printed by the well-known firm of G. Löwensohn (f. 1844), which specialised in illustrated children's books.[15] My examination of surviving flap anatomies revealed that the imported chromolithographic flaps employed for *Dr. Minder's* and *Philips'* circulated across national borders in this period: the same female manikin appears in Dr Galtier-Boissière's *La femme* (c.1905), *Vinton's Anatomical Model of the Human Body (Female)* (19—), and Dr Ellen Sandelin's *Planscher öfver kvinnokroppen och dess organ* (1904). The original use of the figure may be in a German work by Dr Meyer, *Der weibliche Körper in ungefähr ¼ Lebensgrösse: anatomische Darstellung sämtlicher Organe* (c.1903–21), which appeared the same year as *Philips'*. Slight variations in colour and detail between the various editions suggest that they may have been printed using the same lithographic stone, but by different printers.[16] Despite these minor differences, the manikin's widespread use and longevity, as well as the possibility that it was pirated, suggest its broad and enduring appeal for contemporary audiences.

The audience for flap anatomies

There is abundant evidence that *Dr. Minder's* was employed in medical contexts. A copy in the collection of the Drexel Legacy Center, for example, bears the ex-libris of the Woman's Medical College of Pennsylvania, one of the first medical schools in the US founded specifically to train female physicians. Advertisements for *Dr. Minder's* and similar works also appeared regularly in professional publications from the 1890s through to the 1930s.[17] Many advertisements highlight the work's usefulness for students, physicians and curious members of the public alike. A 1906 announcement in the *Publishers Weekly*, for example, asserts that 'The Dr. Minder's Anatomical Manikins are made for people who wish to know more about their body', but quickly adds, 'In use to-day by thousands of Students and Nurses'.[18]

Much of the marketing targeting popular audiences emphasised readers' moral obligation to study and comprehend their own anatomy. In an American context, the imperative 'know thyself' often bore religious dimensions, urging readers to view their own corporeality as a divine creation. Thus Henry H. Rassweiler, author of a popular medical treatise illustrated with flap anatomies, writes, 'Our bodies are dwelling houses ... leased to us by the Creator on the very simple condition that we use them with care and protect every part belonging to the premises against injury or abuse'.[19] For women in this era, such knowledge was inextricably linked to the maternal role. Thus Myer Solis-Cohen, author of *Woman in Girlhood, Wifehood, Motherhood* (1906), introduced his heavily illustrated marriage manual by stating, 'It is to supply the information that keeps a woman well and happy and guides her in bringing up a family strong in body, in mind and in morals, that this book has been written'.[20] Solis Cohen's work included a 'Manikin Chart', a detailed flap anatomy depicting the female body in cross-section, suggesting that visual imagery was viewed as central to this project.

Flap anatomies also played an important role in mediating between 'professional' and 'popular' conceptions of the body by reinscribing older modes of embodied knowledge within an anatomical framework. The flap anatomy thus offered physicians a visual aid with which to explain their diagnoses to patients. A review of *Whittaker's*, for example, recommends the work to physicians, arguing that 'in this age of intelligent patients, where it is an advantage to demonstrate the organ, its appearance in health and the nature of its diseased condition, Whittaker's models will be found more satisfactory than any chart or drawing'.[21]

The visual language of flap anatomies, which presented matters related to sexuality and human reproduction according to the conventions of anatomical illustration, helped to render them suitable for use in both educational settings and in the home. Indeed, flap anatomies were often marketed to secondary schools, as they provided an economical and convenient form of anatomical illustration free from any controversial contact with bodies living or dead.[22] When used in an educational context, *Dr. Minder's* was viewed as especially well-suited to teaching young women about human reproduction. The flap anatomy written by Swedish doctor Ellen Sandelin, which employs the same figure as *Dr. Minder's*, thus declares on its cover that it is 'Especially intended for use in higher elementary schools for girls and in seminaries for the training of female teachers'.[23]

Like most flap anatomies, *Dr. Minder's* presented the body as a composite of systems and structures: its anatomical description of processes such as conception served primarily to *map* or locate such phenomena, rather than describe them in physiological terms. Many reviewers found this to be a suitably modest approach, one that avoided discussion of sexuality in favour of focusing on the culturally valued act of *reproduction*. An anonymous teacher writing in 1924 describes such an exercise: 'While talking to the boys and girls separately, I use Minder's Anatomical Manikin of the Female Body to show the location of the reproductive organs and the normal position of the child in the mother's body at the time of birth. ... It helps to remove unclean thoughts from the minds of those who have heard these things discussed in an unclean way'.[24] The author of this account frames sexuality within the context of reproduction by distinguishing between 'clean' acts related to motherhood and 'unclean' acts related to sexuality. The process of translating students' understanding of the body into anatomical terms is thus described as an act of cleansing, one that restores order to the body by viewing it within a medicalised and scientific framework. Within the explanatory text, this approach at times entailed curiously misleading statements, such as 'The tube from the bladder opens into the vagina just above its entrance', which omits discussion of the vulva in favour of those organs most associated with conception.[25] Similarly, Furneaux's discussion of conception includes 'semen' and 'spermatozoa', but no mention of coitus or the male 'generative organs'.[26]

In addition to its scientific imagery, the colourful format of the flap anatomy may have rendered its contents more acceptable for use in the home and the classroom. Nineteenth-century flap anatomies such as *Dr. Minder's* bore more than a passing similarity to illustrated children's books of the time. By the early nineteenth century publishers were producing large numbers of miniature theatres, paper doll books, vista books and early pop-up books – all with moving parts.[27] It is surely no coincidence that the genre of flap anatomies lives on today in widely read children's publications such as Louie Stowell's *Look Inside Your Body* (2013).

Unveiling the female reproductive body

The title of *Dr. Minder's Anatomical Manikin of the Human Body*, like many anatomical treatises before it, established an idea of the universal 'human' as male. Within this discursive framework, the female sex is understood as an imperfect variation on the human form, and works such as *Dr. Minder's* locate gender difference in women's ability to reproduce. While otherwise identical in format to Furneaux's male manikin, his female figure is overlaid with a panel that obscures her body from the shoulder to mid-thigh. Once the reader turns aside this flap and those beneath it, the interior of the gravid uterus and the foetus within are revealed, associating the undeniably erotic overtones of the work not with sexuality but with the act of reproduction.

This 'modesty panel' effectively creates a veil or screen that invites the viewer to visually 'undress' the figure by turning over the flap (Figure 11.3). In Galtier-Boissière's version, however, the flap is placed just below the level of the figure's eyes, lending a slightly risqué 'peekaboo' appearance to the work (Figure 11.4). Some flap anatomies in popular medical treatises such as Frederick Hollick's *The Origin of Life* (1878) made this symbolic act of disrobing even more explicit by depicting a fully clothed pregnant woman who is subsequently 'undressed' in order to reveal the foetus within.

Once its 'modesty panel' is lifted,[28] Furneaux's figure appears with a loose white cloth draped around her hips – a convention that dates back to the earliest flap anatomies of the sixteenth century.[29] The multiple layers protecting and screening the figure from view – the book's cover, folding panel and depiction of drapery – evoke themes of veiling and unveiling here linked to the production of corporeal knowledge. Evelyn Fox Keller points to the centrality of such metaphors in scientific epistemology, writing, 'The ferreting out of nature's secrets, understood as the illumination of a female interior, or the tearing of nature's veil, may be seen as expressing one of the most unembarrassedly stereotypic impulses of the scientific project',[30] an approach Ludmila Jordanova terms 'physiognomic'.[31] Perhaps nowhere is this idea of penetrating nature's secrets more apparent than in the study of anatomy, traditionally understood as a practice that explored the most forbidden of all realms – the interior of the human body itself. Indeed, as Katharine Park has theorised in her history of the origins of dissection, the 'unveiling' of the female body's reproductive secrets has been a privileged metaphor for the acquisition of more general anatomical knowledge since at least the late Middle Ages.[32]

In the early modern period, anatomical texts often depicted figures peeling back their own flesh in order to reveal their organs, visually equating the 'unveiling' of the body with its anatomical investigation. A well-known image from Adriaan van den Spiegel's work *De humani corporis* (1645), for example, depicts a living female figure delicately pulling aside the exterior wall of her uterus to expose the foetus within (Figure 11.5). Unlike these early modern anatomical figures, Furneaux's model does not participate in her own revelation. Nor does she attempt to cover her nudity: through her frank glance, she appears to acquiesce to

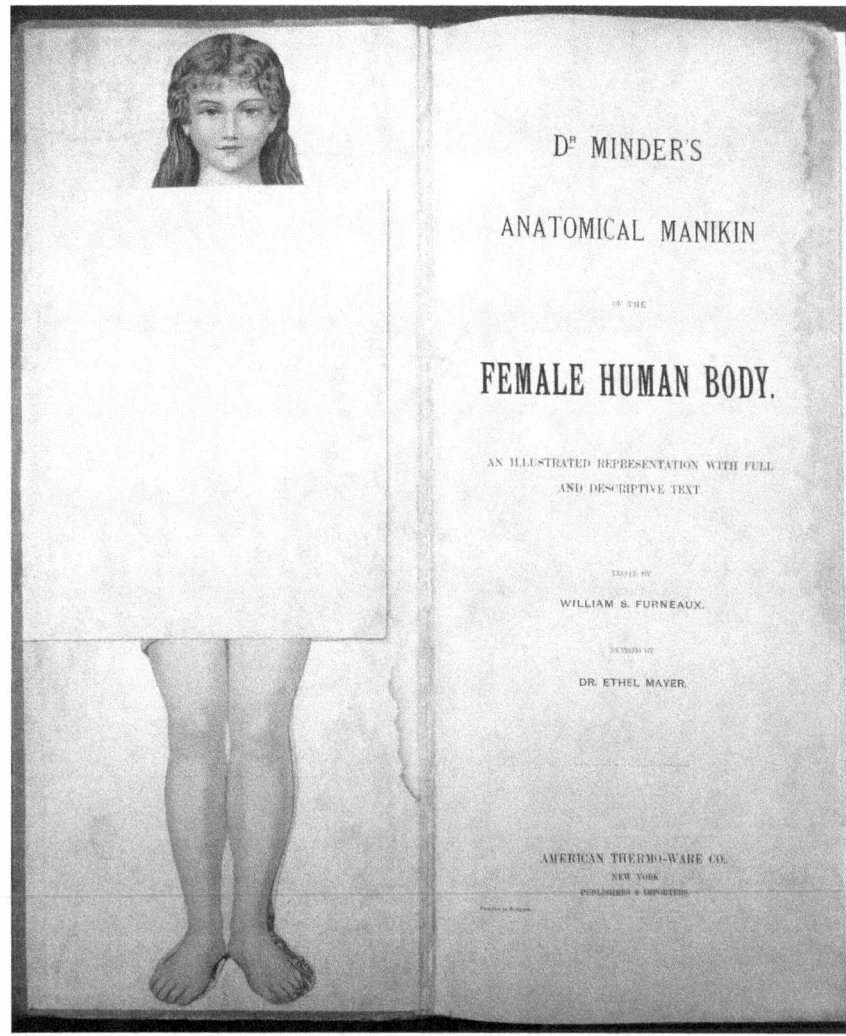

Figure 11.3 Furneaux (ed.), *Dr. Minder's Anatomical Manikin of the Female Human Body*. Drexel University Legacy Center.

our gaze, signalling her status as an anatomical 'specimen' through her symmetrical, frontal pose.

In Furneaux's manikin, the folds of drapery highlight the figure's flowing curves but also create a V-shape that evokes what it also obscures – namely, the pudendum. The presence of this cloth conceals the external sexual organs, while turning the flap reveals the *internal* structures of the uterus, ovaries and vagina. By creating a pictorial work that screens the exterior of

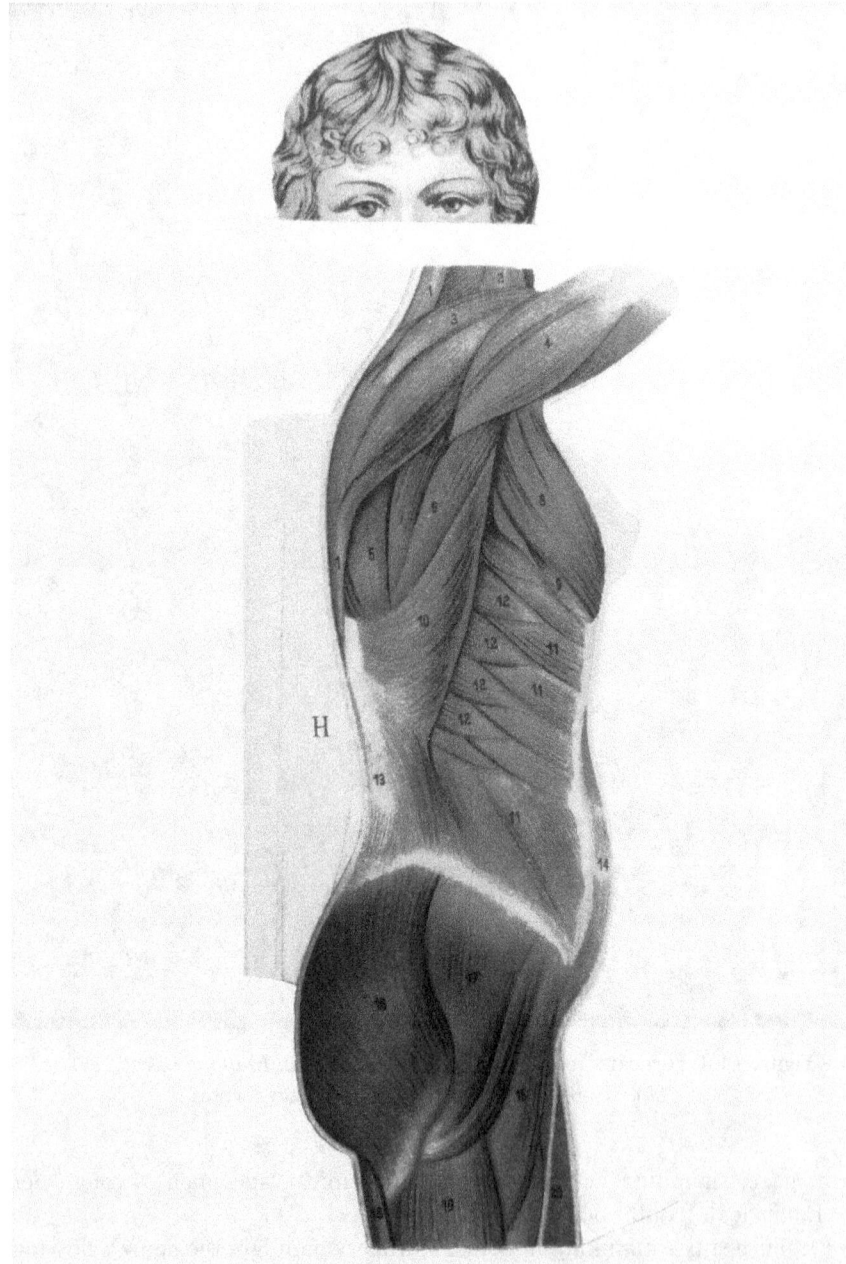

Figure 11.4 Dr. Galtier-Boissière, *La femme: conformation, fonctions, maladies & hygiènes spéciales* (Paris: Schleicher Frères & Cie., Editeurs, [1905]). UCLA.

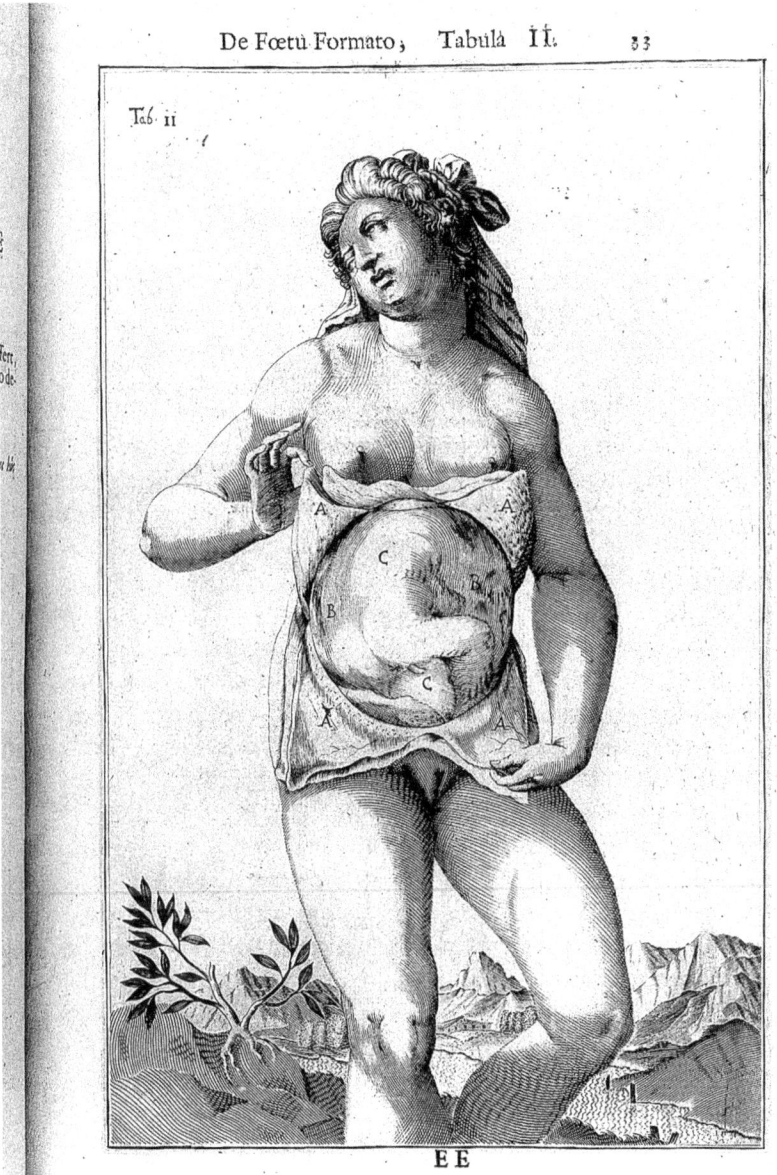

Figure 11.5 Adriani Spigelii, Tabula II, *Opera quae extant omnia. Ex recensione Joh, Antonidae vander Linden* (Amsterdami: Johannem Blaeu, 1645). Wellcome Collection.

the 'generative organs' from view only to reveal their interior once the user has penetrated deeper into the book, *Dr. Minder's* effectively reasserted the 'shameful' and yet ultimately desirable qualities attributed to the female body in popular culture of the time. Moreover, in guiding the viewer's understanding of corporeality as defined by a dialectic between exterior and interior,[33] *Dr. Minder's* and similar works both invite and define knowledge of the body as an act of visual, tactile, and above all anatomical, penetration.

Classical anatomies

The figure's white drapery, as well as her small waist, large hips, and well-defined musculature, strongly evokes classical antecedents such as the Venus de Milo (150–125 BCE). Through the use of classical references, Furneaux aligns his figure with the aesthetics of neoclassicism, which since the time of Johann Joachim Winckelmann (1717–68) had conflated notions of beauty, purity and race.[34] By alluding to the white marble of classical and neoclassical sculpture, Furneaux no doubt sought to defuse some of the tensions inherent in anatomical representation, for illustrations of the female body were vulnerable to accusations that they represented not ideal form, but mere 'flesh'. As Charmaine A. Nelson has argued, 'Flesh was a reminder of bodily functions and secretions, but it was also a reminder of physical desire and sexual contact and was understood as a dangerous trigger to the incitement of passion or desire in the viewing body'.[35]

Reference to classical antecedents also provided an alibi for the potentially indecorous depiction of the nude or partially nude body, as goddesses and historical figures such as the female warriors of Sparta offered a pretext for associating female nudity with youth, vitality and fitness. The contemporary Physical Culture Movement likewise found in ancient works a paradigm for health and beauty,[36] and flap anatomies were employed to illustrate works by proponents of the movement such as the American reformer Susanna Cocroft (1862–1940).[37] The associations thus forged between classical aesthetics and notions of health, whiteness and reproductive fitness – all themes also explored in *Dr. Minder's* – would continue to inform theories around the 'science' of eugenics well into the twentieth century.

The prevalence of classical statuary with missing limbs, meanwhile, offered a visual precedent for the truncated bodies of anatomical illustration, helping to reconcile beauty and disgust. *Baillière's Popular Atlas of the Anatomy and Physiology of the Female Human Body* (1917–44) foregrounded this association by prominently featuring the Venus de Milo on its cover. Familiarity with such classical works would have prepared viewers

Popular consumption of flap anatomies 231

to combine the fragmentary depictions of human anatomy contained in flap anatomies with an imagined notion of their wholeness.[38]

The anatomical gaze

As with the Venuses of classical antiquity, Furneaux's manikin clearly conforms to visual conventions that eroticise the nude female form. Many of the elements that signified the figure's 'natural' state, such as her long, flowing hair, were by contemporary standards highly sexualised.[39] The manikin's topmost flap visually conflates paper and skin, suggesting that as users turned the paper flap, they also touched the figure's bare flesh. The use of colour extends beyond description, moreover, to create an idealised and highly sexualised figure: the manikin's red lips, blushing cheeks and pink nipples evoke good health, but also heightened arousal. This creates a more attractive image, surely, but also one that casts anatomy itself as alluring, more appealing to popular audiences and even pleasurable. This pleasure is as much about touching as it is about seeing: users of flap anatomies explore the human form by manipulating the works' pages as though touching the body itself. Moreover, the status of the flap anatomy as a book-like object lent itself to reading practices that are at once private and discreet, so that the use of such works entailed processes of disrobing, exploration and discovery similar to those involved in the act of sexual reproduction itself.

Indeed, turning aside the flap that conceals the manikin's hips almost immediately produces a shocking sense of intimacy: the figure now appears truncated, shown from neck to mid-thigh, with its arms unexpectedly raised and its striking scarlet musculature shown in profile (Figure 11.6). Lifting this layer in turn reveals a set of paired images, one depicting the skeleton and the other the spine and internal organs – including the gravid uterus – in cross-section (Figure 11.7). The shape of the left-most flap follows the curve of the figure's breast, emphasising its rounded contour, which Furneaux terms the 'beautiful roundness and softness of form' characteristic of the female body.[40] The depiction of the skeleton against a backdrop of peach-coloured pigment circumscribed by a sinuous contour line further accentuates the suggestion of soft, yielding flesh.

Like Furneaux's male manikin, his female figure holds one palm facing the viewer while the other hand points towards the ground. This reflects a longstanding convention in anatomical illustration dating back at least to the Renaissance. In the frontispiece to Giulio Casseri's *Tabulæ anatomicæ* (1632), for example, a female allegory of Ingenium points towards her head, evoking the intellectual aspects of anatomical study, while Diligentia points downwards towards the earth, emphasising the manual dimensions

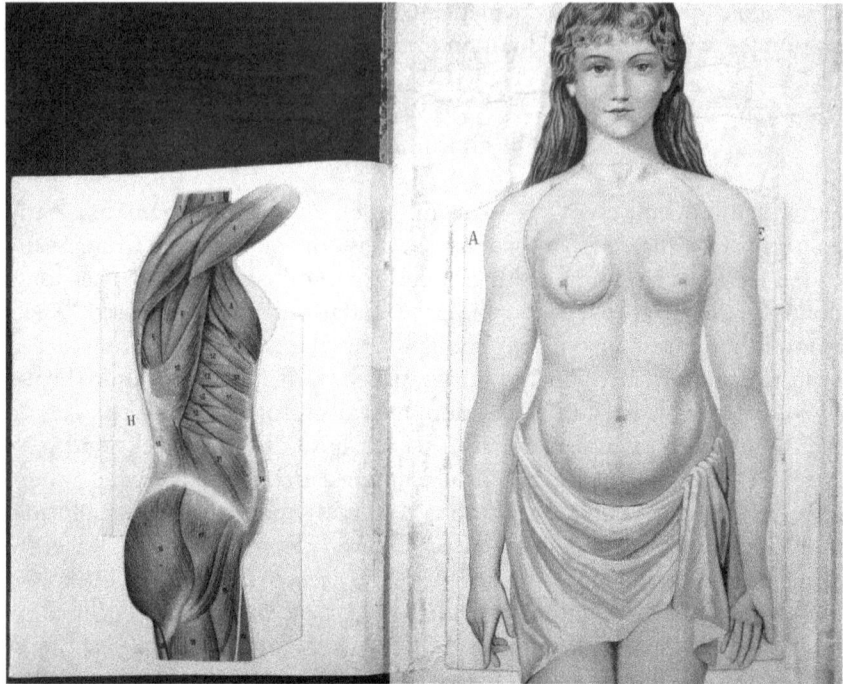

Figure 11.6 Furneaux (ed.), *Dr. Minder's Anatomical Manikin of the Female Human Body*. Drexel University Legacy Center.

of anatomical investigation.[41] Furneaux's figure likewise evokes anatomy's reliance on dissection as a means to knowledge. However, her reference to all things earthly also recalls contemporary theories that associated men with the higher faculties of reason and intellect, and women with the physical and sensual realm.[42] This association is underscored by the fact that Furneaux's male manikin is depicted with a tab that lifts to reveal the contents of his skull, while his female counterpart instead bears a tiny flap illustrating her left breast.

Other references to the figure's origin in anatomical dissection are more subtle. Unlike the male manikin, who appears with his rib cage visibly sectioned, the female figure's torso lifts off smoothly to reveal only the outline of sectioned bone (Figure 11.8). The red and cream stripe depicting the layers of skin, fat and fascia severed to provide this access forms a clean, flowing line that echoes the curves of her silhouette. Colour functions here to suggest life, preserving the fiction that it is possible to 'peer' inside the living human body: the figure's organs appear in brilliant, saturated hues that match the colours of living tissue rather

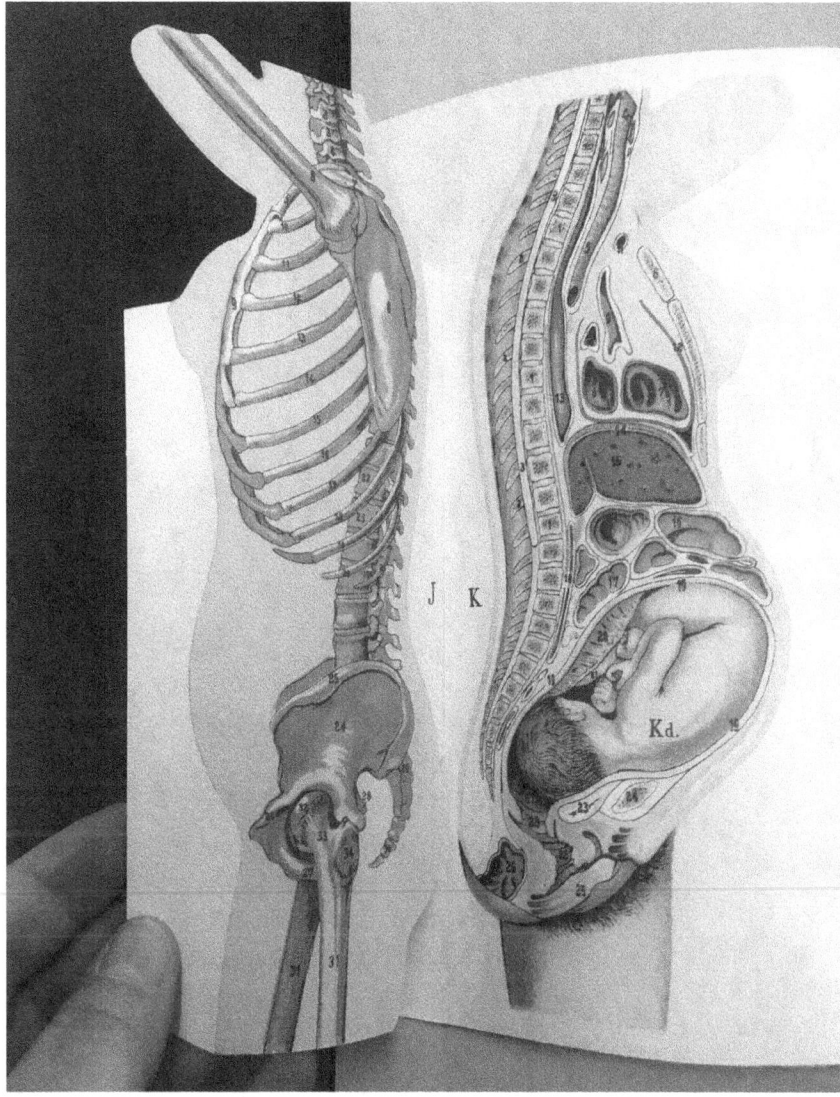

Figure 11.7 Furneaux (ed.), *Dr. Minder's Anatomical Manikin of the Female Human Body*. Drexel University Legacy Center.

than the greys, yellowish whites and browns revealed during anatomical dissection.

By distancing his female model from associations with death and dissection, however, Furneaux also removes the moralising associations present in early modern flap anatomies, which associated knowledge of the body

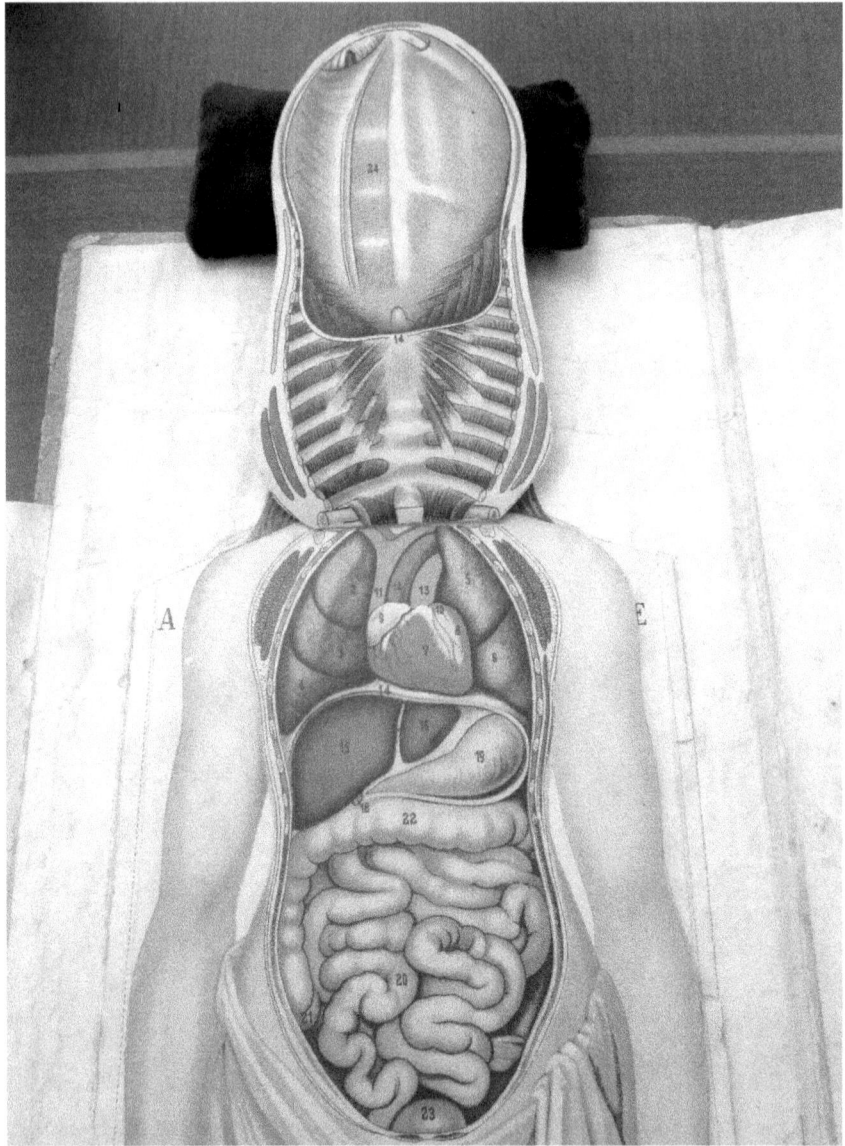

Figure 11.8 Furneaux (ed.), *Dr. Minder's Anatomical Manikin of the Female Human Body*. Drexel University Legacy Center.

with the Fall and its inevitable aftermath – pain in childbirth, shame, death and decay.[43] Furneaux's manikin thus evades potentially controversial associations with the surgical penetration of the body, but also destabilises the figure's meaning: is she a classical statue, a living and desirable woman, or an anatomical specimen? By positioning his paper model at the intersection of these multiple, overlapping points of reference, Furneaux simultaneously drew upon the authority of classical antecedents, invited viewers' curiosity and circumvented controversy. In the process, he strengthened his own claim to scientific objectivity and, at the same time, contributed to the growing discursive power of medicine.

Dissecting the page

It is significant that vividly coloured anatomical atlases with superimposed flaps proliferated during a period when anatomical dissection was a central component of medical education. 'Flap anatomies sought to dramatise and make durable the live performance of anatomical knowledge', Jules Odendahl-James and Mark Olson have argued, but also to 'archive it in book form, opening it to broader economies of circulation'.[44] While the layered dimensions of *Dr. Minder's* evoke the gradual penetration and exploration of the body characteristic of anatomical dissection, there is an important distinction: no cutting is required on the part of the user.[45]

The type of chromolithographic image used in *Dr. Minder's* is commonly called a 'die-cut', a term which refers to the process of stamping out the image using a brass die.[46] The act of cutting out the image parallels the incisions employed in dissection,[47] but offers an alternative that is at once mechanical, crisp and bloodless. Moreover, the paper bodies 'dissected' by the user of flap anatomies, unlike the cadavers of the dissecting room, can be made whole again simply by returning the flaps to their original position. Nor is the flap anatomy prone to the same processes of decay that rendered anatomical dissection an endeavour to be undertaken only in the colder months. The flap anatomy's sublimated references to dissection thus reinforced the authority of anatomical discourse, while also symbolically placing control of this process into the hands of the book's users. This rhetorical strategy not only functioned to render anatomical science, long associated with the controversial practice of dissection, more amenable to contemporary lay audiences, but in the process it may also have encouraged some readers, including women, to pursue the study of medicine.

Works such as *Dr. Minder's* resembled the corporeal form in visual terms but departed from it radically in material terms. The flaps that compose the work are bloodless, paper thin and offered viewers not a specific living or once living body but a composite image. By cleanly separating organs from their surrounding tissues, mapping and labelling structures, working to order and render legible the body, and arresting time and decay, such works impose the language of anatomy upon the unruly materiality[48] of the living, moving and constantly changing human form.

In this way, flap anatomies create a myth of the 'anatomical body', a body that can be disassembled in order to be studied, described in terms of normal and pathological anatomy, and subjected to a clinical gaze that recasts curiosity as 'knowledge'. This anatomical 'body' could also travel: in their flatness and reproducibility, flap anatomies conform to Bruno Latour's definition of the 'immutable mobile',[49] a form of representation that enabled anatomical science to gain ascendancy in both professional and popular contexts as a privileged mode for describing and understanding the body. As printed paper objects, then, flap anatomies were both economical and abundant, moving easily between different spheres of knowledge. While such works reflected earlier traditions of displaying the body, their ability to speak to a multiplicity of audiences and to mobilise a range of diverse meanings dependent on context permitted the broad diffusion of standardised anatomical principles and images. Through their persuasive power, appeal to classical authority, and processes of replication, then, nineteenth-century flap anatomies succeeded in constructing a new myth of the body – one defined by the language of anatomy.

Notes

1 Advertisement, *Protestant Episcopal Review* 7:7 (1894): 7.
2 Katharine Park, *Secrets of Women: Gender, Generation, and the Origins of Human Dissection* (Cambridge, MA: MIT Press, 2006).
3 Theresa Smith, 'Moveable Anatomies and Print Shop Practice in Sixteenth-Century Strasbourg', in David Saunders, Marika Spring and Andrew Meek (eds), *The Renaissance Workshop: The Materials and Techniques of Renaissance Art* (London: Archetype Publications, 2013), pp. 121–129, at p. 122. See also Suzanne Karr Schmidt, *Interactive and Sculptural Printmaking in the Renaissance* (Leiden and Boston: Brill, 2018).
4 See Andrea Carlino, *Paper Bodies: A Catalogue of Anatomical Fugitive Sheets, 1538–1687* (London: Wellcome Institute for the History of Medicine, 1999).
5 Smith, 'Moveable Anatomies', p. 127; L. H. Wells, 'Anatomical Fugitive Sheets with Superimposed Flaps, 1538–1540', *Medical History* 12:4 (1968): 406–407.
6 Meg Brown, 'Flip, Flap, and Crack: The Conservation and Exhibition of 400+ Years of Flap Anatomies', *Book and Paper Group Annual* 32:6 (2013): 6–14, at 8.

7 David Smith, 'Map Publishers of Victorian Britain: The Philip Family Firm 1834–1902', *Map Collector* 38 (1987): 31–32.
8 Furneaux's *Anatomical Model of the Female Human Body*, published by Whittaker, sold for $1.75 in 1902, while *Philips'* retailed for 4 shillings, the equivalent of roughly $1, in 1903. Marion E. Potter (ed.), *The United States Catalog Supplement: Books Published 1902–1905* (Minneapolis, MN: H. W. Wilson Company, 1906), p. 48; *Bookseller: The Organ of the Book Trade* (10 September 1903), p. 801. Baillière, another London publisher, appears to have issued a version of Furneaux's text as *Anatomical Model of the Female Human Body* by 1904. It also sold for 4 shillings. 'Books of the Year', *Medical Annual* 23 (1905), p. 652.
9 Dr Minder, *Der kindliche Körper: Anschauliche Darstellung seines Baues und seiner Organ mit erläuterndem Text* (Fürth: G. Löwensohn, c.1901).
10 Like *Philips' Anatomical Model*, Whittaker's *Anatomical Model* is a translation of a German work, *Der menschliche Körper: Anschauliche Darstellung seines Baues und seiner Organe* (Fürth: [G. Löwensöhn?], [1898?]).
11 Michael R. Thompson, 'Miscellany', Michael R. Thompson Rare Books (Spring/Summer 2021), available at https://www.mrtbooksla.com/images/uplo ad/mrtbooks-miscellany-ss21.pdf, last accessed 23 July 2021. Thompson cites as his source: 'Third Annual Commencement', *Cornell Alumni News* 3:36 (12 June 1910): 1 and *University of the State of New York: Higher Education Bulletin* 17 (1901–02): 67.
12 For more, see Susan Wells, *Out of the Dead House: Nineteenth-Century Women Physicians and the Writing of Medicine* (Madison, WI: University of Wisconsin Press, 2001) and Regina Markell Morantz-Sanchez, *Sympathy and Science: Women Physicians in American Medicine* (New York and Oxford: Oxford University Press, 1985).
13 Michael Sappol, *A Traffic of Dead Bodies: Anatomy and Embodied Social Identity in Nineteenth-Century America* (Princeton, NJ and Oxford: Princeton University Press, 2002), pp. 62, 90.
14 One early twentieth-century source estimates that nearly 90 per cent of Christmas cards sold in England were printed in Germany. *How to Capture German Trade* (London: Hodder and Stoughton, 1914), p. 64.
15 According to Jo Tisinger, many books marked 'Printed in Bavaria' were printed by Lowensöhn. Jo Tisinger, 'G. Löwensohn – Children's Books – Fürth', Vintage Popup Books, https://www.vintagepopupbooks.com/movable-book-history-s/1858.htm, last accessed 6 January 2022. The firm was founded by Gerson Löwensohn (1817–71) in 1844.
16 I am indebted to Russell A. Johnson, Curator for History of Medicine and the Sciences, UCLA Library Special Collections for this observation.
17 See, for example, *Journal of the American Medical Association* 79:27 (1922): 28; *Southern Medical Journal* 15:3 (1922): 39; *The American Physician* (March 1922): 240; and *The Modern Hospital* 15:6 (December 1920): 96.
18 Advertisement, *Publishers Weekly* 69:1778 (24 February 1906): 776.

19 Henry H. Rassweiler, *Portfolio of Life* (Chicago, IL: Western Publishing House, 1891), p. xiv.
20 Myer Solis-Cohen, *Woman in Girlhood, Wifehood, Motherhood: Her Responsibilities and Her Duties at All Periods of Life* (Philadelphia, Chicago and Toronto: John C. Winston Co., 1906), p. 4.
21 'The Reviewers Table: Whittaker's Anatomical Model', *Medical Fortnightly* 10:8 (1896): 562.
22 See, for example, Advertisement, *American School Board Journal* 33:5 (1906): n.p. and Advertisement, *Michigan School Moderator* 14:16 (1894): 505.
23 Ellen Sandelin, *Planscher öfver kvinnokroppen och dess organ* (Stockholm: AB Ljus förlag, 1904).
24 *Proceedings of the High School Conference*, 21:25 (Urbana: University of Illinois, 1924), p. 110.
25 William S. Furneaux (ed.), *Dr. Minder's Anatomical Manikin of the Female Human Body: An Illustrated Representation with Full and Descriptive Text*, rev. Ethel Mayer (New York: American Thermo-Ware, [*c*.1905]), p. 11.
26 Ibid., p. 11.
27 Kathy Piehl, 'Books in Toyland', *Children's Literature Association Quarterly* 12:2 (1987): 79.
28 The panel itself is missing from many extant copies, suggesting that some readers found it necessary to censor the work even further by eliminating those parts of the image that addressed sexuality and reproduction.
29 See anatomical fugitive sheet with female figure, University of Michigan, possibly published by Nicolai (Nicolo) de Sabio in Venice, 1539, and illustrated in L. H. Wells, 'A Remarkable Pair of Anatomical Fugitive Sheets in the Medical Center Library, University of Michigan', *Bulletin of the History of Medicine* 38:5 (1964): 470–476, at 472.
30 Evelyn Fox Keller, 'From Secrets of Life to Secrets of Death', in Mary Jacobus, Evelyn Fox Keller and Sally Shuttleworth (eds), *Body/Politics: Women and the Discourses of Science* (New York: Routledge, 1990), pp. 177–191, at p. 178.
31 Ludmilla Jordanova, *Sexual Visions: Images of Gender in Science and Medicine between the Eighteenth and Twentieth Centuries* (Madison, WI: University of Wisconsin Press, 1989), p. 92.
32 Park, *Secrets of Women*.
33 Karen Rosoff Encarnación, 'The Proper Use of Desire: Sex & Procreation in Reformation Anatomical Fugitive Sheets', in Anne L. McClanan and Karen Rosoff Encarnación (eds), *The Material Culture of Sex, Procreation, and Marriage in Premodern Europe* (New York: Palgrave, 2001), pp. 221–249 at p. 223.
34 Amelia Rauser, *The Age of Undress: Art, Fashion, and the Classical Ideal in the 1790s* (New Haven, CT and London: Yale University Press, 2020), p. 127.
35 Charmaine A. Nelson, *The Color of Stone: Sculpting the Black Female Subject in Nineteenth-Century America* (Minneapolis, MN: University of Minnesota Press, 2007), p. 65.

36 Fae Brauer, 'Eroticizing Lamarckian Eugenics: The Body Stripped Bare during French Sexual Neoregulation', in Fae Brauer and Anthea Callen (eds), *Art, Sex and Eugenics: Corpus Delecti* (Aldershot: Ashgate Publishing, 2008), pp. 97–136 and Anthea Callen, *Looking at Men: Anatomy, Masculinity and the Modern Male Body* (New Haven, CT: Yale University Press, 2018).

37 Susanna Cocroft, *Body Manikin and the Position of Vital Organs* (Chicago, IL: Physical Culture Extension Society, 1905). Advertisements for *Dr. Minder's* appeared with some regularity in publications aimed at physical culture proponents. See, for example, *American Physical Education Review* (1925): 109 and *Physical Training* 17:4 (1920): 95.

38 Lennard J. Davis, 'Nude Venuses, Medusa's Body, and Phantom Limbs: Disability and Visuality', in D. T. Mitchell and S. L. Snyder (eds), *The Body and Physical Difference: Discourses of Disability* (Ann Arbor, MI: University of Michigan Press, 1997), pp. 51–70, at p. 56.

39 For more on women's hair and sexuality, see Elisabeth G. Gitter, 'The Power of Women's Hair in the Victorian Imagination', *PMLA/Publications of the Modern Language Association of America* 99:5 (1984): 936–954.

40 Furneaux, *Dr. Minder's Anatomical Manikin*, p. 6.

41 Viktoria von Hoffmann, '*Ingeniosa peritia*: The Languages of Ingenuity in Italian Renaissance Anatomy', in Richard J. Oosterhoff, José Ramón Marcaida and Alexander Marr (eds), *Ingenuity in the Making: Matter and Technique in Early Modern Europe* (Pittsburgh, PA: University of Pittsburgh Press, 2021), pp. 94–111.

42 For more on the history of these associations, see Sherry B. Ortner, 'Is Female to Male as Nature is to Culture?' *Feminist Studies* 1:2 (1972): 5–31.

43 Encarnación, 'Proper Use of Desire', pp. 223, 230.

44 Jules Odendahl-James and Mark Olson, 'Flap and Click: The Performance of Embodiment in Anatomy and the Archive', paper presented at Animated Anatomies: The Human Body in Anatomical Texts from the 16th through 21st Centuries, Duke University, 18 April 2011.

45 Hannah Wiepke, 'Cut & Paste: An Attempt to Construct Johannes Remmelin's 1754 Flap Anatomy Restrike', paper presented at Union Pacific Fellows Roundtable, University of Minnesota Twin Cities, 19 March 2021.

46 Erika Mosier, Dianne van der Reyden and Mary Baker, 'The Technology and Treatment of an Embossed, Chromolithographic "Mechanical" Victorian Valentine Card', *Book and Paper Group Annual* 11 (1992), n.p.

47 See Rosemary Moore, 'Paper Cuts: The Production of Knowledge in Early Modern Anatomical Prints', PhD thesis, University College London (2016) for a discussion of the links between the act of cutting the body and creating prints in the early modern period. The process of lithography, unlike the creation of an intaglio print, does not involve incision. However, as noted, the stamping of chromolithographic die-cut images could be considered a form of cutting, and carries a similar suggestion of symbolic violence enacted upon the 'body'.

48 Ibid., p. 47.

49 Bruno Latour, 'Visualization and Cognition: Thinking with Eyes and Hands', *Knowledge and Society* 6 (1986): 1–40.

12

'You taught us that which you knew *not* to be the truth': the anti-vaccination medical doctor in Henry Rider Haggard's *Doctor Therne* (1898)

Carlotta Fiammenghi

'My only novel with a purpose': genesis and reception of Henry Rider Haggard's *Doctor Therne*

Henry Rider Haggard (1865–1925) was a prolific author, having written a total of fifty-eight works of fiction which were issued almost yearly for thirty-eight years, as Morton Cohen notes in his biography *Rider Haggard: His Life and Works*.[1] His many adventure novels were also popular, filling the imagination of his contemporaries with fascinating characters who experienced exciting adventures set in exotic lands; some of these adventure novels are still widely read. However, one of Haggard's novels is unique for its plot, setting and moral: *Doctor Therne* (1898), a fictional autobiography of a medical doctor who decides to embrace the anti-vaccination cause in order to win an election as a Radical, despite being a firm believer in the safety and effectiveness of vaccines. Notwithstanding its modest commercial success following publication in 1898 and a positive reception by the scientific and medical authorities of the time, the book is still relatively neglected; Cohen himself mentions it only once, fleetingly and unceremoniously: 'Of the fifty-eight volumes, forty-seven are conventional Rider Haggard adventure romances, and twelve are novels of contemporary life. One is a propagandist novel'.[2] Only in an endnote does he clarify that this 'propagandist' novel is '*Dr Therne* (1898), dedicated to the Jenner Society and issued in the heat of the vaccination controversy of the time'.[3] Cohen's choice of the adjective 'propagandist' is worth exploring, particularly because he does not explain what he means by it and does not otherwise discuss the novel in his biography. It seems possible to speculate that Cohen regarded *Doctor Therne* as a chiefly political enterprise, which sits awkwardly with the literary, entertaining character of Haggard's other novels. Indeed, Haggard was actively and consciously entering the public vaccination debate with *Doctor Therne*, propounding his own views about the necessity and effectiveness of vaccinations; these views are made explicit by the writer himself in his autobiographical works (discussed later in this section). This, however, far from reducing the novel to the status of a propagandistic pamphlet, arguably makes it a fascinating example of the complex intertwining of facts and fiction, and of the potential of fiction to shape social and political reality.

Haggard himself discusses this potential, which appears to be the main reason he was fond of this work, which he calls 'my only novel with a purpose' in his autobiography, *The Days of My Life*:

> I will dwell for a moment upon my only novel with a purpose, which appeared about a year previous to my journeyings in the Near East. It is called 'Doctor Therne,' and deals with the matter of the Anti-Vaccination craze – not, it may be thought, a very promising topic for romance. I was led to treat of it, however, by the dreadful things I had seen and knew of the ravages of smallpox in Mexico and elsewhere, and the fear, not yet realised, that they should repeat themselves in this country. ... Although so different in matter and manner from my other works, this tale has been widely read .... I dedicated it (without permission) to the Jenner Society. The Executive Committee of this society on December 22, 1898, passed a warm and unanimous resolution thanking me for the work.[4]

As this passage demonstrates, *Doctor Therne* was indeed warmly and widely appreciated at the time, and this success was due precisely to the 'purpose' of the novel, which Haggard phrases as an attempt to prevent a renewed smallpox epidemic in England by countering the anti-vaccination movement (which he significantly describes as a 'craze').

The author's direct involvement in contemporary anti-vaccination debates and his firm pro-vaccination position emerge in several other of his writings: for example, in an entry for 20 July 1898 of his diary *A Farmer's Year*, he describes vaccination as a 'boon'.[5] In the same entry he also comments on the introduction of the Conscientious Objection clause to the Vaccination Bill,[6] which made it possible for parents to exempt their children from vaccination on 'conscientious grounds' – a clause that considerably reduced the uptake of the vaccine in various areas of England, and that Haggard feared would gravely undermine the English vaccination campaign.[7] In his own words:

> I see in the paper today that the Government has given way suddenly on the Vaccination Bill, and that henceforth 'conscientious objection' on the part of parents is to entitle them to disregard the law and neglect the vaccination of their children. ... Among tens of thousands of the population, by consent of the State, vaccination, in my belief one of the greatest boons that the century has brought to mankind, will henceforth cease to exist. ... In future an

indolent, or a prejudiced, or a 'conscience-stricken' father or guardian is to be licensed at will to expose children to the ravages of a fearful sickness and the risk of death, and, helpless though they are, it is by Act of Parliament decreed that no hand shall be held up to save them.[8]

Haggard also makes his position very clear in the Author's Note accompanying *Doctor Therne*, where he harshly condemns the leaders of the Government, who 'dismayed their supporters and astonished the world by a sudden surrender to the clamour of the anti-vaccinationists … under the guise of a "graceful concession," the health of the country was given without appeal into the hand of the "Conscientious Objector"' (vii). He also justifies his choice of an unusual medical topic as the subject for his novel by underlining its timely relevance: 'The importance of the issue to those helpless children from whom the State has thus withdrawn its shield, is this writer's excuse for inviting the public to interest itself in a medical tale. As for the moral, each reader can fashion it to his fancy' (viii).

Not only does Haggard appear as an advocate of the benefits of vaccination, and his novel *Doctor Therne* as an active attempt to influence contemporary debates about smallpox vaccination and its enforcement by the Government, his writings also reveal his reflections on the potential of fiction for engaging in the vaccination debate. In his view, English people are unable to foresee the dire consequences of this Conscientious Objection clause because they lack imagination. He concedes that anti-vaccinationists may be honest and well-meaning, albeit misguided, and concludes that their anti-vaccination belief may stem from a lack of experience with the illness: they cannot accurately assess the true risks of smallpox because they have not yet experienced its ravages directly. Most importantly, he is convinced that this void may effectively be filled through works of fiction:

> It seems a pity that the leaders of the anti-vaccination party, who, no doubt, are very honest in their faith, and therefore can scarcely be blamed for endeavouring to enforce it, cannot, as I have done, when a smallpox epidemic is raging travel in foreign parts where that prophylactic is unknown or little practised. I think that they would come back with their views much modified. At present they think little of the disease because they have scarcely seen it at its dreadful work. What they lack is imagination.[9]

Haggard posits here that imagination – and imaginative works – provide a powerful, and possibly unique, means for authors to describe and for readers to encounter the tragic potential of illnesses and ill-managed epidemics. Thus, despite Haggard's claim in his Author's Note that the moral of the novel is left open to the reader's interpretation, *Doctor Therne*'s pro-vaccination stance is quite clear, so much so that the prestigious medical journal the *Lancet*, in commenting favourably on the book, states that

[W]e must commend Mr. Haggard's courage in thus entering the lists against the Anti-Vaccination party. As a novelist and a politician alike[10] it is evidently to his advantage to take no step that would be likely to alienate him from any large body of possible supporters. Yet he has risked losing many readers and creating a fanatical opposition to whatever he may do in a public or private capacity for the sake of telling the truth'.[11]

The *Lancet* here seems to legitimise Haggard as a brave hero in the vaccination campaign, and consequently to endorse fiction as a means of assisting and promoting a national health campaign. Implicitly, it is also affirming the power of the novel to influence the vaccination debates of the time, a power which has possibly remained underappreciated in scholarship so far.

Therefore, the aim of the present chapter is to explore the way Haggard exploited the form of the novel – and thus, of fiction – to accurately represent the various instances of the anti-vaccination movement among his contemporaries. The chapter will present a close reading of select passages in the novel, and a comparison between them and various tracts and pamphlets of the anti-vaccination movement in Victorian England. The analysis also aims to highlight the similarities between past and present anti-vaccination instances, both in the content and in the language used. This investigation is informed by an overarching reflection on the power of literature to reproduce and understand the complexities underlying medico-scientific as well as sociopolitical debates, and therefore to effectively enter controversies where facts and fiction, information and misinformation, may be closely – sometimes inextricably – intertwined.

Late Victorian anti-vaccination movements and their fictional representation

Doctor Therne is a fictional autobiography of James Therne, a medical doctor belonging to the lower middle class who tries to build a name and a career for himself in a fictional suburb called Dunchester. His rival, Doctor James Bell, falsely accuses him of neglect and of having caused the death of an influential upper-class patient. During the trial, Therne is helped by Mr Stephen Strong, a rich tradesman who bails him out of prison; however, his reputation as a medical doctor is now irremediably ruined. Mr Strong thus convinces Therne to begin a political career by participating in the upcoming election as a Radical. In order to gain votes, especially among the working classes, he persuades him to fully embrace and promote the anti-vaccination cause. Despite secretly believing that vaccination is safe and effective, Therne accepts; he starts delivering anti-vaccination speeches and producing anti-vaccination pamphlets, thus winning the election. He continues to act as a fierce anti-vaccinationist throughout his political career, which ensures him unwavering support from his voters; he even decides not to vaccinate his only daughter against smallpox, in order not to leave on her body a visible mark that would betray him, since the vaccine against smallpox leaves a permanent scar on the patient's arm. When a smallpox epidemic strikes Dunchester, however, he decides to secretly vaccinate himself. He is discovered by his daughter, who later dies of smallpox, and by her fiancé, who exposes him in front of the whole town. Thus he loses his family, his reputation and his seat, and is forced to spend his remaining days in exile.

The elements of myth and misinformation represented in the novel, and on which Haggard so effectively focuses, may be examined at various levels, especially for their interaction with historically as well as scientifically accurate details. The present analysis begins with an exploration of the novel's main characters, then proceeds to analyse Haggard's masterful representation of the anti-vaccination rhetoric and its appeal to the public, concluding by discussing the writer's successful representation of precise medical details about the process of vaccination. I deal with each of these topics in turn in the following subsections.

Stephen Strong, Dr Therne, the Government, and the clamour of anti-vaccinationists

'"Look here, doctor," [Stephen Strong] said, "I am honest, I am; right or wrong I believe in this anti-vaccination business, and we are going to run the election on it. If you don't believe in it – and you have no particular call to, since every man can claim his own opinion – you'd better let it alone"' (138). Stephen Strong is a tenacious and sincere character, a 'good-hearted, though misguided, man' (128) – he is probably the fictional counterpart of those 'honest' leaders of the anti-vaccination party that Haggard mentions in his diary. Moreover, Strong's anti-vaccination opinions are deeply rooted in his religious faith, as he himself explains to Therne after bailing him out of prison: 'I do it because I will not see folk locked up for this sort of nonsense about diseases and the like, as though the Almighty who made us don't know when to send sickness and when to keep it away, when to make us live and when to make us die' (83–84). Indeed, this was a common belief among Victorian anti-vaccinationists, who saw vaccination as contrary to the will of God. One of the most famous and influential anti-vaccinationists of the time, John Gibbs, published a pamphlet in 1856 entitled *Compulsory*

Vaccination Briefly Considered in its Scientific, Religious, and Political Aspects, where he expounded his views that the practice of vaccination served to spread, rather than prevent, disease, consequently claiming that vaccination was an attack on the religious beliefs of British citizens who 'have a conscientious conviction that voluntarily to propagate disease is to fly in the face of God, and to violate that precept which says, "Do thyself no harm"'.[12] Gibbs further defines vaccination as 'a *deceitful, disgusting, and unnatural practice* – a practice alike debasing to man and dishonouring to God';[13] he also explicitly criticises the introduction of compulsory vaccination – in his words, an 'unchristian legislation' – by stating that '[t]housands object to vaccination on religious grounds. Are they to be dragooned out of their objections?' (Gibbs was here pleading for a Conscientious Objection clause exempting objectors from vaccination, which was finally introduced in 1898).[14]

Haggard insists on the fact that Stephen Strong's beliefs are genuine, if unfounded, and that he is sincerely expecting authenticity from Therne, who, however, knowingly misinforms him about his true beliefs. In the writer's view, these anti-vaccinators are misguided but also honest in their beliefs, and therefore they may be justified in their battle against compulsory vaccination; much worthier of contempt are those who deliberately deceive them by spreading lies and misinformation, often for personal gain, like Doctor Therne. There appears to be little doubt that, in Haggard's intentions, Therne, with his wilful opportunism, is the real villain of the novel; consequently, lies – and not mistaken beliefs – are the true root causes of the anti-vaccination problem. Indeed, in the novel, the doctor willingly exploits Stephen Strong's good faith and principles by accepting his request to become a Radical and to embrace the anti-vaccination cause in exchange for money and career prospects; but to himself, and to the reader, he reveals:

> Had I spoken the truth, indeed, I should have confessed my inability to support the anti-vaccinationist case, since in my opinion few people who have studied this question with an open and impartial mind can deny that Jenner's discovery is one of the greatest boons – perhaps, after the introduction of antiseptics and anaesthetics, the very greatest – that has ever been bestowed upon suffering humanity. If the reader has any doubts upon the point, let him imagine a time when, as used to happen in the days of our forefathers, almost everybody suffered from smallpox at some period of their lives … . Let him imagine a state of affairs – and there are still people living whose parents could remember it – when for a woman not to be pitted with smallpox was to give her some claim to beauty, however homely might be her features. Lastly, let him imagine what all this means: what terror walked abroad when it was common for smallpox to strike a family of children … . (123)

Haggard's own voice resonates in these lines, where the writer, through his character, appeals directly to the readers to impress upon them the horrors of smallpox and the benefits of vaccination. Haggard's previous, non-fiction writings as well as his Author's Note ('in my belief one of the greatest boons that the century has brought to mankind') echo in this passage: vaccination is 'one of the greatest boons – perhaps ... the very greatest', and the reader only has to think of a world where smallpox is left free to roam in order to understand its benefits. This world can be evoked both through imagination ('let him imagine a time when') and through remembrance, as a world struck by smallpox is not purely fictional, but also a historical truth ('as used to happen in the days of our forefathers'; 'there are still people living whose parents could remember it'). According to Therne (in the novel) and to Haggard (in his autobiographical works), when the memory of the past fades, imagination succeeds in describing the horrors that should not be forgotten nor repeated.

Elsewhere in the novel Therne weighs the consequences of his acts and shows some remorse: 'I have sinned against the code of my profession, and have preached a doctrine I knew to be false, using all my skill and knowledge to confuse and pervert the minds of the ignorant' (43). However, the outcomes of the lies and the misinformation he has willingly spread among his fellow citizens are too dire to be forgotten or forgiven:

> I suppose that in this one city there were very many of these – young people mostly – who owed their deaths to me, since it was my persuasion, my eloquent arguments, working upon the minds of their prejudiced and credulous elders, that surely, if indirectly, brought their doom upon them. 'A doctor is not infallible, he may make mistakes.' ... But if it does not happen to have been a mistake, if, for instance, all those dead, should they still live in any place or shape, could say to me, 'James Therne, you are the murderer of our bodies, since, for your own ends, you taught us that which you knew *not* to be the truth.' How then? I ask. (3)

Indeed, Therne claims to be writing an autobiography where he wishes 'to gloze [sic] over nothing' (22): by uncovering the lies propagated to his electorate he is finally being honest with his readers, and is also actively reflecting on the consequences of misinformation and the responsibilities of the doctor who willingly spreads it (as opposed to the honest practitioner who may yet be fallible). Nonetheless, the character shows both a self-deprecating and at the same time a self-exculpatory attitude.[15] He regrets his anti-vaccination crusades (which eventually led to the death of his unvaccinated daughter during a smallpox epidemic), but also justifies them by depicting himself as a victim, whose medical career had been ruined by the unfounded accusations of his rival Doctor James Bell. According to Therne, Bell was first in lying about him to the people of Dunchester, falsely depicting him as a negligent doctor.

Thus, Therne is one of many characters in the novel who shed their personal beliefs in favour of convenient lies. In his work, Haggard recounts the historical events leading to the addition of the Conscientious Objection clause to the Vaccination Act, ascribing this to the ideological power of anti-vaccinationists (which he fictionally represents through Therne's speeches) and also explicitly blaming the members of parliament who surrendered to their pressure for fear of losing their seats, echoing the judgement he had expressed in his Author's Note. He describes the events that led to the approval of the Conscientious Objection clause, trying to explain them using Therne's voice:

> [A]n eminent leader ... pressing upon an astonished House of Commons the need of yielding to the clamour of the anti-vaccinationists, and of inserting into the Bill, framed upon the report of a Royal Commission, a clause forbidding the prosecution of parents or guardians willing to assert before a bench of magistrates that they objected to vaccination on conscientious grounds. (154)

> [A]lthough about ninety out of every hundred of the individuals who then constituted the House of Commons were strong believers in the merits of vaccination, hardly one of them rose in his place to support the Bill. ... [W]hatever their private faith might be, they were convinced that if they did so it would lose them votes at the next election. ... [T]he First Lord of the Treasury rose and offered to insert a clause by virtue of which any parent or other person who under the Bill would be liable to penalties for the non-vaccination of a child, should be entirely freed from such penalties if within four months of its birth he satisfied two justices of the peace that he conscientiously believed that the operation would be prejudicial to that child's health. The Bill passed with the clause. ... Thus the whole policy of compulsory vaccination, which for many years had been in force in England, was destroyed at a single blow by a Government with a great majority, and a House of Commons composed of members who, for the most part, were absolute believers in its virtues. ... It was a very triumph of opportunism, for the Government, aided and abetted by their supporters, threw over their beliefs to appease a small but persistent section of the electors. (168–169)

Thus, the novel denounces not only the responsibility of the single citizen or single politician, but also – and perhaps most importantly – the political responsibility of a government that disregards the scientists' opinions to appease a vocal, but misguided, part of its electorate.

Doctor Therne, the anti-vaccinators' inflammatory rhetoric, and its antidote

In asking Therne to join the Radicals, Strong already sets their agenda: the aim is to foment the masses' dissatisfaction with the Government and with the medical profession, and to exhort them to demonstrate against compulsory vaccination. This will be achieved by appealing to their anger and their fear (through Therne's 'appeals to the people to rise up in their thousands and save their innocent children' [134]) and by using shocking visuals ('enlarged photographs of nasty-looking cases, and the rest of it' [134]) instead of rational facts and figures (which Strong tellingly calls 'scientific finicking' [134]). Therne follows these instructions obediently, expertly and shrewdly:

> We flooded the constituency with tracts headed "What Vaccination Does," "The Law of Useless Infanticide," "The Vaccine Tyranny," "Is Vaccination a Fraud?" and so forth, and with horrible pictures of calves stretched out by pulleys, gagged and blindfolded, with their under parts covered by vaccine vesicles. Also we had photographs of children suffering from the effects of improper or unclean vaccination ... one or two such children themselves were taken round to meetings and their sores exhibited. (151)

Haggard here reiterates genuine anti-vaccination slogans of the time; it is possible to find evidence that the phrase 'the law of useless infanticide' was used by George S. Gibbs (brother of the above-mentioned John) in six letters he addressed to members of parliament in 1898.[16] Anti-vaccination activists in Victorian England also made wide use of posters and prints, which they sold, hanging them in the streets or in shop windows; they also habitually showed photographs of cases of injury and death – allegedly caused by vaccination – during their lectures,[17] as Therne does in the novel. One famous collection of these photographs was later published by W. J. Furnival, another prominent anti-vaccinationist, in 1906.

Haggard is also very sensitive to the language used by activists and their leaders, an ability he instils into his character James Therne:

> I knew my subject thoroughly, and understood what points to dwell upon and what to gloze [sic] over, how to twist and turn the statistics, and how to marshal my facts in such fashion as would make it very difficult to expose their fallacy. Then, when I had done with general arguments, I went on to particular cases, describing as a doctor can do the most dreadful which had ever come under my notice, with such power and pathos that women in the audience burst into tears. Finally, I ended by an impassioned appeal to all present to follow my example and refuse to allow their children to be poisoned. I called on them as free men to rise against this monstrous Tyranny, to put a stop to

this system of organised and judicial Infanticide, and to send me to Parliament to raise my voice on their behalf. (149–150)

The structure of Therne's speech closely resembles the way John Gibbs typically arranges his tracts, from *Our Medical Liberties* of 1854 to the aforementioned *Compulsory Vaccination Briefly Considered* of 1856: he usually starts with a long list of facts and figures that he uses to demonstrate the ineffectiveness and possible danger of vaccination; then he accumulates examples of children allegedly harmed by vaccination; and finally he concludes with powerful appeals to the people, often inciting them to rebel against the Government's enforcement of compulsory vaccination. As Gibbs's tracts are quite lengthy, it is not possible to reproduce them fully here; however, the following is a typical example of his appeals to the people to rebel against compulsory vaccination: 'Our streets are daringly placarded, and our churches desecrated, with insulting, revolutionary notices, headed "COMPULSORY VACCINATION!" Will Englishmen tamely allow themselves to be thus *bullied* by the tools of a medical faction?'[18]

This kind of anti-vaccination rhetoric was so effective that the then editor of the *British Medical Journal*, Ernest Hart, lamented the 'extremely energetic system of distributing tracts, inflammatory postcards, grotesquely drawn envelopes, and other means of disseminating their views'.[19] Conversely, he continued, '[t]here is nothing on the other side ... as an accessible antidote to these productions'.[20] We could say that *Doctor Therne* was indeed trying to be an effective and accessible antidote, remarkable, once again, precisely because it is expressed in the form of a novel, in the form of fiction.

Fictional, accurate medical details: *Doctor Therne*'s investigation of the question of vaccination

The medical doctor William Thomson, writing for the *Journal of the Royal Society of Medicine* in 1984, praised *Doctor Therne* for the accuracy of its medical details.[21] Indeed, one key scene of the novel, in which Therne decides to vaccinate in order to escape smallpox, is dense with meticulous medical descriptions:

> I took off my coat and rolled up my shirt sleeve, fastening it with a safety-pin to the linen upon my shoulder. After this I lit a spirit-lamp and sterilised my lancet by heating it in the flame. Now, having provided myself with an ivory point and unsealed the tiny tube of lymph, I sat down in a chair so that the light from the electric lamp fell full upon my arm, and proceeded to scrape the skin with the lancet until blood appeared in four or five separate places.

> Next I took the ivory point, and, after cleansing it, I charged it with the lymph and applied it to the abrasions, being careful to give each of them a liberal dose. The operation finished, I sat still awhile letting my arm hang over the back of the chair, in order that the blood might dry thoroughly before I drew down my shirt sleeve. (240)

The process of vaccination at the time was not closely regulated, however, as the exact biological process that made it successful was still unclear (Louis Pasteur was only then starting to elaborate his germ theory, allowing doctors and scientists to thoroughly understand the principles of vaccination); most importantly, rules of hygiene and sanitation were only beginning to be codified scientifically and to be applied consistently. What is more, not everyone could afford to be vaccinated at home. On the contrary, vaccination was often performed arm-to-arm in public vaccination stations, a practice that exposed people to the risk of blood infections, as the lymph used was sometimes impure and the stations themselves were often unsanitary.[22] These incidents were widely reported in the anti-vaccination press; in his 1856 pamphlet, Gibbs lists four cases where children contracted erysipelas (a bacterial infection of the skin) following vaccination, and also mentions cases of scrofula (a lymphadenopathy of the neck) together with a variety of other infectious diseases that could have been caused by contaminated vaccine matter.[23]

Haggard does not wish to gloss over these episodes. In the novel, before standing for Parliament, Doctor Therne visits the child of a bootmaker who suffers precisely from erysipelas. Therne himself suspects that the infection may have been caused by vaccination, forces the authorities to examine the tube of lymph with which he had been vaccinated, and discovers that it was indeed contaminated with streptococcus; the child later dies (1898: 118–121). Following this tragic case, he decides – once again spurred on by Stephen Strong – to investigate episodes in which vaccination was alleged to have caused harm. His analyses prove that in some cases vaccination using impure lymph or performed in inadequate sanitary conditions has been the cause of infection; nevertheless, he remains convinced of the safety and effectiveness of the practice when performed using pure lymph and following the necessary precautions. Therne's studies may thus be considered the – fictional, but arguably very convincing – response to Gibbs's plea: '"Demand investigation!" Does not the whole question of vaccination "demand investigation"?'[24]

Unsurprisingly, though, the doctor in the novel is not vocal in his defence of vaccination, as he refuses to divulge his real views for fear of alienating the anti-vaccinationists who have funded his analyses. Consequently, the conclusions the character delivers in front of the Royal Commission on Vaccination remain deliberately vague and non-committal:

> During a search of two years I established to my satisfaction that vaccination, as for the most part it was then performed, that is from arm to arm, is occasionally the cause of blood poisoning, erysipelas, abscesses, tuberculosis, and other dreadful ailments. These cases I published without drawing from them any deductions whatever, with the result that I found myself summoned to give evidence before the Royal Commission on Vaccination which was then sitting at Westminster. ... [S]ome members of the Commission attempted to draw me into general statements as to the advantage or otherwise of the practice of vaccination to the community. To these gentlemen I replied that as my studies had been directed towards the effects of vaccination in individual instances only, the argument was one upon which I preferred not to enter. (122–123)

But to the reader of his autobiography, Therne explains:

> Indeed, in those days I told neither more nor less than the truth. Evil results occasionally followed the use of bad lymph or unclean treatment after the subject had been inoculated. ... The danger is perfectly preventable, and ought long ago to have been prevented, by making it illegal, under heavy penalties, to use any substance except that which has been developed in calves and scientifically treated with glycerine, when, as I believe, no hurt can possibly follow. This is the verdict of science. (125–126)

Despite his assertion that he has spoken 'neither more nor less than the truth', his purposeful concealment of parts of the truth enables anti-vaccinationists to appropriate his results for their propagandist ends and lays the ground for his own subsequent deceitful speeches and deliberate misinformation. It seems ironic that the character's only authentic work relating to vaccination was ethically unsound in its application. It may be possible that Haggard is here reflecting on the nature of misinformation, suggesting that it can be nuanced, overcoming the dichotomic difference between truth and lies to include the deliberate manipulation of portions of the truth. If Therne's studies had been used properly, they could have contributed to the improvement of the practice of vaccination. Moreover, they might even have contributed to the building of a relationship of trust between the medical profession and the public, who at the time resented the claims of infallibility that doctors sometimes made, which were at odds with the citizens' often negative experience with their methods.[25] Still, the novel itself can be said to provide reassurances to the anxious reader who fears possible negative side-effects of vaccination, accurately listing its risks and balancing them with its benefits. Therefore, *Doctor Therne* can be said to transmit accurate medico-scientific knowledge through the form of fiction, and at the same time to warn its readers against misinformation and dishonesty which could proliferate among the medical, but above all political, class.

What's past is prologue: *Doctor Therne* between the nineteenth and the twenty-first centuries

Many authors have pointed out that there are various similarities between anti-vaccination discourses in Victorian England and anti-vaccination claims today. In her 2005 account of the Victorian anti-vaccination movement, historian Nadja Durbach mentions the controversy surrounding the measles, mumps and rubella vaccine (MMR) that arose in Britain in 1998, causing a sharp decrease in the uptake of the vaccine in various areas of Britain. This drew attention to three major themes that echo Victorian protests: namely the claim that vaccines are unsafe, ineffective and experimental, that the Government abuses its power in forcing vaccination upon its citizens, and that alternative health practices are possible and preferable.[26] Similarly, the American medical doctor Paul Offit, in his influential 2011 book *Deadly Choices*, argues that past and present anti-vaccination movements share remarkably similar beliefs and practices: the claim that doctors are evil; the organisation of public rallies; a diffuse feeling of paranoia; the spreading of false claims of harm caused by vaccines; the belief that vaccines are unnatural; the rejection of germ theory; the lure of alternative medicine; the fear of medical advances; the belief that vaccines are an act against God; and finally, what he calls a 'mass-marketing' of anti-vaccination ideas through the publication and distribution of vast quantities of propagandist materials.[27] Likewise, writing at the height of the Covid-19 pandemic, Erica Eisen states:

> Two hundred years [after Jenner], attempts to discredit the safety and reliability of vaccination – whether against measles or against COVID – persist. The arguments made by today's anti-vaxxers often echo those put forth by their nineteenth-century antecedents: claims of inefficacy, allegations of ghastly side effects, appeals to religion. Jenner seems likely to have assumed that the benefits of vaccination would be so self-evident that they would shut down all debate. That many continue to assail the safety and reliability of the method he pioneered, not only decades but centuries later, is something that, in all likelihood, the doctor never could have imagined.[28]

It could be argued that many, if not all, of these points are accurately represented in Henry Rider Haggard's *Doctor Therne* (although only a few of them could be explored in this chapter, for reasons of space), and that herein lies the real value of the novel, which manages to resonate strongly with contemporary readers who are familiar with (anti-)vaccination discourses as they currently unfold in the press as well as on social media.

Even more remarkable are some of the writer's linguistic choices, which find almost direct correspondence in contemporary vaccination discourses: as an example, let us analyse the noun phrase 'false prophet'. Mrs Strong (Stephen Strong's wife), when talking to Doctor Therne, asserts that their money is well spent if it is going to 'help a clever man to break down the tyranny of wicked governments and false prophets' (173), meaning pro-vaccinators. However, Therne himself uses this same expression to denigrate himself and his choice to become an anti-vaccinator when thinking about his daughter, who died of smallpox because she was not vaccinated: 'the virgin martyr sacrificed on the altar of a false prophet and a coward' (5). In more recent times, Paul Offit published a book with the title *Autism's False Prophets* (2008), criticising scientists who claim to have discovered a link between vaccines and autism, and who go so far as to suggest they have found an alternative cure for autism. Additionally, it is striking that Haggard was able to foresee one peculiar characteristic of twenty-first-century anti-scientific thinking and anti-intellectualism, that is to say, the belief in conspiracy theories. In the novel, Therne wonders: '[L]et [the reader] consider how it comes about, if vaccination is a fraud, that some nine hundred and ninety-nine medical men out of every thousand, not in England only, but in all civilised countries, place so firm a belief in its virtue. Are the doctors of the world all mad, or all engaged in a great conspiracy to suppress the truth?' (125). Curiously, this is exactly what Victorian anti-vaccinators merely ventured to suggest, while their twenty-first-century descendants firmly and vocally proclaim it.[29]

These lexical correspondences prove once again the modernity and relevance of *Doctor Therne* – a book that deserves to be studied, if not for its literary artistry, then surely for its accuracy and insight in depicting anti-vaccination movements, their discourses and their motives. Using Thomson's words again, the novel 'still has a lesson for us today, when medical matters – especially if mishandled by the media and politicians, as they so often are – can assume such strong antisocial feelings'.[30] Moreover, the novel shows how literature may be used effectively to convey scientific facts, by avoiding obscure 'scientific finicking' and appealing directly to the readers' feelings. Indeed, Haggard's insights on the power of imagination to impress upon anti-vaccinationists the dangers of preventable infectious diseases can possibly be considered a precursor of some branches of the medical humanities that see illness narratives as a powerful way to create empathy.[31] Therefore, it can be said that scientists who lament the impossibility of conveying accurate medical facts and at the same time counteracting emotionally loaded, anti-scientific rhetoric may find in *Doctor Therne* a powerful ally in their quest for effective scientific popularisation.

Acknowledgements

I would like to thank Professor Paolo Caponi, from the University of Milan, for his valuable comments on a preliminary version of this essay.

Notes

1. Morton Norton Cohen, *Rider Haggard: His Life and Works* (New York: Walker and Company, 1968), p. 219.
2. Ibid., p. 219.
3. Ibid., p. 301.
4. Henry Rider Haggard, *The Days of My Life* (London: Longman, 1911), pp. 346–347.
5. Henry Rider Haggard, *A Farmer's Year: Being His Commonplace Book for 1898* (New York: Cambridge University Press, 1899), p. 280.
6. Compulsory vaccination was first introduced in England and Wales in 1853. In 1867, a new vaccination act further enforced compulsory vaccination for all children under 14. The 1871 Vaccination Act mandated the employment of vaccination officers. Finally, the 1898 Vaccination Bill introduced exemptions for conscientious objectors.
7. In an endnote to the novel, Haggard writes: '[T]he author has read in the press that in Yorkshire a single bench of magistrates out of the hundreds in England has already granted orders on the ground of "conscientious objection," under which some 2000 children are exempted from the scope of the Vaccination Acts ... At Iperwich also about 700 applications, affecting many children, have been filed'; Henry Rider Haggard, *Doctor Therne* (London: Longman, 1898), p. 110. (From this point onwards all citations to *Doctor Therne* will appear within the text in parentheses.) Historical records seem to confirm that a very high number of exemption certificates was being issued at the time in various cities: for example, magistrates in Oldham were said to have issued 40,000 certificates by December 1898, and in some districts like Southwark and Heywood coverage was said to have decreased from 95 per cent to 2 per cent following the introduction of the clause (see Nadja Durbach, *Bodily Matters: The Anti-Vaccination Movement in England, 1853–1907* (Durham, NC and London: Duke University Press, 2005), pp. 186–187.
8. Haggard, *A Farmer's Year*, pp. 280–281.
9. Ibid., p. 280. Haggard discusses this point again years later in his autobiography: while admitting that no smallpox epidemic has yet occurred in England, he is still worried that this could happen in the future; and once again he blames the falling rates of smallpox vaccination on 'our national lack of imagination: we cannot embody in our minds or provide against that of which we have had no recent experience'. Haggard, *My Life*, p. 318.
10. In 1895, Haggard stood for Parliament as a Conservative candidate for the Eastern division of Norfolk, although he lost by 197 votes (this experience is

recounted in detail by Cohen, *Rider Haggard*, pp. 156–178). Throughout his life he was also deeply involved in reforming agriculture in Britain and was a member of many commissions on land use (a role that led to the publication of his *Farmer's Year* in 1899, *Rural England* in 1906, and *Rural Denmark and its Lessons* in 1913).
11 Quoted in Haggard, *My Life*, p. 347.
12 John Gibbs, *Compulsory Vaccination Briefly Considered in its Scientific, Religious, and Political Aspects* (London: Sotheran and Willis, 1856), p. 5.
13 Ibid., p. 22; italics in the original.
14 Ibid., pp. 59, 46; italics in the original.
15 Richard Reeve, 'Henry Rider Haggard's Debt to Anthony Trollope: *Doctor Therne* and *Doctor Thorne*', *Notes & Queries* 63:2 (2016): 274–278, doi:10.1093/notesj/gjw024.
16 George S. Gibbs, *The Law of Useless Infanticide Miscalled Vaccination; Being the Substance of Six Letters Addressed to Members of Parliament, etc.* (London: Allen, 1989).
17 Durbach, *Bodily Matters*, p. 48.
18 Gibbs, *Compulsory Vaccination*, p. 52; small capitals and italics in the original.
19 Quoted in Durbach, *Bodily Matters*, p. 50.
20 Ibid.
21 William A. R. Thomson, 'Rider Haggard and Smallpox', *Journal of the Royal Society of Medicine* 77:6 (1984): 445–536, at 510.
22 Durbach, *Bodily Matters*, pp. 113–149.
23 Gibbs, *Compulsory Vaccination*, pp. 12–13.
24 Ibid., p. 12.
25 As stated by Gibbs, 'Deficient in modesty, logic, and common sense, is it strange that compulsory vaccinators should find their arrogance repulsed, their claims to infallibility derided?' Gibbs, *Compulsory Vaccination*, p. 58.
26 Durbach, *Bodily Matters*, pp. 204–205.
27 Paul Offit, *Deadly Choices: How the Anti-Vaccine Movement Threatens Us All* (New York: Basic Books, 2011), pp. 107–119.
28 Erica X. Eisen, '"The Mark of the Beast": Georgian Britain's Anti-Vaxxer Movement', *Public Domain Review* (2021), available at https://publicdomainreview.org/essay/the-mark-of-the-beast-georgian-britains-anti-vaxxer-movement, last accessed 27 January 2023.
29 See, for example, Richard A. Stein, 'The Golden Age of Anti-Vaccine Conspiracies', *GERMS* 7:4 (2017): 168–170.
30 Thomson, 'Rider Haggard and Smallpox', 510.
31 See, for example, Rita Charon, 'The Narrative Road to Empathy', in Howard M. Spiro, Mary G. McCrea Curnen and Enid Peschel (eds), *Empathy and the Practice of Medicine: Beyond Pills and the Scalpel* (New Haven, CT: Yale University Press, 1993), pp. 147–159.

Afterword

Allan Ingram

Misinformation and ignorance are clearly not the same thing, though equally clearly – and many of the chapters in this volume have demonstrated this – there is considerable overlap. This is particularly true in the field of medical information, where current medical knowledge, and especially advances in medical knowledge, may find itself in friction with established religious or political positions, or even with prevailing superstitions and long-held, but not necessarily justified, folk wisdom. While this is by no means confined to the period covered by this book – we only have to recall the heatedness of positions taken on Covid-19 vaccination, and the strength, not least in the United States, of the anti-vax movement, to appreciate this – it was particularly so in the eighteenth century, an era of remarkable medical advances and of equally remarkable medical ignorance and disbelief. These were therefore the perfect conditions for the breeding of misinformation and new myths, many of which lingered into the following century, or gave birth to fresh successors. Entrenched positions, not all of them medical in origin, had a serious knock-on effect on the acceptability or otherwise of advances in medicine, and in consequence medical facts, or 'facts', were subject to fresh interpretations, many of them impossibly far from the original medical evidence. These then became part of the entrenchment that justified the belief or principle being defended. It is hard, especially from the distance of two centuries, to condemn such reinterpretation as ignorance: for many sincere Christians, the word of God naturally overruled so-called evidence brought forward by a mere human scientist, just as Isaac Newton's advances in the understanding of the nature of the universe were slanted in different ways to prevent them from undermining the myth of the Creation, among other things. Misinformation is not necessarily ignorance.

Equally, misinformation can effectively play upon ignorance, ignorance that is sometimes wilful. For a writer or orator, or public figure of any kind, one of the easiest routes to garnering public endorsement is to feed the prejudices of readers and listeners, even though the feeder may well be aware that those prejudices are based on ignorance or misunderstanding, or indeed on misinformation originally provided by interested parties such as the feeder him or herself. An obvious instance from the contemporary scene would be the QAnon conspiracy theory, which has been a growing movement in US politics since 2017 – a theory that brings together the attractive idea of heroic resistance against sexual exploitation of the most vulnerable by the most privileged and the implausible figure of one saviour as the ideal leader. And QAnon was only fortified when vaccination against Covid-19 came along and was regarded as equally conspiratorial. As the magazine *Rolling Stone* put it, QAnon members 'increasingly see vaccination as part of a diabolical plot by the "deep state" to enslave humanity'.[1] Such a position might be too extreme even for the eighteenth century, but equally vehement views were widely held and exploited, not the least of the issues drawn upon being, once more, vaccination – or inoculation, as it was in its first phase. As Kelly McGuire puts it, regarding what was seen as the potential of inoculation to place a greater degree of control in the hands of humans themselves, rather than of the Almighty: 'Of course, this power of self-determination proved problematic from a religious standpoint because clerics and many physicians objected that the practice usurped the divine prerogative to inflict disease as a punishment for sin and excess'. And she cites 'One of the first clergymen to express his vehement opposition to the practice of inoculation, Edmund Massey'. Here is Massey preaching in 1722:

> No doubt but Providence has a good and beneficial Design in all those Deaths, which we improperly call untimely; either the Good is taken to his Reward, or the Wicked hindred from increasing his Punishment. What Reason then for this saving, this anti-providential Project, this pretended art of Preserving, which thus tends in a great Measure to prevent that religious Watchfulness, which Christianity, as a Warfare, requires?[2]

One physician on the opposing side, she notes, John Arbuthnot, who is discussed in this volume by John Baker, 'sarcastically invokes Edmund Massey's equation of inoculation with atheism'.[3] It is, of course, impossible to determine the sincerity of such proponents as Massey, or how far the 'Misrepresentation' by a physician like William Wagstaffe, attacked by Arbuthnot along with Massey, was genuinely based on some kind of understanding of medical evidence, or merely on a mix of playing to popular prejudice and the desire to cash in and to protect the status quo where their own standing and incomes were concerned. The same is true of those pressing against Covid-19 vaccinations or on behalf of the QAnon conspiracy. One's instinct, both regarding the early eighteenth century – and indeed later in the period when Edward Jenner's development of vaccination from the example of inoculation also led to antagonism and mockery – and the twenty-first, is to judge that not all adherents were 100 per cent sincere, or 100 per cent ignorant.

Perhaps the clearest case of insincerity is found in the closing chapter in this volume, Carlotta Fiammenghi's '"You taught us that which you knew *not* to be the truth": the anti-vaccination medical doctor in Henry Rider Haggard's *Doctor Therne* (1898)', a piece that points the way strikingly clearly to our own recent experiences, as well as picking up on so much in the history and cultural context of medicine in the Western world. As she puts it at the outset, the novel is 'a fictional autobiography of a medical doctor who decides to embrace the anti-vaccination cause in order to win an election as a Radical, despite being a firm believer in the safety and effectiveness of vaccines'. In other words, Therne is shamelessly ignoring all his own medical and personal ethics for the sole cause of self-advancement. Misinformation, it would seem, is a small price to pay for personal gain. As well as reviving interest in a little-known novel by a writer mostly familiar for adventure stories, her chapter makes a fitting point of closure, gathering as it does the momentum of past centuries of myth and misinformation and propelling it towards our own time with markedly uncomfortable relevance.

Not all misinformers and myth-spreaders in the volume have been so starkly unprincipled, and some have even been guided by the highest motives, or unsuspectingly fallen victim to modes of presentation. Others have made genuine advances to medical understanding through a shift in perspective beyond the standard for their time. The flap anatomies presented by Jessica Dandona are a case in point here, in terms of medical education through a new and particularly instructive medium. Some who were not misinformers at all, or not by choice, like satirist and polymath John Arbuthnot, or the highly personal, and highly fashionable, physician George Cheyne, as written about by Clark Lawlor, found their distinctive modes of presentation cast a strong slant over their views of medicine, which might well have been considered misinforming by their many detractors. Other presentations, not least fictional ones, have shown the power and effectiveness of lay practitioners, as well as the public perception of them, such as those discussed by Laurence Sullivan and Declan Kavanagh – particularly relevant because of the medical qualification and background of their author, Tobias Smollett. The same can be said of Elizabeth Gaskell's presentation of unqualified but effective lay practice in *Mary Barton*, brought out by Barbara Witucki. Modes of labelling and modes of marking for ownership, analysed by Helen Williams and Laura Robson-Mainwaring respectively, expanded on routes for misinformation and its correction, while such specialist branches as skincare (Katherine Aske) and even dog care and its reputation for exploitation (Stephanie Howard-Smith) were potential victims for accusations of misinformation, some of them justifiable and some quite clearly not. Above all, though, there remains the question of ignorance, less now the ignorance of the presenters, writers and commercial interests as of the consuming public. Hence the importance of such educational undertakings as Sir Anthony Carlisle's *The Horrors of Oakendale Abbey*, as discussed by Bethany Brigham. Misinformation and ignorance are not the same thing, but the latter massively facilitates the spread and credibility of the former – frighteningly so. Even if one removes the potentially toxic potency of the strongest religious or political views – which of course frequently overlap and reinforce each other – and their capacity to slant and to infect the ways in which medical issues are interpreted and either adopted or deplored, there still remains consumer ignorance.

One of the most enduringly popular works from the whole span of the eighteenth century, one discussed by Declan Kavanagh and also cited by Barbara Witucki, in connection, significantly, with Elizabeth Gaskell almost one hundred years later, was William Buchan's *Domestic Medicine: or, a Treatise on the Prevention and Cure of Diseases by Regimen and Simple Medicines*. This was first published in 1769 and continuously republished over half of the nineteenth century, and even, in the United States, into the twentieth. One attraction of Buchan's work was that it was written in plain English, but also that it was addressed to plain people, consumers who lived ordinary down-to-earth lives and welcomed straightforward ways of retaining, or regaining, the kind of health that their lifestyles demanded and without the necessity for exotic and expensive medical purchases. That is what Buchan's work gave them, that and the confidence that here was a writer, a real doctor with real patients, whose practice was based in lived experience. Almost as a side issue, but supremely relevant as far as the present volume is concerned, *Domestic Medicine*, within its own parameters and the parameters of its time, also educated. As such, it, and the similar works that followed it and were inspired by it, were the perfect antidote to medical myth and misinformation and to those people who made it their business to exploit such qualities for their own non-medical purposes.

Notes

1 Tim Dickinson, 'How the Anti-Vaxxers Got Red-Pilled', *Rolling Stone* (10 February 2021).
2 Kelly McGuire, 'Death by Inoculation: The Fashioning of Mortality in Eighteenth-Century Smallpox Pamphlets', in Allan Ingram and Leigh Wetherall Dickson (eds), *Disease and Death in Eighteenth-Century Literature and Culture: Fashioning the Unfashionable* (London, Palgrave Macmillan, 2016), pp. 189–206 (at p. 192), citing Edmund Massey, *A Sermon Against the Dangerous and Sinful Practice*

of Inoculation. Preach'd at St. Andrew's Holborn, on Sunday, July 8th, 1722 (London: Meadows, 1722), p. 27.
3 McGuire, 'Death by Inoculation', p. 191, citing John Arbuthnot, *Mr. Maitland's Account of Inoculating the Small Pox Vindicated, from Dr. Wagstaffe's Misrepresentation of that Practice, with Some Remarks on Mr. Massey's Sermon* (London: Peele, 1722), p. 49.

Bibliography

Archival material in manuscript

Bodleian Library, The, Oxford, Robert Hale, Letter to Dr. Charlett, Ballard MSS 24, f. 149.
British Library, The, London, John Arbuthnot, 'An *English* poem by Dr. Arbuthnott. *Autograph*.' Department of Manuscripts, Add.MS.22625, f.31.
London Metropolitan Archives, Insured: John Cox 11 Berners Street Oxford Street bookseller, Records of the Sun Fire Office, 4 April 1822, Policy Register, MS 11936/493/989752.
National Archives, The, Kew (TNA):
    Census for England and Wales, RG10/1659/69/21; RG 10/3180/11/16/88; RG11/582/11/20; RG12/1646/48/45; RG13/1993/69/3; RG14/269/18.
    Letter from William Gilbert, Assistant Poor Law Commissioner to the Poor Law Commission, regarding the Death of a Child [Henry Love] in the Workhouse in consequence of an improper medicine having been administered by mistake. Plymouth, 7 March 1839 (Devon Poor Law Unions: Axminster 76), [MS] MH12-1-2096.
    Mitchinson, The National Archives, ADM 196/9/532.
    Officer's Service Records, Browning, The National Archives, ADM 196/9/258.
    'Preparations for publication of the Trade-Marks Journal', *STAT 12/1/19*, 25 February 1876.
    Will of Benjamin Rane Cox, 11 October 1828, Medical Bookseller and Publisher of Saint Thomas Street, The National Archives, PROB 11/1746/276.
    Will of Elizabeth Cox, 6 February 1841, Medical Bookseller of Brewers Court Saint Thomas Street Southwark, The National Archives, PROB-11-1940-300.
    Will of Thomas Cox, Bookseller and Engraver of Southwark, Surrey (1806), The National Archives, PROB-11-1444-260.
National Library of Scotland, George Cheyne, *Essay of Health*, NLS, Acc. 9345.
Wellcome Collection, The, London, Medical Directories 1845–1942 Collection.

Periodicals

American Physical Education Review
American Physician, The

American School Board Journal, The
Atlas, The
Bell's Weekly Messenger
Blackwood's Edinburgh Magazine
Bookseller: The Organ of the Book Trade
British Medical Journal
Caledonian Mercury
Chemist and Druggist
Derby Mercury
Examiner, The
Friend of India and Statesman
Globe
Hereford Journal
Inverness Courier
Journal of the American Medical Association
Journal of the House of Commons
Kentish Gazette
Lancet, The
London and China Express
London Courier and Evening Gazette
London Evening Standard
London Gazette
London Medical Gazette, or Journal of Practical Medicine
London Morning Herald
Medical Annual, The
Medical Directory
Medical Fortnightly, The
Medical Press and Circular
Medical Register
Medical Times and Gazette
Michigan School Moderator
Modern Hospital, The
Morning Advertiser
Morning Chronicle
Morning Herald
Morning Journal (Kingston)
Morning Post
New Times
Northampton Mercury
Nottingham and Newark Mercury
Nuneaton Advertiser
Oxford Journal
Physical Training
Post Boy
Proceedings of the High School Conference
Protestant Episcopal Review, The
Public Advertiser
Publishers Weekly, The
Roscommon & Leitrim Gazette

Saunders's News-Letter
Scotsman, The
Southend Standard and Essex Weekly Advertiser
Southern Medical Journal
Times, The

Printed Primary Material

Anderson, M. F., *Phosphates: Their Chemical Composition and Uses in the Different Tissues of the Body* (Coventry: Robertson and Gray, 1877).
Anon., *An Epistle to G—ge Ch—ne M.D. F.R.S. upon his Essay of Health* (J. Roberts, 1725?).
Anon., *Der menschliche Körper: Darstellung S. Baues u. S. inneren Organe* (Fürth: [G. Löwensöhn?], [1898?]).
Anon., *Dr. Minder's Anatomical Manikin of the Human Body: An Illustrated Representation with Full and Descriptive Text*, rev. Ethel Mayer (New York: American Thermo-Ware, [c.1900]).
Anon., *Hammond's Anatomical Model of the Female Human Body: An Illustrated Representation with Full and Descriptive Letterpress* (New York: Hammond, c.1899).
Anon., *Hammond's Popular Manikin; or, Model of the Human Body* (New York: Hammond, c.1919).
Anon., *How to Capture German Trade* (London: Hodder and Stoughton, 1914).
Anon., 'Imaginary Interview: George Orwell and Jonathan Swift', *BBC African Service*, 6 November 1943.
Anon., *Philips' Anatomical Model: A Pictorial Representation of the Human Frame and its Organs* (London: G. Philip, [c.1893–1900]).
Anon., *Philips' Anatomical Model of the Female Human Body: An Illustrated Representation with Full and Descriptive Letterpress* (London: G. Philip, c.1903).
Anon., *The Catalogue of the Fellows and other members of the Royal College of Physicians* [Broadside] (London: The Statutes of the College of Physicians, 1696).
Anon., *The Parliamentary Register; or, The History of the Proceedings and Debates of the House of Commons*, 44 (London: Printed for J. Debrett, Piccadilly, 1796).
Anon., *Whittaker's Anatomical Model: An Illustrated Representation of the Human Frame and its Organs* (New York: Thomas Whittaker, [c.1893]).
Anon., *Whittaker's Anatomical Model of the Female Human Body* (New York: Thomas Whittaker, [c.1906]).
Arbuthnot, John, *An Essay on the Usefulness of Mathematical Learning: in a Letter from a Gentleman in the City to his Friend in Oxford* (Oxford: Peisley, 1701).
Arbuthnot, John, *Gnothi Seauton. Know Your Self* (London: J. Tonson, 1734).
Arbuthnot, John, *Mr. Maitland's Account of Inoculating the Small Pox Vindicated, from Dr. Wagstaffe's Misrepresentation of that Practice, with Some Remarks on Mr. Massey's Sermon* (London: Peele, 1722).
Arbuthnot, John, *Proposals for Printing A very Curious Discourse, in Two Volumes in Quarto, Intitled, ΨΕΥΔΟΛΟΓΙΑ ΠΟΛΙΤΙΚΗ; or, A Treatise on the Art of Political Lying, with An Abstract of the First Volume of the said Treatise* (London: Morphew, 1712).

Arbuthnot, John, et al., *A Collection of Poems. By Several Hands* (London: Dodsley, 1748).
Armstrong, John, *'The Art of Preserving Health': Eighteenth-Century Sensibility in Practice*, ed. Adam Budd (Farnham: Ashgate, 2011).
Bailey, James Blake, *The Diary of a Resurrectionist, 1811–1812: To which are Added an Account of the Resurrection Men in London and A Short History of the Passing of the Anatomy Act* (London: Swan Sonnenschein & Co., 1896).
Barker, Jane, *A Patch-Work Screen for the Ladies* (London: Curll, 1723).
Bate, George, *Pharmacopoeia Bateana* (London: Sam Smith, 1688).
Bate, George, *Pharmacopoeia Bateana* (London: Sam Smith, 1691).
Bate, George, *Pharmacopoeia Bateana: or, Bate's Dispensatory*, with additions by William Salmon (London: Sam Smith and Benj. Walford, 1694).
Bell, Jacob and Theophilus Redwood, *Historical Sketch of the Progress of Pharmacy in Great Britain* (London: Pharmaceutical Society, 1880).
Biss, Hubert E. J., *Baillière's Popular Atlas of the Anatomy and Physiology of the Female Human Body*, 3rd edn (London: Baillière, Tindall, & Cox, 1921).
Blackmore, Richard, 'Essay upon Writing', in *Essays upon Several Subjects. By Sir Richard Blackmore, Kt. M.D. and Fellow of the College of Physicians in London*, Vol. II (London: Wilkins, 1717), pp. 241–287.
Blaine, Delabere Pritchett, *A Domestic Treatise on the Diseases of Horses and Dogs* (London: Boosey, 1803).
Bloom, Edward A. and Lillian Bloom (eds), *The Piozzi Letters: The Correspondence of Hester Lynch Piozzi 1784–1821*, 6 vols (Newark, DE: University of Delaware Press, 1989).
Boswell, James, *Boswell's London Journal, 1762–1763*, ed. Frederick A. Pottle (Melbourne: Heinemann, 1950).
Boswell, James, *The Life of Samuel Johnson, LL.D*, 4 vols, 3rd edn (London: Dilly, 1799).
Bretherton, James, after Henry William Bunbury, *The Dog Barber. La Francia* (1772), coloured etching, 24 × 15.8 cm. Wellcome Collection.
Brockbank, Edward Mansfield, *Sketches of the Lives and Works of the Honorary Medical Staff of the Manchester Infirmary from its Foundation in 1752 to 1830 When it Became the Royal Infirmary* (Manchester: Manchester University Press, 1904).
Buchan, William, *Domestic Medicine; or, the Family Physician [...] Chiefly Calculated to Recommend a Proper Attention to Regimen and Simple Medicines* (Edinburgh: Balfour, 1769).
Buchan, William, *Observations Concerning the Prevention and Cure of the Venereal Disease. Intended to Guard the Ignorant and Unwary against the Baneful Effects of that Insidious Malady*, with an appendix (Dublin: Wogan, 1796).
Bunbury, Henry William (after), *The Dog Barber* (1771), etching, 22.4 × 13.8 cm, Metropolitan Museum of Art.
Bunbury, Henry William (after), *View on the Pont Neuf at Paris* (1771), etching, 25.1 × 37.7 cm, British Museum.
Burney, Frances, *Cecilia, or Memoirs of an Heiress*, 5 vols (London: Payne and Cadell, 1782).
Carver, Mrs, *The Horrors of Oakendale Abbey* (London: Minerva Press, 1797).
Carver, Mrs, *The Horrors of Oakendale Abbey* (Zittaw Press, 2006).

Chapple, J. A. V. and Arthur Pollard (eds), *The Letters of Mrs. Gaskell* (Manchester: Manchester University Press, 1967).

Cheyne, George, *An Essay of Health and Long Life* (London: printed for George Strahan and J. Leake, Bath, 1724).

Cheyne, George, *The English Malady: or. a Treatise of Nervous Diseases of all Kinds: as Spleen, Vapours, Lowness of Spirits, Hypochondriacal and Hysterical Distempers [...] with the Author's Own Case at Large*, ed. Roy Porter (London: Routledge, 1991 [1733]).

Cheyne, George, *The Letters of George Cheyne to Samuel Richardson*, ed. and published by Charles F. Mullett (Columbia, MO: University of Missouri Press, 1942).

Cocroft, Susanna, *Body Manikin and the Position of Vital Organs* (Chicago, IL: Physical Culture Extension Society, 1905).

Coke, Mary, *The Letters and Journals of Lady Mary Coke*, ed. James Archibald Home, 4 vols (Edinburgh: David Douglas, 1896).

Coleridge, Samuel Taylor, *The Collected Works of Samuel Taylor Coleridge. Biographia Literaria or Biographical Sketches of My Literary Life and Opinions* (1817), vol. II, ed. James Engells and W. Jackson Bate (Princeton, NJ: Princeton University Press, and London: Routledge & Kegan Paul, 1983).

Cox, Elizabeth, *Companion to the Family Medicine Chest*, 33rd edn (London: Simpkin, 1845).

Cox, Elizabeth, *Companion to the Medicine Chest* (London: Cox, 1843).

Cox, Elizabeth, *Companion to the Medicine Chest*, 15th edn (London: Cox, 1836).

Cox, Elizabeth, *Companion to the Medicine Chest*, 32nd edn (London: Simpkin, 1845).

Cox, Elizabeth, *Companion to the Medicine Chest: with Plain Rules for Taking the Medicines in the Cure of Diseases*, 13th edn (London: Cox, 1830).

Cox, Elizabeth, *Companion to the Medicine Chest, with Plain Rules for Taking the Medicines in the Cure of Diseases*, 15th edn (London: Cox, 1832).

Cox, Elizabeth, *Companion to the Medicine Chest with Plain Rules for Taking the Medicines in the Cure of Diseases*, 17th edn (London: Cox, 1833) [pharmecutical remedy booklet], Accession Number, 1954.3.2, Kingston Museum of Healthcare University Health Network, Academy of Medicine Collection, available at https://mhc.andornot.com/en/permalink/artifact15264, last accessed 20 October 2023.

Cox, Elizabeth, *Companion to the Sea Medicine Chest*, 20th edn (London: Simpkin, 1844).

Cox, Elizabeth, *Cox's Catalogue of Dispensing Labels, as per Specimens, at 2s. 6d. per Thousand, Gummed at the Back, and Ready for Immediate Use* (London: Cox, 1828). (Wellcome Trust b31909401.)

Cox, Elizabeth, *Cox's Catalogue of Dispensing Labels, at 2s. 6d. per thousand, Gummed for Immediate Use* (London: Cox, 1836). (Wellcome Library b30387826.)

Cox, Elizabeth, *Cox's Companion to the Family Medicine Chest*, 48th edn (London: Simpkin, 1887), available at https://wellcomecollection.org/works/dz6e4qvv, last accessed 22 July 2022.

Cox, Elizabeth, *Cox's Companion to the Sea Medicine Chest*, 1st American from the 33rd London edn (London: Simpkin, 1851).

Cox, Elizabeth, *Cox's Companion to the Sea Medicine Chest*, 'new edition' (London: Cox, 1836).

Cox, Elizabeth, *Druggists' Price Book* (London: Cox, 1836).
Cox, Elizabeth et al., 'DRAFT Trade card of Christopher Woodhouse, Chemist', British Museum, Museum Number Heal,35.84.
Cullen Project, The, *The Consultation Letters of Dr William Cullen (1710–1790 at the Royal College of Physicians*, available at https://www.cullenproject.ac.uk/, last accessed 5 April 2023.
de Styrap, Jukes, *A Code of Medical Ethics* (London: J. & A. Churchill, 1878).
Edwards, Henry Sutherland, *Malvina*, 3 vols (London: Hurst and Blackett, 1871).
Fletcher, John, *The Mad Lover, in Comedies and Tragedies written by Francis Beaumont and John Fletcher* (London: Robinson and Moseley, 1647).
Ford, John, *The Lover's Melancholy* (London: Seile, 1629).
Fothergill, Anthony, 'On the Premature Death of Cloe Snappum, a Lady's Favourite', *An Asylum for Fugitive Pieces, in Prose and Verse, Not in Any Other Collection: With Several Other Pieces Never before Published*, 3 vols (London: Debrett, 1789).
Fox, Joseph, *Natural History of the Human Teeth* (London: Cox, 1803).
Furneaux, William S. (ed.), *Dr. Minder's Anatomical Manikin of the Female Human Body: An Illustrated Representation with Full and Descriptive Text*, rev. Ethel Mayer (New York: American Thermo-Ware, [*c*.1905]).
Gaskell, Elizabeth, *Mary Barton: A Tale of Manchester Life* (New York: Penguin, 1996).
Gaskell, Elizabeth, *The Works of Elizabeth Gaskell in Eight Volumes*, Knutsford Edition, (1906; Reprint, New York: AMS Press, 1972).
Gibbs, George S., *The Law of Useless Infanticide Miscalled Vaccination; Being the Substance of Six Letters Addressed to Members of Parliament, etc.* (London: Allen, 1989).
Gibbs, John, *Compulsory Vaccination Briefly Considered in Its Scientific, Religious, and Political Aspects* (London: Sotheran and Willis, 1856).
Graham, Thomas John (1826), *Modern Domestic Medicine*, 3rd edn, much enlarged (London: published for the author, 1827).
Gregory, Henry, *A Companion to the Medicine* Chest (London: Butler, 1837).
Haggard, Henry Rider, *A Farmer's Year: Being His Commonplace Book for 1898* (New York: Cambridge University Press, 1899).
Haggard, Henry Rider, *Doctor Therne* (London: Longman, 1898).
Haggard, Henry Rider, *The Days of My Life* (London: Longman, 1911).
Hamilton, Robert, *Remarks on the Means of Obviating the Fatal Effects of the Bite of a Mad Dog* (Ipswich: Shave and Jackson, 1785).
Hanger, George, *To All Sportsmen, Farmers, And Gamekeepers* (London: Stockdale, 1814).
Harington, Henry, 'The Following Diploma Lately Obtained by the Celebrated Canine Professor of Physic in this City' [broadside] (Bath: 1786).
Haywood, Eliza, *The Invisible Spy*, 4 vols (London: Gardner, 1755).
Herriot, James, *If Only They Could Talk* (London: Joseph, 1970).
James, Robert, *A Treatise on Canine Madness* (London: Newberry, 1765).
Jonson, Ben, *The Alchemist* (London: Burre, 1612).
Kerby-Miller, Charles (ed.), *Memoirs of the Extraordinary Life, Works, and Discoveries of Martinus Scriblerus. Written in Collaboration by the Members of the Scriblerus Club: John Arbuthnot, Alexander Pope, Jonathan Swift, John*

Gay, Thomas Parnell and Robert Harley, Earl of Oxford (New Haven, CT: Yale University Press, 1950; Reissued New York: Russell & Russell, 1966).
Locke, John, 'The Epistle to the Reader', *An Essay concerning Human Understanding*, ed. Peter H. Nidditch (Oxford: Clarendon Press, 1975), pp. 6–14.
Markham, Gervase, *The Dumbe Knight* (London: Bache, 1608).
Massey, Edmund, *A Sermon Against the Dangerous and Sinful Practice of Inoculation: Preach'd at St. Andrew's Holborn, on Sunday, July 8th, 1722* (London: Meadows, 1722).
McDowell, Paula (ed.), *Elinor James: Printed Writings 1641–1700* (London: Routledge, 2005).
Meyler, William, *Poetical Amusement on the Journey of Life; Consisting of Various Pieces in Verse: Serious, Theatric, Epigrammatic and Miscellaneous* (Bath: Meyler, 1806).
Milton, John, *Paradise Lost* (London: Parker, 1667).
More, Sir Antonio, after Robert Thew (engraver), *Sir Thomas Gresham, Founder of the Royal Exchange* [engraving, uncoloured] (London: Elizabeth Cox, 1823).
Mullett, Charles F. (ed.), *The Letters of Dr George Cheyne to Samuel Richardson (1733–1743)* (Columbia, MO: University of Missouri Studies, 1943).
Nabbes, Thomas, *The Bride* (London: Blaikelocke, 1640).
Orwell, George, *Essays*, ed. Peter Davison (London, New York and Toronto: Everyman's Library, 2002).
Patent Office, The, *A Century of Trade Marks 1876–1976* (London: HMSO, 1976).
Pitt, Robert, *The Craft and Frauds of Physick Expos'd* (London: Tim Childe, 1702).
Pomet, Pierre, *A Complete History of Druggs* (London: R. Bonwicke et al., 1712).
Pope, Alexander, *The Dunciad*, ed. James Sutherland (London: Methuen, 1963).
Pope, Alexander and John Gay, 'Memoirs of P. P.: Clerk of this Parish', in *Miscellanies*, 3 vols (London: Motte, 1727), vol. 2, pp. 268–284.
Potter, Marion E. (ed.), *The United States Catalog Supplement: Books Published 1902–1905* (Minneapolis, MN: H. W. Wilson Company, 1906).
Price, Roger and Frazer Swift (eds), *Catalogue of Nineteenth-Century Medical Trade Marks 1800–1880* (London: Science Museum, 1988).
Radcliffe, John, *Some Memoirs of the Life of John Radcliffe, M.D.* (London: Printed for E. Curll, 1715).
Rassweiler, Henry H., *Portfolio of Life* (Chicago, IL: Western Publishing House, 1891).
Reece, Richard, *Domestic Medical Guide* (London: Stower, 1803).
Rivirii, Lazari, *Praxis medica cum theoria* (Lypsiae [Leipzig]: Matthiam Trinkberg, 1660).
Ross, Angus (ed.), *The Correspondence of Dr John Arbuthnot* (Munich: Fink, 2006).
Rowlandson, Thomas, *The Cobbler: Tom Stichwell Dog Wormer And Cat Gelder* (1789), watercolour, 27.9 × 35.6 cm, Paul Mellon Photographic Archive (PA-F02122-0003).
Rowlandson, Thomas, *The Coblers Cure for a Scolding Wife* (1809), hand-coloured etching, 36.9 × 26.5 cm, Royal Collection Trust (RCIN 810778).
Rowlandson, Thomas, *Tommy Stichwell, Cobbler and Dog-Doctor* (*c.*1789), pen, ink and watercolour over pencil, 24 × 30.25 cm, Lot 85, Old Masters, British & European Paintings, Wednesday 6th March 2019, Woolley & Wallis, p. 32.

Rowlandson, Thomas, *Wit's Last Stake, or the Cobbling Voters and Abject Canvassers* (1784), hand-coloured etching, 26.3 × 36.2 cm, Metropolitan Museum of Art (59.533.62).
Royal College of Physicians, The, *Pharmacopoeia Londinensis* (London, 1618).
Sandelin, Ellen, *Planscher öfver kvinnokroppen och dess organ* (Stockholm: AB Ljus förlag, 1904).
Schröder, Johann (John), *Zoologia: or, The History of Animals as they are Useful* (London: E. Coats, 1659).
Smollett, Tobias, *An Essay on the External Use of Water*, ed. Claude E. Jones (Baltimore, MD: Johns Hopkins Press, 1935).
Smollett, Tobias, *The Adventures of Roderick Random*, 2 vols (London: J. Osborn, 1748).
Smollett, Tobias, *The Adventures of Roderick Random*, ed. Paul Gabriel-Boucé (Oxford: Oxford University Press, 1999 [1748]).
Smollett, Tobias, *The Adventures of Sir Launcelot Greaves*, 2 vols (London: Coote, 1762).
Smollett, Tobias, *The Expedition of Humphry Clinker*, 2 vols (London: Johnston, 1771).
Smollett, Tobias, *The Letters of Tobias Smollett*, ed. Lewis M. Knapp (Oxford: Clarendon Press, 1970).
Solis-Cohen, Myer, *Woman in Girlhood, Wifehood, Motherhood: Her Responsibilities and Her Duties at All Periods of Life* (Philadelphia, Chicago and Toronto: John C. Winston Co., 1906).
Solomon, Samuel, *A Guide to Health, or, Advice to Both Sexes, to Obtain a Radical and Permanent Cure for those Secret Infirmities of Nature which Delicacy often Forbid to Disclose* (London: printed for the author, [1796?]).
Southey, Robert, *Poems, by Robert Southey* (London: Cottle, 1797).
Spurzheim, J. G., *Phrenology, in Connexion with the Study of Physiognomy*, 1st American edn (Boston, MA: Capen & Lyon, 1833).
Strother, Edward, *The Family Companion for Health* (London: Fayram, 1729).
Swift, Jonathan, *Gulliver's Travels*, ed. with an introduction by Paul Turner (Oxford and New York: Oxford University Press, 1986 [1726]).
Swift, Jonathan, *Journal to Stella*, ed. Harold Williams (Oxford: Blackwell, 1974).
Swift, Jonathan, 'The Battle of the Books', in Marcus Walsh (ed.), *A Tale of A Tub and Other Works, The Cambridge Edition of the Works of Jonathan Swift* (Cambridge: Cambridge University Press, 2010), pp. 137–164.
Temple, Sir William, *Miscellanea*, 3 vols (London, 1680, 1692 and 1702).
Thompson, Michael R., 'Miscellany', *Michael R. Thompson Rare Books* (Spring/Summer 2021), https://www.mrtbooksla.com/images/upload/mrtbooks-miscellany-ss21.pdf, last accessed 23 July 2021.
Thrale, Hester Lynch, *Thraliana; The Diary of [...] Mrs Piozzi*, ed. K. C. Balderston, 2 vols (Oxford: Clarendon, 1942).
Turner, Daniel, *Apologia Chyrurgica: a Vindication of the Noble Art of Surgery* (London: J. Whitlock, 1695).
Turner, Daniel [A London Physician], *The Modern Quack* (London: J. Roberts, 1718).
Turner, Daniel, *De Morbis Cutaneis* (London: R. Bonwicke et al., 1714).
Turner, Daniel, *Syphilis: A Practical Dissertation on the Venereal Disease* (London: Walthoe, 1724).

Turner, Daniel, *Syphillis: A Practical Dissertation on the Venereal Disease* (London: R. and J. Bonwicke, et al., 1724).
Vane-Tempest-Stewart, Edith Helen and H. M. Hyde (eds), *The Russian Journals of Martha and Catherine Wilmot, 1803–1808* (London: Macmillan, 1935).
W., T., 'Elegy on the Death of Bungy', *Gentleman's Magazine* (August 1784), p. 614.
Wake, Joan and Deborah Champion Webster (eds), *The Letters of Daniel Eaton to the Third Earl of Cardigan, 1725–1732* (Kettering: Northamptonshire Record Society, 1971).
Warner, Richard [Peter Paul Pallet], *Bath Characters: Or, Sketches from Life* (London: Wilkie and Robinson, 1807).
Wilkinson, Robert Oliver, *Druggists' Price Book*, 3rd edn (London: Cox, 1836). (British Library RB23.a.12230.)
Wilkinson, Robert Oliver, *The Druggist's Price-Book, or a Catalogue of the Drugs, Chemicals, and Perfumery Generally Sold by Chemists & Druggists, with the Doses and Old Names Annexed*, 2nd edn (London: Cox, 1832).
Williams, Ralph, *Physical Rarities* (London: J. M. for George Calvert, 1651).
Wilson, Carol Shiner (ed.), *The Galesia Trilogy and Selected Manuscript Poems of Jane Baker* (Oxford: Oxford University Press, 1997).
Wolcot, John [Peter Pindar], *Pindariana; Or Peter's Portfolion* (London: T. Salisbury, 1794).
Wollstonecraft, Mary, *Letters Written in Sweden, Norway and Denmark* (Oxford: Oxford University Press, 2009).
Wood, John George, *Petland Revisited* (London: Longman, 1884).
Woodward, John, *An Essay toward a Natural History of the Earth and Terrestrial Bodies, especially Minerals: as also of the Sea, Rivers, and Springs: with an Account of the Universal Deluge: and of the Effects that it had upon the Earth* (London: Printed for Richard Wilkin, 1695).
Woolley, Hannah, *A Supplement to The Queen-like Closet* (London: Richard Lownds, 1674).
Z., A., *An Address to the College of Physicians, and to the Universities of Oxford and Cambridge* (London: M. Cooper, 1747).

Secondary Material

Ahmed, Sara, *Queer Phenomenology: Orientations, Objects, Others* (Durham, NC and London: Duke University Press, 2006).
Aitken, George A., *The Life and Works of John Arbuthnot M.D., Fellow of the Royal College of Physicians* (Oxford: Clarendon, 1892).
Alberti, Samuel J. M., *Morbid Curiosities: Medical Museums in Nineteenth-Century Britain* (Oxford: Oxford University Press, 2011).
Amato, Sarah, *Beastly Possessions: Animals in Victorian Consumer Culture* (Toronto: University of Toronto Press, 2015).
Anderson, Stuart, 'From "Bespoke" to "Off-the-Peg": Community Pharmacists and the Retailing of Medicines in Great Britain 1900 to 1970', *Pharmacy in History* 50:2 (2008): 42–69.
Anderson, Stuart, *Pharmacy and Professionalization in the British Empire, 1780–1970* (Switzerland: Palgrave Macmillan, 2021).

Andrews, Jonathan, 'History of Medicine: Health, Medicine and Disease in the Eighteenth Century', *Journal for Eighteenth Century Studies* 34:4 (2011): 503–515.

Andrews, Jonathan and James Kennaway, 'Experiencing, Exploiting, and Evacuating Bile: Framing Fashionable Biliousness from the Sufferer's Perspective', *Literature and Medicine* 35:2 (207): 292–333.

Arnold-Forster, Kate and Nigel Tallis, *The Bruising Apothecary: Images of Pharmacy and Medicine in Caricature* (London: Royal Pharmaceutical Society, 1989).

Aske, Katherine, 'Sharing Skincare Secrets in Eighteenth-Century Popular Culture', in Katherine Aske et al. (eds), *Participation, Collaboration, Association: Communities, Exchanges, Politics and Philosophies in the Eighteenth-Century* (Paris: Honoré Champion, 2023).

Aston, Jennifer, *Female Entrepreneurship in Nineteenth-Century England: Engagement in the Urban Economy*, Palgrave Studies in Economic History (Basingstoke: Palgrave, 2016).

Baker, Cathleen A. and Rebecca M. Chung (eds), *Making Impressions: Women in Printing and Publishing* (Ann Arbor, MI: Legacy, 2020).

Barker, Hannah, 'Medical Advertising and Trust in Late Georgian England', *Urban History* 36:3 (2009): 379–398.

Barker, Hannah, *The Business of Women: Female Enterprise and Urban Development in Northern England, 1760–1830* (Oxford: Oxford University Press, 2006).

Bartrip, P. W. J., 'Churchill, John Spriggs Morss (1801–1875), *Oxford Dictionary of National Biography*, ed. H. C. G. Matthew and Brian Harrison (Oxford: Oxford University Press, 2004), vol. 11, pp. 634–635.

Beattie, Lester M., *John Arbuthnot, Mathematician and Satirist* (Cambridge, MA: Harvard University Press, 1935).

Bently, Lionel, 'The First Trade Mark Case at Common Law? The Story of Singleton V. Bolton (1783)', *UC Davis Law Review* 47:3 (2014): 969–1013.

Bertucci, Paula, 'Shocking Subjects: Human Experiments and the Material Culture of Medical Electricity in Eighteenth-Century England', in Erika Dyck and Larry Stewart (eds), *The Uses of Humans in Experiment: Perspectives from the Seventeenth to the Twentieth Century* (Leiden: Brill, 2016), pp. 111–138.

Beswick, Thomas, 'Local Associations with Mrs. Gaskell', *Knutsford and Mrs. Gaskell.* Issued by The Gaskell Committee, 1960 (Derby: New Centurion).

Bewell, Alan, *Romanticism and Colonial Disease* (Baltimore, MD: Johns Hopkins University Press, 1999).

Birnbaum, Martin, *Jacovleff and Other Artists: Alexandre Jacovleff, William Blake and Other Illustrators of Dante, Thomas Rowlandson, Aubrey Beardsley, Marcus Behmer, Arthur Rackham, Hermann Struck, Anne Goldthwaite* (New York: Struck, 1946).

Blackwood, Ashleigh, Allan Ingram and Helen Williams (eds), *Writing Doctors and Writing Health in the Long Eighteenth Century*, Special Issue of *Journal for Eighteenth-Century Studies*, 46:1 (2023).

Blakey, Dorothy, *The Minerva Press, 1790–1820* (Oxford and London: Bibliographical Society, 1939).

Bock, Carol A., 'Elizabeth Gaskell's "Useful" Relatives: Katharine and Anthony Todd Thomson and the Society for the Diffusion of Useful Knowledge', *Gaskell Journal* 22 (2008): 72–85.

Bolaki, Stella, *Illness as Many Narratives: Arts, Medicine and Culture* (Edinburgh: Edinburgh University Press, 2016).

Brack, O M, Jr., 'Smollett and the Authorship of "Memoirs of a Lady of Quality"', in O M Brack, Jr. (ed.), *Tobias Smollett, Scotland's First Novelist* (Newark, DE: University of Delaware Press, 2007), pp. 35–73.

Brauer, Fae, 'Eroticizing Lamarckian Eugenics: The Body Stripped Bare during French Sexual Neoregulation', in Fae Brauer and Anthea Callen (eds), *Art, Sex and Eugenics: Corpus Delecti* (Aldershot: Ashgate, 2008), pp. 97–136.

British Book Trade Index, The, available at http://bbti.bodleian.ox.ac.uk/#, last accessed 28 July 2022.

Brown, Laura, *Homeless Dogs and Melancholy Apes: Humans and Other Animals in the Modern Literary Imagination* (Ithaca, NY: Cornell University Press, 2010).

Brown, Meg, 'Flip, Flap, and Crack: The Conservation and Exhibition of 400+ Years of Flap Anatomies', *Book and Paper Group Annual* 32:6 (2013): 6–14.

Brown, P. S., 'Herbalists and Medical Botanists in Mid-Nineteenth-Century Britain with Special Reference to Bristol', *Medical History* 26:4 (1982): 405–420.

Brunton, Deborah, *The Politics of Vaccination: Practice and Policy in England, Wales, Ireland, and Scotland 1800–1874* (Rochester, NY: University of Rochester Press, 2008).

Burrell, Robert and Catherine Kelly, 'Myths of the Medical Methods Exclusion: Medicine and Patents in Nineteenth-Century Britain', *Legal Studies* 38:4 (2018): 607–626.

Bynum, W. F. and Roy Porter (eds), *Medical Fringe and Medical Orthodoxy, 1750–1850* (Kent: Croom Helm, 1987).

Bynum, William F., *Gastroenterology in Britain: Historical Essays* (London: Wellcome Institute, 1997).

Callen, Anthea, *Looking at Men: Anatomy, Masculinity and the Modern Male Body* (New Haven, CT: Yale University Press, 2018).

Cambau, E. and M. Poljak, 'Sniffing Animals as a Diagnostic Tool in Infectious Diseases', *Clinical Microbiology and Infection* 26:4 (2020): 431–435.

Carlino, Andrea, *Paper Bodies: A Catalogue of Anatomical Fugitive Sheets, 1538–1687* (London: Wellcome Institute for the History of Medicine, 1999).

Center for Countering Digital Hate, *Failure to Act: How Tech Giants Continue to Defy Calls to Rein in Vaccine Misinformation* (1 December 2020), available at https://counterhate.com/research/failure-to-act/, last accessed 5 April 2020.

Chadwick, Mrs Ellis H., *Mrs. Gaskell, Haunts, Homes & Stories* (New York: Frederick A. Stokes, 1911).

Chakrabarti, Pratik, *Materials and Medicine: Trade, Conquest and Therapeutics in the Eighteenth Century* (Manchester: Manchester University Press, 2010).

Chakrabarti, Pratik, *Medicine and Empire, 1600–1960* (Basingstoke: Palgrave Macmillan, 2011).

Chapple, John, *Elizabeth Gaskell: The Early Years* (Manchester: Manchester University Press, 1997).

Charon, Rita, 'The Narrative Road to Empathy', in Howard M. Spiro, Mary G. McCrea Curnen, and Enid Peschel (eds), *Empathy and the Practice of Medicine: Beyond Pills and the Scalpel* (New Haven, CT: Yale University Press, 1993), pp. 147–159.

Chico, Tita, *The Experimental Imagination: Literary Knowledge and Science in the British Enlightenment* (Stanford, CA: Stanford University Press, 2018).

Child, Paul W., "The Case of the Author": George Cheyne's Providential Medical Autobiography', *AnaChronisT* 11 (2005): 70–84.

Christensen, Allan Conrad, *Nineteenth-Century Narratives of Contagion: 'Our Feverish Contact'* (London: Routledge, 2005).

Class, Monika, 'Introduction: Medical Case Histories as Genre: New Approaches', *Literature and Medicine* 32:1 (2014): ii–xvi.

Cock, Emily, '"He would by no means risque his Reputation": Patient and Doctor Shame in Daniel Turner's *De Morbis Cutaneis* (1714) and *Syphilis* (1717)', *Medical Humanities* 43:4 (2017): 231–237.

Cohen, Morton Norton, *Rider Haggard: His Life and Works* (New York: Walker and Company, 1968).

Cole, R. J., 'Sir Anthony Carlisle F.R.S.', *Annals of Science* 8:3 (1952): 255–270.

Coleborne, Catharine, 'Exhibiting "Madness": Material Culture and the Asylum', *Health and History* 3:2 (2001): 104–117.

Colman, Eric, 'The First English Medical Journal: *Medicina Curiosa*', *Lancet* 354:9175 (1999): 324–326.

Connor, Henry, 'Medieval Uroscopy and its Representation on Misericords – Part 1: Uroscopy', *Clinical Medicine* 1:6 (2001): 507–509.

Coventry, Francis, *The History of Pompey the Little* (London: Cooper, 1751).

Cox's Companion to the Sea Medicine Chest (London: Simpkin, Marshall & Co., 1845), available at https://www.abebooks.co.uk/servlet/BookDetailsPL?bi=30870412362&searchurl=kn%3Dcox%2Bmedical%2Bbookseller%26sortby%3D17&cm_sp=snippet-_-srp1-_-title14, last accessed 22 July 2012.

Crellin, J. K. and J. R. Scott, 'Pharmaceutical History and its Sources in the Wellcome Collections: II. Drug Weighing in Britain, *c*.1700–1900', *Medical History* 13:1 (1969): 51–67.

Curth, Louise Hill (ed.), *From Physick to Pharmacology: Five Hundred Years of British Drug Retailing* (Aldershot: Ashgate, 2006).

Curwen, Henry, *A History of Booksellers, the Old and the New* (London: Chatto & Windus, 1874).

Davis, Lennard J., 'Nude Venuses, Medusa's Body, and Phantom Limbs: Disability and Visuality', in D. T. Mitchell and S. L. Snyder (eds), *The Body and Physical Difference: Discourses of Disability* (Ann Arbor, MI: University of Michigan Press, 1997), pp. 51–70.

Davis, Lennard J., *Obsession: A History* (Chicago, IL and London: University of Chicago Press, 2008).

Debus, Allen G., *The English Paracelsians* (New York: Watts, 1966).

deVries, Leonard, *Victorian Advertisements* (London: John Murray, 1968).

Dickinson, Tim, 'How the Anti-Vaxxers Got Red-Pilled', *Rolling Stone* (10 February 2021).

Digby, Anne, *Making a Medical Living: Doctors and Patients in the English Market for Medicine, 1720–1911* (Cambridge: Cambridge University Press, 1994).

Dopson, Laurence, 'St Thomas's Parish Vestry Records and a Body-Snatching Incident', *British Medical Journal* 2:4618 (1949): 69.

Dorner, Zachary, *Merchants of Medicines: The Commerce and Coercion of Health in Britain's Long Eighteenth Century* (Chicago, IL: University of Chicago Press, 2020).

Douglas, Aileen, *Uneasy Sensations: Smollett and the Body* (Chicago, IL: University of Chicago Press, 1995).

Duden, Barbara, *The Woman Beneath the Skin: A Doctor's Patients in Eighteenth-Century Germany*, trans. Thomas Dunlap (Cambridge, MA: Harvard University Press, 1998).

Duguid, Paul, 'Developing the Brand: The Case of Alcohol, 1800–1880', *Enterprise & Society* 4:3 (2003): 405–441.

Dupree, Marguerite W., 'Other Than Healing: Medical Practitioners and the Business of Life Assurance during the Nineteenth and Early Twentieth Centuries', *Society for the Social History of Medicine* 10:1 (1997): 79–103.

Durbach, Nadja, *Bodily Matters: The Anti-Vaccination Movement in England, 1853–1907* (Durham, NC and London: Duke University Press, 2005).

Earl of Ilchester, *Lord Hervey and his Friends: 1726–38* (London: Murray, 1950).

Eccles, Audrey, 'The Reading Public, the Medical Profession, and the Use of English for Medical Books in the 16th and 17th Centuries', *Neuphilologische Mitteilungen* 75:1 (1974): 143–156.

Eisen, Erica X., '"The Mark of the Beast": Georgian Britain's Anti-Vaxxer Movement', *Public Domain Review* (2021), available at https://publicdomainreview.org/essay/the-mark-of-the-beast-georgian-britains-anti-vaxxer-movement, last accessed 27 January 2023.

Ellis, Markman, 'Suffering Things: Lapdogs, Slaves and Counter-Sensibility', in Mark Blackwell (ed.), *The Secret Life of Things: Animals, Objects, and It-Narratives in Eighteenth-Century England* (Lewisburg, PA: Bucknell University Press, 2007), pp. 93–113.

Encarnación, Karen Rosoff, 'The Proper Use of Desire: Sex & Procreation in Reformation Anatomical Fugitive Sheets', in Anne L. McClanan and Karen Rosoff Encarnación (eds), *The Material Culture of Sex, Procreation, and Marriage in Premodern Europe* (New York: Palgrave, 2001), pp. 221–249.

Engels, Friedrich (1845), *The Condition of the Working Class in England* (London, Panther, 1969).

Estes, J. W., 'The Pharmacology of Nineteenth-Century Patent Medicines', *Pharmacy in History* 30:1 (1988), 3–18.

Fairley, Michael and Tony White, *The History of Labels: The Evolution of the Label Industry in Europe* (London: Tarsus, 2014).

Fashionable Diseases Leverhulme Trust, *Fashionable Diseases*, available at http://www.fashionablediseases.info/, last accessed 24 April 2023.

Faubert, Michelle, *Rhyming Reason: The Poetry of Romantic-Era Psychologists* (London: Routledge, 2009).

Fitzwilliam, Marie, 'Mr. Harrison's Confessions: A Study of the General Practitioner's Social and Professional Disease', *Gaskell Society Journal* 12 (1998): 28–36.

Flynn, Carol Houlihan, *The Body in Swift and Defoe* (Cambridge: Cambridge University Press, 1990).

Foster, Janet and Julia Sheppard (eds), 'Society of Apothecaries Archives', *British Archives*, 4th edn (Basingstoke: Palgrave, 2002), pp. 462–463.

Foucault, Michel, *Discipline and Punish: The Birth of the Prison* (London: Penguin, 1991).

Fox, Christopher, *Locke and the Scriblerians: Identity and Consciousness in Early Eighteenth-Century Britain* (Berkeley, Los Angeles, London: University of California Press, 1988).

Frampton, Sally, 'Honour and Subsistence: Invention, Credit and Surgery in the Nineteenth Century', *Owning Health: Medicine and Anglo-American Patent Cultures*, Special Issue of *British Journal for the History of Science* 49:4 (December 2016): 561–576.

Frampton, Sally, 'Patents, Priority Disputes and the Value of Credit: Towards a History (and Pre-History) of Intellectual Property in Medicine', *Medical History* 55:3 (2011): 319–324.

Frampton, Sally and Jennifer Wallis, 'Reading Medicine and Health in Periodicals', *Media History* 25:1 (2019): 1–5.

French, Roger, *Ancients and Moderns in the Medical Sciences: From Hippocrates to Harvey* (Aldershot: Ashgate, 2000).

Furdell, Elizabeth Lane, 'Bate, George [pseud. Theodorus Veridicus] (1608–1668)', *Oxford Dictionary of National Biography* (January 2008), https://doi.org/10.1093/ref:odnb/1661, last accessed 13 January 2023.

Furdell, Elizabeth Lane, *Publishing and Medicine in Early Modern England* (Rochester, NY: University of Rochester Press, 2002).

Gabbard, D. Christopher, 'The Compleat, Common Form': Disability and the Literature of the British Enlightenment', in Clark Lawlor and Andrew Mangham (eds), *Literature and Medicine: The Eighteenth Century* (Cambridge: Cambridge University Press, 2021), pp. 219–241.

Gabriel, Joseph M., *Medical Monopoly: Intellectual Property Rights and the Origins of the Modern Pharmaceutical Industry* (Chicago, IL: University of Chicago Press, 2014).

Gallagher, Noelle, *Itch, Clap, Pox: Venereal Disease in the Eighteenth-Century Imagination* (New Haven, CT: Yale University Press, 2018).

Gardiner, Andrew, 'The "Dangerous" Women of Animal Welfare: How British Veterinary Medicine Went to the Dogs', *Social History of Medicine* 23:3 (2014): 466–487.

Garside, Peter, James Raven and Rainer Schowerling, *The English Novel 1770–1829: A Bibliographical Survey of Prose Fiction Published in the British Isles* (Oxford: Oxford University Press, 2000).

Gaskell, Peter, *Artisans and Machinery: The Moral and Physical Condition of the Manufacturing Population Considered with Reference to Mechanical Substitutes for Human Labour* (1836; Reprints of Economic Classics, New York: Kelly, 1968).

Gasperini, Anna, *Nineteenth-Century Popular Fiction, Medicine and Anatomy* (London: Palgrave, 2019).

Gentilcore, David, *Medical Charlatanism in Early Modern Italy* (Oxford: Oxford University Press, 2006).

Gillam, Sarah, 'Sir Samuel Garth's poem, "The Dispensary"', *Royal College of Physicians Blog*, 22 September 2017, https://history.rcplondon.ac.uk/blog/sir-samuel-garths-poem-dispensary, last accessed 3 November 2023.

Gitter, Elisabeth G., 'The Power of Women's Hair in the Victorian Imagination', *PMLA/Publications of the Modern Language Association of America* 99:5 (1984): 936–954.

Goldstein, David B., 'A Guide to Ladies: Hannah Woolley's Missing Book emerges from the Archives', *Shakespeare and Beyond Blog*, 29 March 2019, https://shakespeareandbeyond.folger.edu/2019/03/29/a-guide-to-ladies-hannah-woolley-missing-book/, last accessed 17 October 2023.

Golightly, Jennifer, *The Family, Marriage, and Radicalism in British Women's Novels of the 1790s: Public Affection and Private Affliction* (Lewisburg, PA: Bucknell University Press, 2012).
Green, David G., *Working-Class Patients and the Medical Establishment* (Aldershot: Gower, 1985).
Grell, Ole Peter, Andrew Cunningham and Jon Arrizabalaga (eds), *Centres of Medical Excellence: Medical Travel and Education in Europe, 1500–1789* (Farnham: Ashgate, 2009).
Griffenhagen, George B. and Mary Bogard, *History of Drug Containers and Their Labels* (Madison, WI: American Institute of the History of Pharmacy, 1999).
Griggs, Barbara, *Green Pharmacy: A History of Herbal Medicine* (New York: Viking, 1981).
Grogan, Suzie, *Death, Disease & Dissection: The Life of a Surgeon-Apothecary, 1750–1850* (South Yorkshire: Pen & Sword, 2017).
Guerrini, Anita, *Obesity and Depression in the Enlightenment: The Life and Times of George Cheyne* (Norman, OK: University of Oklahoma Press, 2000).
Hacking, Ian, 'Kinds of People: Moving Targets: British Academy Lecture', in P. J. Marshall (ed.), *Proceedings of the British Academy*, Volume 151: *2006 Lectures (1)* (Oxford: British Academy, 2007), pp. 285–318.
Harner, Christie, 'Physiognomic Discourse and the Trials of Cross-Class Sympathy in *Mary Barton*', *Victorian Literature and Culture* 43:4 (2015): 705–724.
Harris, Michael, 'Printed Ephemera', in Michael F. Suarez, S.J. and M. R. Woudhuysen (eds), *The Oxford Companion to the Book*, 2 vols (Oxford: Oxford University Press, 2010), vol. 1, pp. 120–128.
Harrison, Mark, *Medicine in an Age of Commerce and Empire: Britain and its Tropical Colonies 1660–1830* (Cambridge: Cambridge University Press, 2010).
Hatfield, Gabrielle, *Memory, Wisdom, and Healing: The History of Domestic Plant Medicine* (Stroud: Sutton, 1999).
Hayley, Heather, '"Convenient in Any Exigency": The Transcendence of the Medicine Chest from the Professional to the Domestic in the Early Nineteenth Century', *Global Maritime History*, July 2017, available at https://globalmaritimehistory.com/convenient-exigency-transcendence-medicine-chest-professional-domestic/, last accessed 22 July 2022.
Hilton, Christopher, 'Elizabeth Gaskell and Mesmerism: An Unpublished Letter', *Medical History* 39:2 (1995): 219–235.
Hogarth, Rana A., *Medicalizing Blackness: Making Racial Difference in the Atlantic World, 1780–1840* (Chapel Hill, NC: University of North Carolina Press, 2017).
Hollander, Stanley C., *History of Labels: A Record of the Past Developed in the Search for the Origins of an Industry* (New York: Hollander, 1956).
Holloway, Sydney W. F., *Royal Pharmaceutical Society of Great Britain, 1841–1991* (London: Pharmaceutical Press, 1991).
Howard-Smith, Stephanie, 'The First Dog Doctors: Canine Healthcare Practitioners in the Eighteenth-Century Medical Marketplace', *Social History of Medicine* (forthcoming at the time of writing).
Howard-Smith, Stephanie, 'In the Dog House: British Canines at Home, 1688–1832', *Home Cultures* 18:2 (2021): 129–149, available at https://doi.org/10.1080/17406315.2021.1963610, last accessed 19 October 2023.
Howsam, Leslie, 'In My View: Women and Book History', *SHARP News* (1998).

Hughes, Linda K., '"Cousin Phillis", *Wives and Daughters*, and Modernity', in Jill L. Matus (ed.), *The Cambridge Companion to Elizabeth Gaskell* (Cambridge: Cambridge University Press, 2007), pp. 98–101.

Hunting, Penelope, *A History of the Society of Apothecaries* (London: Worshipful Society of Apothecaries of London, 1998).

Hurren, Elizabeth T., *Dissecting the Criminal Corpse: Staging Post-Execution Punishment in Early Modern England* (London: Palgrave Macmillan, 2016).

Hurren, Elizabeth T., *Dying for Victorian Medicine: English Anatomy and its Trade in the Dead Poor, c.1834–1929* (Basingstoke: Palgrave Macmillan, 2012).

Ingram, Allan, *Boswell's Creative Gloom: A Study of Imagery and Melancholy in the Writings of James Boswell* (London and Basingstoke: Macmillan, 1982).

Ingram, Allan and Leigh Wetherall Dickson (eds), *Disease and Death in Eighteenth-Century Literature and Culture: Fashioning the Unfashionable* (London: Palgrave, 2016).

Jenner, Mark and Patrick Wallis (eds), *Medicine and the Market in England and its Colonies, c.1450–1850* (Basingstoke: Palgrave Macmillan, 2007).

Jones, Claire L., 'A Barrier to Medical Treatment? British Medical Practitioners, Medical Appliances and the Patent Controversy, 1870–1920', *British Journal for the History of Science* 49:4 (2016): 601–625.

Jones, Claire L., *The Medical Trade Catalogue in Britain, 1870–1914* (London: University of Pittsburgh Press, 2013).

Jones, Roger, 'Thomas Wakley, Plagiarism, Libel, and the Founding of *The Lancet*', *Lancet* 371:9622 (2008): 1410–1411.

Jones, Susan D., *Valuing Animals: Veterinarians and Their Patients in Modern America* (Baltimore, MD: Johns Hopkins University Press, 2003).

Jonsson, Fredrik Albritton, 'The Physiology of Hypochondria in Eighteenth-Century Britain', in Christopher E. Forth and Ana Carden-Coyne (eds), *Cultures of the Abdomen: Diet, Digestion, and Fat in the Modern World* (Basingstoke: Palgrave Macmillan, 2005), pp. 15–30.

Jordanova, Ludmilla, *Sexual Visions: Images of Gender in Science and Medicine between the Eighteenth and Twentieth Centuries* (Madison, WI: University of Wisconsin Press, 1989).

Jules Odendahl-James and Mark Olson, 'Flap and Click: The Performance of Embodiment in Anatomy and the Archive', paper presented at Animated Anatomies: The Human Body in Anatomical Texts from the 16th through 21st Centuries, Duke University, 18 April 2011.

Kaplan, Fred, '"The Mesmeric Mania": The Early Victorians and Animal Magnetism', *Journal of the History of Ideas* 35:4 (1974): 691–702.

King, Kathryn R., 'Galesia, Jane Barker, and Coming to an Authorship', in Carol J. Singley and Susan Elizabeth Sweeney (eds), *Anxious Power: Reading, Writing, and Ambivalence in Narrative by Women* (New York: State University of New York Press, 1993), pp. 91–104.

King, Kathryn R., 'Jane Barker, *Poetical Recreations*, and the Sociable Text', *ELH* 61:3 (1994): 551–570.

Kraft, Elizabeth, *Women Novelists and the Ethics of Desire, 1684–1814: In the Voice of Our Biblical Mothers* (Aldershot: Ashgate, 2008).

Lane, Joan, 'Farriers in Georgian England', in A. R. Michell (ed.), *The Advancement of Veterinary Science*, Vol. 3: *History of the Healing Professions: Parallels between Veterinary and Medical History* (Wallingford: CAB International, 1993), pp. 99–117.

Latour, Bruno, 'Visualization and Cognition: Thinking with Eyes and Hands', *Knowledge and Society* 6 (1986): 1–40.

Lawlor, Clark, *Consumption and Literature: The Making of the Romantic Disease* (Basingstoke: Palgrave, 2006).

Lawlor, Clark and Andrew Mangham (eds), *Literature and Medicine: The Eighteenth Century* (Cambridge: Cambridge University Press, 2021).

Lawlor, Clark and Andrew Mangham (eds), *Literature and Medicine: The Nineteenth Century* (Cambridge: Cambridge University Press, 2021).

Lawrence, C. J., 'William Buchan: Medicine Laid Open', *Medical History* 19:1 (1975): 20–35.

Lawrence, Susan C., 'Anatomy and Address: Creating Medical Gentlemen in Eighteenth-Century London', in Vivian Nutton and Roy Porter (eds), *The History of Medical Education* (Brill: Rodopi, 1995), pp. 199–228.

Levy, Michelle, 'Do Women Have a Book History?', *Studies in Romanticism* 53:3 (2014): 297–317.

Lewis, Ann and Ellis, Markman, *Prostitution and Eighteenth-Century Culture: Sex, Commerce and Morality* (London: Pickering and Chatto, 2012).

Loeb, Lori, 'Doctors and Patent Medicines in Modern Britain: Professionalism and Consumerism', *Albion: A Quarterly Journal Concerned with British Studies* 33:3 (2001): 404–425.

Loudon, Irvine, *Medical Care and the General Practitioner* (Oxford: Clarendon Press, 1986).

Louis-Courvoisier, Micheline, 'The Soul in the Entrails: The Experience of the Sick in the Eighteenth Century', in Rebecca Anne Barr, Sylvie Kleiman-Lafon and Sophie Vasset (eds), *Bellies, Bowels and Entrails in the Eighteenth Century* (Manchester: Manchester University Press, 2018), pp. 80–98.

MacKay, Michael Hubbard, 'The Rise of a Medical Specialty: The Medicalisation of Elite Equine Care *c*.1680–*c*.1800', PhD thesis, University of York (2009), available at http://etheses.whiterose.ac.uk/14229/1/625453.pdf, last accessed 10 April 2020.

Mackintosh, Alan, *The Patent Medicines Industry in Georgian England: Constructing the Market by the Potency of Print* (Basingstoke: Palgrave, 2016).

Madden, Deborah, *'A Cheap, Safe and Natural Medicine': Religion, Medicine and Culture in John Wesley's Primitive Physic* (Amsterdam and New York: Rodopi, 2007).

Mainwaring, Laura, 'Profit and Paratexts; the Economics of Pharmaceutical Packaging in the Long Nineteenth Century', in Hannah C. Tweed and Diane G. Scott (eds), *Medical Paratexts from Medieval to Modern: Dissecting the Page* (Basingstoke: Palgrave, 2018), pp. 75–90.

Mann, Annika, *Reading Contagion: The Hazards of Reading in the Age of Print* (Charlottesville, VA: University of Virginia Press, 2018).

Manning, Susan, 'Boswell's Pleasures, the Pleasures of Boswell', *British Journal for Eighteenth-Century Studies* 20:1 (1997): 17–32.

Marshall, Tim, *Murdering to Dissect: Grave-Robbing, Frankenstein and the Anatomy Literature* (Manchester: Manchester University Press, 1995).

Maxted, Ian, 'Thomas Cox', in *The London Book Trades 1775–1800: A Preliminary Checklist of Members*, Exeter Working Papers in British Book Trade History (Folkstone: Dawson, 1977).

McDowell, Paula, *The Women of Grub Street: Press, Politics, and Gender in the London Literary Marketplace 1678–1730* (Oxford: Clarendon, 1998).

McNaught, Alison, 'Two Nonconformist Women Printers and Booksellers in the Mid-Eighteenth Century', *Bunyan Studies* 24 (2020): 65–84.

McNeil, Maureen, *Under the Banner of Science: Erasmus Darwin and His Age* (Manchester: Manchester University Press, 1987).

Mercer, John, 'A Mark of Distinction: Branding and Trade Mark Law in the UK from the 1860s', *Business History* 52:1 (2010): 17–42.

Miller, Ian, *A Modern History of the Stomach* (London: Pickering & Chatto, 2011).

Monaghan, Jessica, 'Authenticity and Fashionable Disease in Eighteenth-Century Britain', *Literature and Medicine* 35:2 (2017): 387–408.

Moore, Erika, 'Paper Cuts: The Production of Knowledge in Early Modern Anatomical Prints', PhD thesis, University College London (2016).

Moore, Wendy, 'The Adventures of Roderick Random', *BMJ: British Medical Journal* 343:d5718 [online], updated 14 September 2011 [cited 27 September 2021], available at https://www.bmj.com/content/343/bmj.d5718, last accessed 19 October 2023.

Moore, Wendy, *The Knife-Man* (London: Bantam Press, 2006).

Moores, Teri, 'Woolley, Hannah (c.1623–after 1677)', *Historical Dictionary of British Women*, ed. Cathy Hartley (London: Europa, 2003).

Morantz-Sanchez, Regina Markell, *Sympathy and Science: Women Physicians in American Medicine* (New York and Oxford: Oxford University Press, 1985).

Mosier, Erika, Dianne van der Reyden and Mary Baker, 'The Technology and Treatment of an Embossed, Chromolithographic "Mechanical" Victorian Valentine Card', *Book and Paper Group Annual* 11 (1992): n.p.

Neiman, E. A. and C. Morin, 'Re-evaluating the Minerva Press: Introduction', *Romantic Intertextualities: Literature and Print Culture, 1780–1840* 23 (2020): 11–23.

Neiman, Elizabeth, *Minerva's Gothics: The Politics and Poetics of Romantic Exchange, 1780–1820* (Cardiff: University of Wales, 2019).

Nelson, Charmaine A., *The Color of Stone: Sculpting the Black Female Subject in Nineteenth-Century America* (Minneapolis, MN: University of Minnesota Press, 2007).

Nevett, Terence R., *Advertising in Britain* (London: Heinemann, 1982).

Ngg, Genice, 'The Changing Face of Quack Doctors: Satirizing Mountebanks and Physicians in Seventeenth- and Eighteenth-Century England', in S. M. Hilger (ed.), *New Directions in Literature and Medicine Studies* (Basingstoke: Palgrave Macmillan, 2017), pp. 333–356.

O'Brien, Christopher, 'The Origins and Originators of Early Statistical Societies: A Comparison of Liverpool and Manchester', *Journal of the Royal Statistical Society* 174:1 (2011): 51–62.

Offit, Paul, *Deadly Choices: How the Anti-Vaccine Movement Threatens Us All* (New York: Basic Books, 2011).

Ortner, Sherry B., 'Is Female to Male as Nature is to Culture?', *Feminist Studies* 1:2 (1972): 5–31.

Owens, Deirdre Cooper, *Medical Bondage: Race, Gender, and the Origins of American Gynecology* (Athens, GA: University of Georgia Press, 2017).

Ozment, Kate, 'Rationale for Feminist Bibliography', *Textual Cultures* 13:1 (2020): 149–178.

Park, Katharine, *Secrets of Women: Gender, Generation, and the Origins of Human Dissection* (Cambridge, MA: MIT Press, 2006).
Parssinen, T. M., 'Popular Science and Society: The Phrenology Movement in Early Victorian Britain', *Journal of Social History* 8:1 (1974): 1–20.
Patrick Chalmers, *The Adhesive Postage Stamp* (London: Wilson, 1886).
Pegram, C., E. Raffan, E. White, A. H. Ashworth, D. C. Brodbelt, D. B. Church and D. G. O'Neill, 'Frequency, Breed Predisposition and Demographic Risk Factors for Overweight Status in Dogs in the UK', *Journal of Small Animal Practice* 62:7 (2021): 521–530.
Pemberton, Neil and Michael Worboys, *Mad Dogs and Englishmen: Rabies in Britain, 1830–2000* (Basingstoke: Palgrave, 2007).
Peterson, M. Jeanne, *The Medical Profession in Mid-Victorian London* (Berkeley, CA: University of California, 1978).
Petty, Ross D., 'Pain-Killer: A 19th Century Global Patent Medicine and the Beginnings of Modern Brand Marketing', *Journal of Macromarketing* 39:3 (2019): 287–303.
Piehl, Kathy, 'Books in Toyland', *Children's Literature Association Quarterly* 12:2 (1987): 79–83.
Pope, Alexander, *The Correspondence of Alexander Pope*, ed. George Sherburn, 5 vols (Oxford: Oxford University Press, 1956).
Porter, Dorothy and Roy Porter, *Patient's Progress: Doctors and Doctoring in Eighteenth-Century England* (Palo Alto, CA: Stanford University Press, 1989).
Porter, Roy, *Disease, Medicine and Society in England, 1550–1860* (Cambridge: Cambridge University Press, 1995).
Porter, Roy, *Flesh in the Age of Reason: The Modern Foundations of Body and Soul* (New York: Norton, 2004).
Porter, Roy, *Health for Sale: Quackery in England, 1660–1850* (Manchester: Manchester University Press, 1989).
Porter, Roy, 'John Woodward: "A Droll Sort of Philosopher"', *Geological Magazine* 116:5 (1979): 335–417.
Porter, Roy, *Quacks: Fakers & Charlatans in English Medicine* (London: Tempus Publishing, 2003).
Porter, Roy, *The Greatest Benefit to Mankind* (London: Harper Collins, 1997).
Porter, Roy (ed.), *The Popularization of Medicine 1650–1850* (London: Routledge, 1992).
Quinlan, Maurice J. (ed.), 'Memoir of William Cowper', *Proceedings of the American Philosophical Society* 97.4 (1953): 359–382.
Rauser, Amelia, *The Age of Undress: Art, Fashion, and the Classical Ideal in the 1790s* (New Haven, CT and London: Yale University Press, 2020).
Raven, James, *The Publishing Business in Eighteenth-Century England* (Woodbridge: Boydell, 2014).
Reeve, Richard, 'Henry Rider Haggard's Debt to Anthony Trollope: *Doctor Therne* and *Doctor Thorne*', *Notes & Queries* 63:2 (2016): 274–278.
Reinarz, Jonathan and Kevin Siena, 'Scratching the Surface: An Introduction', in Jonathan Reinarz and Kevin Siena (eds), *A Medical History of Skin: Scratching the Surface*, Studies for the Society for the Social History of Medicine, 10 (London: Routledge, 2016), pp. 1–15.
Richards, Katherine, 'Medical Celebrity in Eighteenth-Century Britain', PhD thesis, West Virginia University (2018).

Richards, Thomas, *The Commodity Culture of Victorian Britain: Advertising and Spectacle 1851–1914* (California: Stanford University Press, 1990).

Richardson, Ruth, *Death, Dissection and the Destitute* (London: Routledge & Kegan Paul, 1987).

Richardson, Ruth, *The Making of Mr. Gray's Anatomy: Bodies, Books, Fortune, Fame* (Oxford: Oxford University Press, 2008).

Riddle, John M., *Eve's Herbs: A History of Contraception and Abortion in the West* (Cambridge, MA: Harvard University Press, 1997).

Rivers, Isabel (ed.), *Books and their Readers in Eighteenth-Century England* (Leicester: Leicester University Press, 1982).

Roberts, Clayton, 'The Fall of the Godolphin Ministry', *Journal of British Studies* 22:1 (1982): 71–93.

Roberts, Marie Mulvey and Roy Porter (eds), *Literature and Medicine During the Eighteenth Century* (London: Routledge, 1993).

Robson-Mainwaring, Laura, 'Branding, Packaging and Trade Marks in the Medical Marketplace *c*.1870–*c*.1920', unpublished PhD thesis, University of Leicester (2019).

Roger Cooter (ed.), *Studies in the History of Alternative Medicine* (Hampshire and London: Macmillan, 1988).

Rosenberg, Charles E., 'Medical Text and Social Context: Explaining William Buchan's *Domestic Medicine*', *Bulletin of the History of Medicine* 57:1 (1983): 22–42.

Ross, J. H., 'Elizabeth Gaskell (1810–1865) and the Medical World', *Journal of Medical Biography* 24:2 (2016): 215–219.

Rovelli, Giulia, 'John Pechey (1654–1718) and the Popularization of Learned Medicine', *Writing Doctors and Writing Health in the Long Eighteenth Century*, Special Issue of *Journal for Eighteenth-Century Studies* 46:1 (2023): 59–73.

Russell, Gillian, *The Ephemeral Eighteenth Century: Print, Sociability, and the Cultures of Collecting* (Cambridge: Cambridge University Press, 2020).

Russell, K. F., 'A Check List of Medical Books Published in English before 1600', *Bulletin of the History of Medicine* 21 (1947): 922–958.

Sappol, Michael, *A Traffic of Dead Bodies: Anatomy and Embodied Social Identity in Nineteenth-Century America* (Princeton, NJ and Oxford: Princeton University Press, 2002).

Schmidt, Suzanne Karr, *Interactive and Sculptural Printmaking in the Renaissance* (Leiden and Boston: Brill, 2018).

Senior, Emily, *The Caribbean and the Medical Imagination, 1764–1834: Slavery, Disease and Colonial Modernity* (Cambridge: Cambridge University Press, 2018).

Seth, Suman, *Difference and Disease: Medicine, Race, and the Eighteenth-Century British Empire* (Cambridge: Cambridge University Press, 2018).

Shapin, Steven, 'Trusting George Cheyne: Scientific Expertise, Common Sense, and Moral Authority in Early Eighteenth-Century Dietetic Medicine', *Bulletin of the History of Medicine* 77:2 (2003): 263–297.

Shelton, Don, 'Anthony Carlisle and Mary Shelley: Finding Form in a *Frankenstein* Fog', *Athens Journal of Philology* 6:2 (2019): 105–130.

Shelton, Don, 'Sir Anthony Carlisle and Mrs Carver', *Romantic Textualities: Literature and Print Culture, 1780–1840* 19 (2009): 54–69.

Shuttleton, D., '"My Own Crazy Carcase": The Life and Works of Dr George Cheyne (1672–1743)', PhD thesis, University of Edinburgh (1993).

Shuttleton, D., '"Pamela's Library": Samuel Richardson and Dr. Cheyne's "Universal Cure"', *Eighteenth-Century Life* 23:1 (1999): 60–80.
Shuttleton, D., *Smallpox and the Literary Imagination 1660–1820* (Cambridge: Cambridge University Press, 2007).
Shuttleton, D., 'The Fashioning of Fashionable Diseases in the Eighteenth Century', *Literature and Medicine* 35:2 (2017): 270–291.
Siena, Kevin P., 'The "Foul Disease" and Privacy: The Effects of Venereal Disease and Patient Demand on the Medical Marketplace in Early Modern London', *Bulletin of the History of Medicine* 75:2 (2001): 199–224.
Silva, Christobal, *Miraculous Plagues: An Epidemiology of Early American Narrative* (New York: Oxford University Press, 2011).
Skipper, Alison, 'Form, Function and Fashion: Health, Disease and British Pedigree Dog Breeding During the Long Twentieth Century', PhD thesis, King's College London (2021).
Skipper, Alison, 'The "Dog Doctors" of Edwardian London: Elite Canine Veterinary Care in the Early Twentieth Century', *Social History of Medicine* 33:4 (2020): 1233–1258, available at https://doi.org/10.1093/shm/hkz049, last accessed 28 February 2023.
Smith, David, 'Map Publishers of Victorian Britain: The Philip Family Firm 1834–1902', *Map Collector* 38 (1987): 31–32.
Smith, Frank, *The Life and Work of Sir James Kay-Shuttleworth* (London: John Murray, 1923).
Smith, Ginnie, '"Prescribing the Rules of Health": Self Help and Advice in the Late Eighteenth Century', in Roy Porter (ed.), *Patients and Practitioners: Lay Perceptions of Medicine in Pre-Industrial Society* (Cambridge: Cambridge University Press, 1985), pp. 249–282.
Smith, Helen, *'Grossly Material Things': Women and Book Production in Early Modern England* (Oxford: Oxford University Press, 2012).
Smith, Hugh, *The Family Physician: Being a Collection of Useful Family Remedies*, 8th edn (London: Printed for the author, 1770–1775?).
Smith, John Thomas, *Nollekens and His Times: Comprehending a Life of that Celebrated Sculptor; and Memoirs of Several Contemporary Artists, from the Time of Roubiliac, Hogarth, and Reynolds, to that of Fuseli, Flaxman, and Blake*, ed. Wilfred Whitten, 2 vols, 2nd edn (London: Lane, 1829).
Smith, Roger, *The Fontana History of the Human Sciences* (London: Fontana, 1997).
Smith, Theresa, 'Moveable Anatomies and Print Shop Practice in Sixteenth-Century Strasbourg', in David Saunders, Marika Spring and Andrew Meek (eds), *The Renaissance Workshop: The Materials and Techniques of Renaissance Art* (London: Archetype Publications, 2013), pp. 121–129.
Solomon, Harry, *Sir Richard Blackmore* (Boston, MA: Twayne, G. K. Hall, 1980).
Souter, Keith, *Medical Meddlers, Mediums and Magicians: The Victorian Age of Credulity* (Stroud: History Press, 2012).
Sparks, Tabitha, *The Doctor in the Victorian Novel: Family Practices* (Aldershot: Ashgate, 2009).
Spence, Joseph, *Observations, Anecdotes and Characters of Books and Men Collected from Conversation*, ed. James M. Osborn, 2 vols (Oxford: Oxford University Press, 1966).
Spencer, Jane, 'Creating the Woman Writer: The Autobiographical Works of Jane Barker', *Tulsa Studies in Women's Literature* 2:2 (1983): 165–181.

St Clair, William, *The Reading Nation in the Romantic Period* (Cambridge: Cambridge University Press, 2004).

Stein, Richard A., 'The Golden Age of Anti-Vaccine Conspiracies', *GERMS* 7:4 (2017): 168–170.

Stephen, Leslie, 'Arbuthnot, John', in *Dictionary of National Biography*, vol. 2 (London: Smith, Elder, and Co., 1885–1900).

Stobart, Anne, *Household Medicine in 17th-Century England* (London: Bloomsbury, 2016).

Storm, Erica M., 'Gilding the Pill: The Sensuous Consumption of Patent Medicines, 1815–1841', *Social History of Medicine* 31:1 (2018): 41–60.

Susser, Mervyn and Zena Stein, 'Germ Theory, Infection, and Bacteriology', in *Eras in Epidemiology: The Evolution of Ideas* (Oxford: Oxford University Press, 2009), pp. 107–122.

Swabe, Joanna, 'Veterinary Dilemmas: Ambiguity and Ambivalence in Human–Animal Interaction', in A. L. Poderscek, E. S. Paul and J. A. Serpell (eds), *Companion Animals and Us* (Cambridge: Cambridge University Press, 2000), pp. 292–311.

Tague, Ingrid, *Animal Companions: Pets and Social Change in Eighteenth-Century Britain* (University Park, PA: Pennsylvania State University, 2015).

Talairach-Vielmas, Laurence, *Gothic Remains: Corpses, Terror and Anatomical Culture, 1764–1897* (Cardiff: Cardiff University Press, 2019).

Tave, Stuart, *The Amiable Humorist: A Study in the Comic Theory and Criticism of the Early Eighteenth and Early Nineteenth Centuries* (Chicago, IL: University of Chicago Press, 1960).

Thackray, Arnold, 'Natural Knowledge in Cultural Context: The Manchester Mode', *American Historical Review* 79:3 (1974): 672–709.

Thomson, William A. R., 'Rider Haggard and Smallpox', *Journal of the Royal Society of Medicine* 77:6 (1984): 445–536.

Tisinger, Jo, 'G. Löwensohn – Children's Books – Fürth', Vintage Popup Books, available at https://www.vintagepopupbooks.com/movable-book-history-s/1858.htm, last accessed 6 January 2022.

Vasset, Sophie, 'Medical Laughter and Medical Polemics: The Woodward–Mead Quarrel and Medical Satire', *XVII–XVIII* (*Autour du rire / Laughing Matters*) 70 (2013): 109–133.

Vasset, Sophie, *Murky Waters: British Spas in Eighteenth-Century Medicine and Literature* (Manchester: Manchester University Press, 2022).

von Hoffmann, Viktoria, '*Ingeniosa peritia*: The Languages of Ingenuity in Italian Renaissance Anatomy', in Richard J. Oosterhoff, José Ramón Marcaida and Alexander Marr (eds), *Ingenuity in the Making: Matter and Technique in Early Modern Europe* (Pittsburgh, PA: University of Pittsburgh Press, 2021), pp. 94–111.

Vretos, Athena, *Somatic Fictions: Imagining Illness in Victorian Culture* (Stanford, CA: Stanford University Press, 1995).

Waddington, Ivan, *The Medical Profession in the Age of the Industrial Revolution* (Dublin: Gill and Macmillan, 1984).

Waddington, Keir, *An Introduction to the Social History of Medicine: Europe Since 1500* (Basingstoke: Palgrave Macmillan, 2011).

Waldstreicher, David, 'The Long Arm of Benjamin Franklin', in Katherine Ott, David Serlin and Stephen Mihm (eds), *Artificial Parts, Practical Lives: Modern Histories of Prosthetics* (New York: New York University Press, 2002), pp. 300–326.

Ward, Richard, 'The Criminal Corpse, Anatomists and the Criminal Law: Parliamentary attempts to Extend the Dissection of Offenders in Late Eighteenth-Century England', *Journal of British Studies* 50:1 (2015): 63–87.
Wear, Andrew, *Knowledge & Practice in English Medicine, 1550–1680* (Cambridge: Cambridge University Press, 2000).
Wells, L. H., 'A Remarkable Pair of Anatomical Fugitive Sheets in the Medical Center Library, University of Michigan', *Bulletin of the History of Medicine* 38:5 (1964): 470–476.
Wells, L. H., 'Anatomical Fugitive Sheets with Superimposed Flaps, 1538–1540', *Medical History* 12:4 (1968): 403–407.
Wells, Susan, *Out of the Dead House: Nineteenth-Century Women Physicians and the Writing of Medicine* (Madison, WI: University of Wisconsin Press, 2001).
Werner, Sarah, 'Working Towards a Feminist Printing History', *Printing History New Series*, 27/28 (2020): 11–25.
Whaley, Leigh, *Women and the Practice of Medical Care in Early Modern Europe, 1400–1800* (London: Palgrave Macmillan, 2011).
Whelan, Timothy, Introduction, *A Tradition of Nonconformist & Dissenting Women Writers, 1650–1850*, available at https://www.nonconformistwomenwriters1650-1850.com/introduction, last accessed 30 June 2022.
Whelan, Timothy, 'Mary Lewis and her Family of Printers and Booksellers, 1 Paternoster Row, 1749–1812', *Publishing History* 85 (2021): 31–67.
Whitley, W. T., 'Turner as a Lecturer', *Burlington Magazine for Connoisseurs* 22 (1913): 255–259
WHO, UN, UNICEF, UNDP, UNESCO, UNAIDS, ITU, UN Global Pulse and IFRC, *Managing the COVID-19 Infodemic: Promoting Healthy Behaviours and Mitigating the Harm from Misinformation and Disinformation* (23 September 2020), available at https://www.who.int/news/item/23-09-2020-managing-the-covid-19-infodemic-promoting-healthy-behaviours-and-mitigating-the-harm-from-misinformation-and-disinformation, last accessed 5 April 2023.
Wiepke, Hannah, 'Cut & Paste: An Attempt to Construct Johannes Remmelin's 1754 Flap Anatomy Restrike', paper presented at Union Pacific Fellows Roundtable, University of Minnesota Twin Cities, 19 March 2021.
Wild, Wayne, *Medicine-By-Post: The Changing Voice of Illness in Eighteenth-Century British Consultation Letters and Literature* (Amsterdam: Rodopi, 2006).
Wilkins, Mira, 'The Neglected Intangible Asset: The Influence of the Trade Mark on the Rise of the Modern Corporation', *Business History* 34:1 (1992): 66–95.
Williams, David Innes, 'Anthony Todd Thomson and the Rise of the General Practitioner', *Journal of Medical Biography* 10:4 (2002): 206–214.
Williams, Helen, 'Family Planning and the Long Eighteenth-Century Pocketbook', *Writing Doctors and Writing Health in the Long Eighteenth Century*, Special Issue of *Journal for Eighteenth-Century Studies* 46:1 (2023): 113–133.
Williams, Helen, *Laurence Sterne and the Eighteenth-Century Book* (Cambridge: Cambridge University Press, 2021).
Williamson, Stanley, *The Vaccination Controversy: The Rise, Reign and Fall of Compulsory Vaccination for Smallpox* (Liverpool: Liverpool University Press, 2007).
Wilson, Philip K., 'Salmon, William (1644–1713)', *Oxford Dictionary of National Biography* (November 2021), available at https://doi.org/10.1093/ref:odnb/24559, last accessed 13 January 2023.

Wilson, Philip K., *Surgery, Skin and Syphilis: Daniel Turner's London (1667–1741)* (Amsterdam and Atlanta, GA: Rodopi, 1999).

Wilson, Philip K., 'Turner, Daniel (1667–1741)', *Oxford Dictionary of National Biography* (January 2008), available at https://doi.org/10.1093/ref:odnb/27844, last accessed 13 January 2023.

Wright, Edgar, *Mrs. Gaskell: A Basis for Reassessment* (London: Oxford University Press, 1965).

Wrigley, Richard and George Revill (eds), *Pathologies of Travel* (Amsterdam: Rodopi, 2000).

Wyett, Jodi L., 'The Lap of Luxury: Lapdogs, Literature, and Social Meaning in the "Long" Eighteenth Century', *Lit: Literature Interpretation Theory* 10:4 (1999): 275–301.

Zigarovich, Jolene, *Sex and Death in Eighteenth-Century Literature* (Abingdon: Routledge, 2013).

Index

Note: literary works can be found under authors' names; page references to illustrations are given in italics.

able-bodiedness 13, 129–131
  see also Boswell, James
ableism 12, 131
Addison, Joseph 4, 5
  Spectator, The 66
  see also Blackmore, Richard (Sir)
advertisements, medical 1, 36, 193–195, 198, 201, 206–212, 224
advertising 158–161, 193–198, 201, 206–212, 222, 223–224
  see also branding, medical; patent medicines; quacks
anatomy 14, 77
  atlases of
    see also flap anatomies
  debates 13, 18, 135–139, 146, 148–149
  female 167
    see also flap anatomies
  knowledge of 77, 84, 232
  legislation concerning 137, 143–144, 148
    see also Anatomy Act, the (1832)
  negative views on 135, 142–143, 147
  notions of 17, 218, 223–224, 231–232, 236
  practices 92, 93, 135–137, 139, 141–142, 144, 148
  study of 77, 84, 135–138, 218, 222–226, 231

  supply issue 135–138, 144–145
    see also body snatching; gothic fiction
Anatomy Act, the (1832) 14, 135–136, 148
anxiety see English Malady, the
apothecaries see medical practitioners
apprenticeships, medical 15, 47, 100, 123, 180, 182–184
  see also education; medical profession
Arbuthnot, Dr John 9–10, 62
  Art of Political Lying, The 10, 46–47
  career of 42, 44–45
  Gnothi Seauton, Know your self, 10, 53–56, 59n.51
  Memoirs of Martinus Scriblerus 10, 43, 49–53, 54
    see also Woodward, Dr John
  religious beliefs of 53–56, 257
  treatments of 42, 51
  and truth 42, 44–48, 258
  works of 42–43, 45–46, 49
  see also Scriblerus Club, the; Swift, Jonathan
Arsenic Act, the (1851) 196
authenticity 3–4, 161, 163–164, 209, 245–246
  see also advertisements, medical; fakery; fashionable disease; labelling, medical; medical misinformation

autopathography 13
  see also Boswell, James; illness narratives

Barber-Surgeons Company, the 25
Barker, Jane 11, 78
  approach to gender conventions, 87–88, 93
  authorial identity of 78, 82–83, 84
  medical practice of 84–85
  Patch-Work Screen for the Ladies, A 11, 78–79, 80–88
  Poetical Recreations 78, 82
  written style of 80–81, 84, 87
Bartholin the Younger, Caspar 84
Bate, George 31–35, 37n.14
  Pharmacopoeia Bateana 9, 32
Bath (city) 10, 62, 65–67, 73, 96, 104, 107
  see also Cheyne, George
Bath Spa 62
Blackmore, Sir Richard 4, 60
  'Essay upon Writing' 4
  medical writings 4–5, 60, 61
    see also medical language, vernacular
  'Of Controversial Writings' 4–8
  religious beliefs of 6, 7, 21n.20
  and truth 4–7
Blaine, Delabere 111
  see also dog doctors
blood 6, 28–29, 55, 69, 84–85, 100, 210, 220, 249–250
  see also humours, bodily; spirits, bodily
body snatching 13–14, 135
  legal reforms of 14, 135, 137, 143–144, 145, 149
  practice of 137, 139, 141–142, 145, 148–149
  public reaction against 136–138, 141–142, 143
  see also Anatomy Act, the (1832); gothic fiction
book history, discipline of 8, 153–154
booksellers see medical marketplace

Boswell, James 12, 13
  life writing of 13, 117, 126–129, 131
  London Journal 12, 13, 118, 126–132
  melancholia of 72, 128–129, 130–131
  venereal disease of 126–128, 131–132
  see also illness narratives; masculinity; venereal disease
botanical periodicals 167
  see also Cox, Elizabeth; medical journals
Bozzi Granville, Augustus, *St. Petersburgh: A Journal of Travels to and from that Capital* 154
branding, medical 16, 165–166, 197–198, 213
  see also consumerism; labelling, medical; medical marketplace; trademarks
British Medical Association 197
Buchan, William 12–13, 119–122, 123–124, 127, 132
  Domestic Medicine 122, 123, 186, 191n.60, 259
    see also medical language, vernacular
  Observations Concerning the Prevention and Cure of the Venereal Disease 12, 119–122, 123–124
  see also Smollett, Tobias; sexual health, male; venereal disease
Bunbury, Henry William 108
  Dog Barber, The 109
  View of the Pont Neuf at Paris 108
  see also dog ownership
Burke, William 136
  see also body snatching; Hare, William
Burney, Frances, *Cecilia* 100

Callow, John 157, 159, 168
  see also Cox, Elizabeth

canine healthcare. *see* veterinary
    medicine
  see also dog doctors
Carlisle, Sir Anthony 13–14, 136–140,
    143, 146–147, 149, 150n.16
  see also anatomy; 'Carver, Mrs';
    gothic fiction
'Carver, Mrs' (Sir Anthony Carlisle)
    13–14, 136–137, 138–140,
    142–143, 145–149
  Horrors of Oakendale Abbey, The
    13–14, 136, 138, 139–140,
    142–149, 259
  see also Minvera Press, the
  see also anatomy; Carlisle, Sir
    Anthony; gothic fiction
Chemist and Druggist 198, 207, 209,
    213
Cheyne, George 8, 10, 51, 258
  celebrity of 10, 19n.7, 67–68
  and diet 51, 69, 106
  English Malady, The 10, 60–61, 64,
    68–74
  Essay of Health and Long Life, An
  Essay on the Gout, An
  neurological theories of 10, 61,
    63–64, 70–72
  readership of 62, 64–65, 67–68
    female 66–67, 70–72
  self-fashioning of 60–61, 64–68,
    70–74, 76n.22
  writing of 60, 62–68
  see also diet; English Malady, the;
    medical writing; Richardson,
    Samuel; sensibility
childbirth 234–235
  see also flap anatomies
cholera 2–3, 175
Church of England, the 61, 87, 91
  see also witchcraft
Churchill, Reverend James 158, 168
celebrity, medical 2, 19n.7, 60, 67, 99
  see also Cheyne, George; dog doctors
circulating libraries 140
consumerism 12, 16, 73, 140, 161,
    198, 213, 259
  see also branding, medical

consumption 4, 61, 210
  see also tuberculosis
contagion 2–3, 125–126
  see also epidemics; medical
    misinformation; pandemics
Cornell Medical College 223
Coventry, Francis, *History of
    Pompey the Little, The* 12,
    101–102
  see also dog doctors; lapdogs
Covid-19 (coronavirus) pandemic 1, 8,
    9, 17, 252, 256, 257
  see also pandemics; vaccination
Cowper, William 158
Cox, Elizabeth Rane 8, 14, 154
  business practices of 14–15,
    157–159, 163, 168
  *Cox's Companion to the Medicine
    Chest* 15, 156, 164–166, 168,
    172n.59, 173–174n.70
  Cox's Druggist's Price Book
    157–158, 166
  medical publishing of 14, 152,
    156–62, 163–168
  see also branding, medical; labelling,
    medical; medical treatises;
    medical knowledge
Cox, Roland, *Manual of Trade Mark
    Cases* 198
Cox, Thomas 156
Crayle, Benjamin 84
creativity 3–4, 71–72, 242
  and gender 7–8
  see also genre; medical language;
    medical treatises; medical
    writing; rhetoric
Critical Review, The 139
  see also Smollett, Tobias
Culpeper, Nicolas 171n.44
  Pharmacopeoia Londinensis 159

death culture 142–143, 146–147
depression *see* English Malady, the
diet 44, 51, 61, 62, 67, 69, 73–74, 77,
    85, 98
  see also Arbuthnot, Dr John; Cheyne,
    George

disability studies 12
Dodd, Reverend William 147
dog doctors
  criticism of 11–12, 96, 103–107, 111–112
  in fiction 96, 101–103, 104–107, 112
    see also Coventry, Francis
  role of 12, 96–97, 98–101, 111–112
  in visual culture 108–111
  see also dog ownership; veterinary medicine
dog ownership 11–12, 97–98, 101–102
  companion dogs 12, 96–98, 101, 103–104, 112
  and diet 98, 104–106
  grooming 99
  lapdogs 98–99, 101–105, 107
  sales 99–100
  and women 96–101, 106–107, 112
  see also dog doctors; *tondeurs de chien*; veterinary medicine
Dr James's Fever Powder. *see* James, Dr Robert
Dr. Minder's Anatomical Manikin of the Female Human Body see Furneaux, William S.

Edinburgh 13, 175
  Royal Infirmary 206
  Royal Medical Society 206
  see also body snatching
education
  medical 1, 11, 13–14, 34, 77, 79, 89–91, 93, 142, 182–183, 193, 222, 224, 235, 258–259
    see also medical knowledge; medical language
  university 77, 89
  of women 11, 29, 78–79, 86, 89
  see also apprenticeships, medical; Barker, Jane; flap anatomies; medical students; Smollett, Tobias
embodiment 123, 224
  see also Smollett, Tobias

Endersby, Richard 99, 104
English Malady, the 69–70, 71, 73–74
  anxiety 13, 55, 79, 126–129, 134n.51
  depression 10, 129
  melancholia 127, 129
  melancholy 71–72, 126–127, 129–30
  spleen, the 61, 69, 72
  vapours, the 69, 72
  see also Arbuthnot, Dr John; Boswell, James; Cheyne, George
Enlightenment, the (British) 6, 7, 61, 120, 128
epidemics 2–3, 117, 241–244, 246–247, 254n.9
  see also pandemics, vaccination
ethics, medical 2, 14–15, 16, 123, 125–126, 131, 195–196, 202, 207, 212, 258
experiments, medical 4, 6, 20, 28–30

fakery 3–4, 71–72
  see also authenticity; medical misinformation
fashionable disease 3, 64, 70, 72, 131, 134n.54
feedback looping 3
  see also creativity; medical language; medical networks; medical practitioners
flap anatomies 218, 220, 222
  design of 220, 222–223, 224–225, 226, 230–31, 236
  distorted gender discourse of 17, 220, 225–226, 230, 231–236
  in education 16–17, 218, 222–224, 235–236, 258
  see also Furneaux, William S.
Fothergill, Anthony 107
Foucault, Michel, *Discipline and Punish: The Birth of the Prison* 145
Frederick, Sir John (MP) 143–144
  see also body snatching
Furneaux, William S. 222–223, 230, 231–233, 235

Dr. Minder's Anatomical Manikin of the Female Human Body 16–17, 218, 220, 222–236
  see also flap anatomies

Galtier-Boissière, Dr Émile, *La femme* 223, 226
Gaskell, Elizabeth 8, 15–16, 174–176, 182, 185, 187–188
  Cranford 175, 183, 185
  Mary Barton 15, 174, 176–179, 184–185, 187–188, 258
  Moorland Cottage, The 184
  Mr. Harrison's Confessions 175, 179
  My Lady Ludlow 186
  Ruth 182–184, 186
  Wives and Daughters 174, 175, 179–181, 182–184, 187–188
  see also herbalism; medical practitioners; traditional healing
Gay, John 43, 49, 62, 104
genre
  literary 2, 4
  medical writing 60–61, 64–66, 68–70, 72–74, 77, 164–166
  see also creativity, gothic fiction; medical treatises; medical writing; self-fashioning
George III, King 147
Gibbs, John
  Compulsory Vaccination Briefly Considered 17, 244–245, 248–250
Godwin, William, *Things as They Are; or, The Adventures of Caleb Williams* 139
Goldsmith, Oliver 1
gothic fiction 13–14, 135–136, 139, 142–143, 149
  see also Carlisle, Sir Anthony; 'Carver, Mrs'; Minerva Press, the
gout 4, 11, 61–63, 82–85
  see also Barker, Hannah; Cheyne, George; Smollett, Tobias

Haggard, Henry Rider 8, 17, 240–243, 246, 248–249, 253, 254–255n.10
  Days of My Life, The 241
  Doctor Therne 17, 240–243, 248–251, 252–253, 258
  Farmer's Year, A 17, 241
  see also vaccination
Hale, Dr Robert 62
Hamilton, Robert 100
Hare, William 136
  see also body snatching; Burke, William
Harvey, William 69, 84–85
Haywood, Eliza 87
  Invisible Spy, The 102
Hazlitt, William 138
herbalism 177–179, 185, 186–187
  see also Gaskell, Elizabeth
Hervey, John (Lord) 67–68, 71
heteronormativity 12–13
heterosexuality 129
Highley, Samuel 157
Holcroft, Thomas, *Adventures of Hugh Trevor, The* 139
Hollick, Frederick, *Origin of Life, The* 226
household management 8, 67, 77, 86–87
  see also Barker, Jane; Strother, Edward
humoral theory 69
humours, bodily 6
  see also blood; spirits, bodily
Hunter, John 147
hypochondria 72, 107, 127
  see also Boswell, James; Cheyne, George; English Malady, the; sensibility

illness narratives 126–128, 131, 253
  see also autopathography; Boswell, James
indigestion 6, 210
influenza 2–3
infodemics 1

inoculation 51, 251, 257–258
  see also Jenner, Edward; vaccination

James, Dr Robert 1, 100
  Dr James's Fever Powder 1, 193
Jenner, Edward 245, 252, 257–258
  see also inoculation; vaccination
Jenner Society, the 240–241
Jodrell, Richard (MP) 143–144
  see also body snatching
Johnson, Samuel 72
Journal of the House of Commons, the 141
  see also body snatching

Kay, James Phillips, *Moral and Physical Condition of the Working Class, The* 175–176
  see also Gaskell, Elizabeth

labelling, medical 15, 18, 65, 153–156, 158–162, 168, 186, 196, 209, 258
  legislation for 156
  manufacture of 161–162, 165–166, 171n.54
  mislabelling 15, 154–156, 163–164, 167
  see also branding, medical; Cox, Elizabeth
Lamb, Charles 139
Lane, William 140
  see also Minerva Press, the
lapdogs see dog ownership
lawsuits, medical 163–164
Leper Hospital, Singapore 206
Lock and Chinese Hospital 206
London and China Express 206
London Company of Surgeons 14
London Evening Standard 162, 206, 211
Lyttelton, George (Lord) 67–68

Macdonald, James 130–131
Manchester 15, 174–177
  Literary and Philosophical Society 176

Royal Manchester Infirmary 175
  see also Gaskell, Elizabeth
Mann, Edward Cox 167
marriage, problems of 87–88, 90, 93
Martyn, John 64
masculinity 12, 108, 119, 125, 130–132
  see also Boswell, James; Smollett, Tobias
maternal imagination, the 26, 37n.18
Mayer, Dr Ethel 222–223
  see also flapbook anatomies; Furneaux, William S.
McDonald Bentley, Arthur James 206
Medical Act, the (1858) 183, 193
medical authority 2, 6–7, 35, 91–92, 93, 98–99, 120–121, 198, 212–213, 234–236
  see also medical knowledge; labelling, medical; Smollett, Tobias
medical journals 180–181, 193–195, 207
  British Medical Journal 193, 195, 249
  Dentist Register, The 199
  Journal of the Royal Society of Medicine 249
  Lancet, the 157, 168, 181, 185–186, 194–195, 207
  London Medical Gazette, The 154
  Medical Press and Circular 194–195, 209
  Medical Register, The 199
  Medical Times and Gazette 197
medical knowledge 13
  advancement of 14–15, 23–24, 36n.2, 38n.36, 136–138, 256
  popularization of 2, 4, 9, 19n.7, 28, 34–35, 61–62, 117, 119
  and women 14, 29–30, 78, 84–88, 93–94, 153–154
  see also education, medical language
medical language 1–2, 9, 31, 44–45, 210, 218–219, 235–236, 243, 248–249

Latin 1, 4, 9–10, 15, 26, 28, 30–35, 61, 65–66, 73, 74n.3, 81, 155–156, 160–161, 166, 184, 186
vernacular 1–4, 7, 9–10, 26, 60–61, 65–66, 73, 74n.3, 155–156, 166, 220
visual 218–219, 224–225
see also Cheyne, George; Haggard, Henry Rider; labelling, medical
medical marketplace, the 1, 16, 196, 194–195, 197–199, 207–208
and booksellers 1–2, 65, 157, 166
medical misinformation 11–12, 60–61, 77–78, 122
medical networks 15, 139–140, 149, 153, 157–158, 187–188
see also creativity; feedback loops; medical practitioners
medical practice 14–16, 23, 53, 79, 135–136, 142, 149, 168, 187, 193–195, 212, 218–219
domestic 8–9, 15, 18, 23–25, 29–30, 35–36, 67, 77–79, 93–94, 121–122, 164–165, 168, 174, 176–179, 185, 187–188, 190n.33
folk 174, 176–179, 187–188, 191n57
see also anatomy; Gaskell, Elizabeth; herbalism; surgery
medical practitioners 1–3, 16, 18, 24–25, 35, 60–61, 79, 93, 102, 137–138, 142, 146, 158, 165–166, 179–180, 190n.38, 194, 197, 199–200, 212–213
apothecaries 7, 8, 24, 31, 52, 81–82, 84, 93, 118, 120–124, 154, 161, 177, 198
chemists 8, 154, 155–156, 161–162, 185, 196, 198–199
doctors 2, 15, 24–26, 35, 61–62, 74, 106–107, 118, 120, 174, 179–181, 184, 187–188, 197, 202, 207–208, 213, 250–253

druggists 155–156, 161, 174, 177, 198, 199
female 24, 67, 78–83, 89, 93–94, 223–224
see also Barker, Jane; dog doctors; Smollett, Tobias
midwives 7, 78, 175, 178–179
pharmacists 154, 161
physicians 2, 16, 24–25, 26, 30–31, 50–53, 78–79, 81–82, 92, 93, 107, 119–121, 183–184, 190n.33, 198–199, 218, 223–224, 257
quacks 13, 26, 121, 190n.33, 193–194
surgeons 24–25, 92, 93, 100, 118, 136–138, 144, 147, 161, 174–175, 183–184, 190n.33, 198, 207
see also anatomy; body snatching; medical networks
medical profession, the 8, 16, 20n.15, 32, 128, 153, 158–159, 175–176, 179–180, 182–183, 193–195, 211–213, 223, 248, 251
see also apprenticeships, medical; education; medical practice; medical practitioners; trademarks
medical students 16, 100, 175, 218
medical treatises 23, 26, 44, 73, 77, 197, 226
see also medical language; medical marketplace, the
medical writing 3–4, 60–61, 65–66
see also Cheyne, George; creativity; genre; medical language; self-fashioning
medicine cabinets 155–156, 164–166
see also Cox, Elizabeth
medicine chests 15, 164–166
medicines 1, 14, 24, 28–29, 31, 77, 154–156, 160–161, 164–166, 177–178, 193–199, 207–209, 211–213
patent 16, 161, 193, 195–199

medicines (*cont.*)
   recipes, medicinal 8, 29–30, 31–35, 81, 186–187
   see also branding, medical; herbalism; labelling, medical
Medicine Stamp Act (1804) 196
melancholia. *see* English Malady, the
melancholy. *see* English Malady, the
Merchandise Marks Act, the (1862) 197
Meyler, William 96, 105
   see also dog doctors
midwifery 76, 167, 179
   see also medical practitioners
Minerva Press, the 13–14, 136–138, 140–142, 149
   see also Lane, William
Morning Chronicle 101, 164
Murder Act, the (1752) 14, 137, 144, 147, 148
   see also body snatching

Nabbes, Thomas, *Bride, The* 101
Naples, Joshua, *Diary of a Resurrectionist, The* 135
   see also body snatching
Newbery, Elizabeth 157
New Times 167
Norborn, John 99, 105, 106
   see also dog doctors

pandemics 1–3, 8–9, 252
   see also Covid-19 (coronavirus) pandemic; epidemics; vaccination
Parliament, British 14, 135, 137, 143–145, 147
Patent Office, the 193, 194, 196, 199, 206
   see also medicines; Trade Marks Registration Act, the
Peel, Sir Robert 137
pharmaceutics. *see* medical practice
Pharmacy Act, the (1868) 196
Philips' Anatomical Model of the Female Human Body 222
   see also flap anatomies
physiognomy 178, 187, 192n.66
   see also Gaskell, Elizabeth

Pitcairne, Archibald 61–62, 64
   see also Cheyne, George
poisons 78, 154–156, 160, 162, 177, 195–196
   see also labelling, medical
polemic 4–5, 7
   see also Blackmore, Sir Richard
Pomet, Pierre, *Complete History of Druggs, A* 30
Poor Law, the (1834) 155, 169n.14, 267
Pope, Alexander 4, 9, 42–43, 49, 56, 60, 62, 64, 66–67, 72, 104
   Epistle to Dr Arbuthnot, An 71
   Essay on Man, An 53–54
   see also Arbuthnot, John; Gay, John; Scriblerus Club, the; Swift, Jonathan
print media, and medical (mis)information 1, 14, 17, 153–154, 166, 168–169n.2, 193, 220–223
   see also Cox, Elizabeth
printing technologies 16, 161–162, 218, 220–223
   chromolithography 220
   colour lithography 16, 218, 239n.47
   halftone printing 16, 218
Publishers Weekly 224

QAnon conspiracy theory 257
queering 13, 18
queer studies 12, 129

Radcliffe, Ann 13, 143
Radcliffe, John 52–53
Rassweiler, Henry H. 224
   see also flap anatomies
Reece, Richard, *Domestic Medical Guide* 165
Reeve, Clara 143
Register of Pharmaceutical Chemists and Chemists and Druggists 199
rhetoric 2, 6–7, 8–9, 21n.20, 53–55, 65, 68, 235–236, 243–244, 248–249, 253
   see also Arbuthnot, Dr John; Blackmore, Sir Richard; Cheyne, George; genre; medical language

Richardson, Samuel 60, 70, 72, 74
  Pamela 67
  see also Cheyne, George
Rose, William 24
  see also Royal College of Physicians, the
Rousseau, Jean-Jacques 68, 70
Rowlandson, Thomas 108–109, *111*
Royal College of Physicians, the 24–25, 32, 34, 44, 171n.44, 201
Royal Society, the 44, 138

Salmon, William 9, 32–35
  see also Bate, George
satire, medical 2, 46, 50, 62, 63, 103, 107
  see also dog ownership
scabies 30
  see also skin
Scott, Walter 140
Scriblerus Club, the 9, 42–43, 49, 57n.4, 62
self-fashioning, of medical practitioners 1–2, 10, 60–61, 66, 68–69, 74, 83
  dialogic 10, 60–61, 65–66, 73–74
  see also Cheyne, George
sensibility 10, 64–65, 70–74, 103
  see also Cheyne, George
sentimentalism 12–13, 64, 97, 103, 123, 125
  see also dog ownership
sexual health 222–225
  female 123–126, 131–132
    see also Smollett, Tobias
  male 12–13, 117, 119, 122, 123–126, 127–128, 131–132
    see also Boswell, James; Smollett, Tobias
  see also flap anatomies; venereal disease
Shelley, Mary 139
  Frankenstein 136
shingles 26
  see also skin
Shipton, James 32–33

skin 23, 36n.2, 38n.36, 231
  distempers of 8–9, 23–26, 30–31, 35–36, 249–250
  freckles 26, 31–33, 38n.36
  pimples 23, 30–31
  skincare 8–9, 23, 31, 35–36, 39n.42, 258
  treatment of 23–26, 30–31, 33–35, 39n.42
  see also Turner, Daniel
smallpox 2–3, 26, 28, 30–31, 50–51, 241–242, 244–247, 249, 253, 254n.9
  see also skin
Smith Gibbes, Dr George 107
Smollett, Tobias 8, 11, 79, 117, 132, 139, 258
  Adventures of Launcelot Greaves, The 100
  Adventures of Roderick Random, The 12–13, 79, 88–92, 123–126
    see also masculinity; medical practitioners; sexual health; venereal disease
  Essay on the External Use of Water, An 126
  Expedition of Humphry Clinker, The 90, 101, 104–105
social status
  and illness 15, 24, 70–73, 112, 137–138, 178, 185
    see also Cheyne, George; fashionable disease; herbalism; hypochondria; Poor Law, the
  and medical practice 25, 78–79, 82, 86, 92, 176, 202, 207
sociopolitical issues, and medicine 17, 243
Solis Cohen, Myer, *Woman in Girlhood, Wifehood, Motherhood* 224
Southey, Sir Robert 139, 149
  'Mary' 139
    see also body snatching
  'Surgeon's Warning, The' 179–180
    see also Carlisle, Sir Anthony
Spectator, The 65–66

spleen *see* English Malady, the
spirits, bodily 6, 69
   see also blood; humours, bodily
Stationery Office, the 196
Strother, Edward 77–78
   Family Companion of Health, The 77
surgery 92, 179, 183
   see also medical practice; medical practitioners
Swift, Jonathan 9, 42, 43–44, 46, 48, 49, 56, 62
   Battle of the Books, The 6
   Examiner 46, 37
   Gulliver's Travels 43–44
   see also Arbuthnot, John; Pope, Alexander; Scriblerus Club, the

Temple, Sir William, 'Essay of Health' 66
Theatre of Anatomy and Medicine, the 157
Thomas Smith, John 105–106
Thomson, Dr Anthony 175
   see also Gaskell, Elizabeth
Thrale, Hester 68
Tibbits, Dr Herbert 201–202, 210
Times, The 144–145, 159
Tindal, James, *Companion to the Medicine Chest* 165
tondeurs de chien 99, 108
   see also dog doctors; dog ownership
Trade Marks Journal 194, 199
trademarks, medical 16, 194–195, 197–213
   legislation for 16, 193, 195, 197, 212
   see also branding, medical; labelling, medical
Trade Marks Registration Act, the (1875) 193–194, 197–199, 212
traditional healing 176–177, 184
tuberculosis 3, 251
   see also consumption

Turner, Daniel 8–9, 23–26, 28, 30–32, 35–36, 37n.18, 40n.53, 117–118, 122, 132
   Apologia Chyrurgica 24
   De Morbis Cutaneis 9, 23–30, 34–35
   Modern Quack, The (attributed) 34–35, 40n.53
   Syphilis: A Practical Dissertation on the Venereal Disease 25, 117–119
typhoid 3
typhus 3, 177, 182

vaccination 1–2, 8, 241–253, 254n.6, 254n.9, 256–258
   anti-vaccination 17–18, 242–253, 258
   anti-vaxxers 252, 256
   Royal Commission on Vaccination 247, 250–251
   Vaccination Act, the 241–242, 247, 254n.6
   see also Gibbs, John; Haggard, Henry Ryder
vapours, the. *see* English Malady, the
venereal disease 3, 12–13, 26, 117–126, 132, 166
   gonorrhoea 117, 121, 126–127, 131
   herpes 28
   pox 12, 117, 121, 124, 132
   see also Boswell, James; medical practitioners; sexual health; Smollett, Tobias
Vesalius, Andreas
   Epitome 220
   De humani corporis fabrica 220
veterinary medicine 11–12, 97, 100, 11–112, 155
   canine healthcare 100, 104, 107, 112. *see also* dog doctors; medical practice
Vogtherr, Heinrich, *Anothomia, oder abconterfettung eines Weybs leyb* 220

Wagstaffe, William 257
Warren, Samuel, *Passages from the Diary of a Late Physician* 135–136, 150n.3
  see also body snatching
Westminster Hospital 138–139
  see also Carlisle, Sir Anthony
Whiggism 4, 7, 47–48
Whittaker's Anatomical Model 222
Whittick, James 96, 105, 107
  see also dog doctors
Wilberforce, William (MP) 144
Wilkinson, Robert Oliver, *Druggists' Price Book* 166
  see also labelling, medical
Willis, Thomas 84–85
wise women 11, 23, 78
  see also medical practitioners
witchcraft 11, 29, 78, 88–89, 90–91, 139
  see also herbalism

Wolcot, John (Peter Pindar) 105
  see also dog ownership
Wollaston, William, *Religion of Nature Delineated, The* 66–67
Wollstonecraft, Mary 139
  Letters Written in Sweden, Norway and Denmark 139, 146
Woman's Medical College of Pennsylvania 223
Woolley, Hannah 29–30, 32
  Queen-like Closet, The 29
  Supplement to The Queen-like Closet, A 29
'Writing Doctors Medical Representation and Personality, ca. 1660–1832' (project) 8, 14

Yale University 25
  see also Turner, William

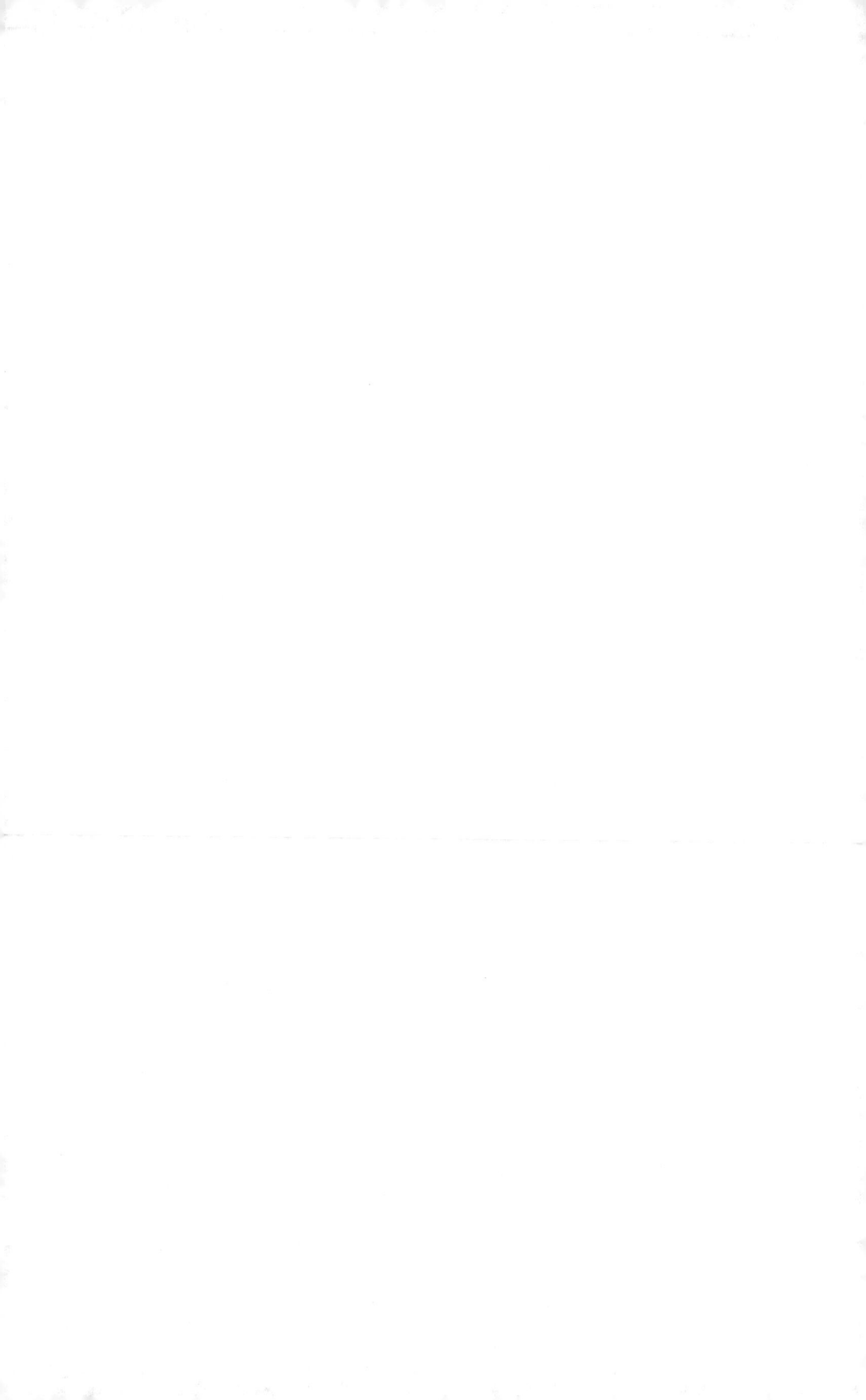

EU authorised representative for GPSR:
Easy Access System Europe, Mustamäe tee 50,
10621 Tallinn, Estonia
gpsr.requests@easproject.com